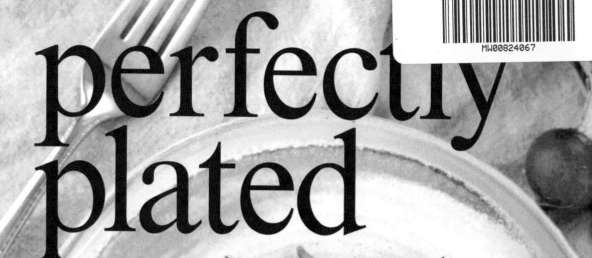

perfectly plated

A HANDS-ON GUIDE TO DIGESTIVE HEALTH AND NUTRITIONAL WEALTH

LAURA GARWOOD

FOREWORD BY BRIAN R. CLEMENT, PhD, LN

Perfectly Plated: A Hands-On Guide to Digestive Health and Nutritional Wealth

As You Wish Publishing, LLC
Connect@asyouwishpublishing.com

ISBN-13: 978-1-951131-09-8

Library of Congress Control Number: 2020919892

Printed in the United States of America.

Nothing in this book or any affiliations with this book is a substitute for medical or psychological help. If you are needing help please seek it.

To the people who suffer in silence, left feeling powerless by the medical establishment, this book is for you.

Disclaimer:

For Educational and Informational Purposes Only. All information contained herein is for educational and informational purposes only.

Not Medical Advice. The information provided is not intended to replace medical care, diagnose, treat, prevent, mitigate, or cure disease. The author is not a medical health professional nor makes any such claims. This book is not intended to provide health care, medical, or nutrition therapy, nor does it attempt to diagnose, treat, or cure in any matter whatsoever any disease, condition, or other physical or mental ailment of the human body.

Consult Your Physician or Health Care Provider. The intent of the author is not to replace any relationship that exists, or should exist, between you and a medical doctor or other health care professional. Always seek the advice of your physician or another qualified health care professional regarding any questions or concerns you have about your specific health situation. As always, consult with a heath care professional before attempting any self-help program. Do not disregard professional medical advice or delay seeking professional advice because of information you have read in this book. Do not stop taking medications without speaking to your physician or health care professional. If you have or suspect that you have a medical problem, contact your health care immediately.

Not Evaluated by the FDA. Any claims to health benefits have not been evaluated by the Food and Drug Administration and are not intended to diagnose, treat, cure, or prevent any disease, nor is it intended to be medical or psychological advice.

No Guarantees. The author believes in the individual's informed right to choose their own self-health program. The author makes no such claims of obtaining particular results. As with any health-related program or service, your results may vary and will be based on many different variables including but not limited to, your individual capacity, life experience, unique health and genetic profile, health-related conditions, or access to resources that may affect your overall results.

Assumption of Risk. There are sometimes unknown individual risks and circumstances that can arise when embarking on a dietary change. Your use or non-use of this information is at your own risk. If you have a known allergy or sensitivity to certain foods, as always, consult your physician.

To the people who suffer in silence,
left feeling powerless by the medical
establishment, this book is for you.

acknowledgements

I'm sure I'm going to miss someone, so please forgive me if I do. These next individuals, groups, or places have encouraged me, supported me, or kept me going in some way, and I thank you.

To my friends who believed me and believe in me. You exercise compassion and understanding. You may never know just how appreciative I am of you. You are the salt of the earth, grounded and instinctively insightful. You offer wisdom, strength, and I love you.

For the countless doctors who tried to put a name to my symptoms. You tried. It's OK. I found another way.

To the Hippocrates Health Institute, for just being in existence. You make a difference in so many people's lives. I am forever grateful for my experience there. Without your program, I would not be well.

To my local community for evolving and changing. For your eyes are open to the amazing wonders of food. I, and so many others, benefit from what you offer.

To Got Sprouts? in West Palm Beach. Without your wheatgrass and sprouts, I could not continue on my wellness journey or help so many others. Thank God for UPS.

To the kindest people I have ever met, the drive-thru employees at McDonald's for serving me, without judgment, on those days, I just felt so shitty. It didn't make me feel better, but it got me through. I am human. It's OK.

To the countless clients I have worked with. What I brought to you pales in comparison to what I learned from you. You make my program better.

And to all of the professionals who helped me create and further my program, my website, my online programs, and this book. I couldn't have a presence without you. Your dedication, time, and work are invaluable.

To my favorite chefs, Drew and Xavier, for always making me laugh! You two just do, no questions asked. You are rockstars in my eye. Life is better with you in it.

Thank you, Kim Kirk, my amazing food photographer. You underestimate your talents. To have you on this project is an honor.

acknowledgements

To Maribel, who draws out my ideas and brings them to life. Your artistic creations are as beautiful as you.

To Rick, who helped me find a name for my business, even in Spanish. I appreciate your continued friendship.

To Kim, who gave me my very first book about toxins. Without that book, I had nowhere to start.

To Stephanie for helping me pull all of my work together in a title. That was probably the most challenging part of this whole process, but you made it fun!

To my favorite local food purveyors who constantly nourish me; Native Sun and GYO Greens. Our community is better because of businesses like you.

To my kids. I really did write a book and wasn't shopping online all this time as you thought. I'm ready to go grocery shopping now.

To my sweet husband. You make all things possible. Without your unwavering support, love, and encouragement, I couldn't have done this. I love you beyond words. I'm ready for our next chapter.

foreword

Perfectly Plated is a genuine and gentle approach to enhance your health and wellbeing. Laura's contribution is meant to move many from the grips of perpetual lifestyle mishaps to a pattern of self-enhancing actions. Woven together like a comforting quilt, she guides you to take the effective steps that have healed her and hundreds of thousands. Expressing the ultimate methods, it becomes apparent that you can move at your own pace to reach these pinnacles of wholeness. On her journey, she gathered an inner strength and comprehensive wisdom that enabled her to help others. From this vast landscape of experience, she was compelled to gather her thoughts and place them on the same paper that manifested "Hands on Health." What I loved the most about Ms. Bushey-Garwood's methods is the abundance of humanity and reflective expression. When relating to her thoughts, you will engage in an exercise that will fulfill your desire to rise above the disorders that tax your very soul. True health is liberating and inviting at the same time. Your ability to leave behind limitations and embrace progress is often tied to the inspiration others afford you. You will certainly be filled with vigor and purpose, which ultimately results in happiness.

Laura's request to write the forward to this book deeply touched me, since I have seen the commitment, hard work, and success she has brought about. Each of our search for mentors who resonate with our sphere of understanding. *Perfectly Plated* throws a large net that will capture any and all who are ready to leave behind premature aging, disease, and pessimism finally. Her proven method will become your mantle of courage, and you will then possess the power to live a purposeful life without pain, suffering, and discord.

Brian Clement, Ph.D., L.N., is the co-Director of the renowned Hippocrates Health Institute, West Palm Beach, Florida (U.S.A.); the world's foremost complementary residential health center. Over the last half-century, he and his team have pioneered clinical research and training in disease prevention using hundreds of thousands of participants who provided volumes of data, giving Clement a privileged insight into the lifestyle required to prevent disease, enhance longevity, and maintain vitality.

Brian Clement has written over 20 books focused on health, spirituality, and natural healing. Among them are EmoSpirit, Dairy Deception, Supplements Exposed, 7 Keys to Lifelong Sexual Vitality, Living Foods for Optimum Health, Longevity, and Lifeforce, which Dr. Colin Campbell calls "One of the most important books ever written on nutrition." Additionally, he has authored three volumes for the scientific community, "Food is Medicine."

Brian Clement co-directs the Hippocrates Health Institute with his wife, Anna Maria Gahns-Clement Ph.D., L.N.

Brian Clement, Ph.D., L.N.

perfectly plated

A HANDS-ON GUIDE TO DIGESTIVE HEALTH AND NUTRITIONAL WEALTH

BY LAURA GARWOOD

table of contents

FOREWORD   vii
ABOUT ME   2
ABOUT KITCHEN OF LIFE   3

INTRODUCTION   **4**

HOW TO USE THIS BOOK   6
UTILIZE SENSIBLE EATING   7
WHERE TO START?   8

CHAPTERS

CHAPTER ONE Digestion and Optimal Health   11
CHAPTER TWO Become a Champion Grocery Shopper   25
CHAPTER THREE Blood, the Sustenance of Life   37
CHAPTER FOUR Phytochemicals, Antioxidants and the Controversy Over Soy 47
CHAPTER FIVE Omega Oils 3, 6, 9 and Saturated Fats   57
CHAPTER SIX Superfoods   65
CHAPTER SEVEN Where's the Beef?   77
CHAPTER EIGHT Dairy Farms and the 'Got Milk' Campaign   87
CHAPTER NINE Eating Fish? There's a Catch!   91
CHAPTER TEN The "All-Natural" Chicken   99
CHAPTER ELEVEN Water   108

INTRODUCING KALE & QUINOA   **115**

Quinoa & Arugula Salad Dressed in Cumin-Lime Vinaigrette   117
Kale Caesar with Faux Parmesan Crumbles   119
Kale Salad with Toasted Pine Nuts and Avocado   121
Grilled Eggplant with Quinoa & Red Pepper Salsa   123
Tuscan White Bean Soup with Kale Threads & fresh Thyme   125
Roasted Acorn Squash with Pine Nuts, Grapes, and Quinoa   127

CRUCIFEROUS VEGETABLES 129

Raw Broccoli Salad 131
Thai Collard Wraps with Peanut Sauce 133
Watercress Salad with Asian Pear and Tahini Dressing 137
Detoxifying Slaw 138
Chicory-Leek Soup with Black Caviar Lentils 139
Collard Wraps with Pesto and Broccoli Sprouts 141

VEGETABLE JUICING 143

The Southwestern 151
Roots and Shoots 153
The Daily Green 153
Tums Away! 155
Glow 157
Sour Apple 157

COLORS OF THE RAINBOW 159

KITCHEN GADGETS AND SMALL APPLIANCES 161
Miso Soup 167
Root Vegetable Salad with Organic Sweet Sauce 168
Indian Spiced Root Vegetable Curry with Creamy Coconut 169
Curried Lentils and Sweet Potatoes 171
Baingan Ka Bharta 173
Rainbow Salad in Rice Paper with Sesame Tahini Dipping Sauce 175

DETOXIFYING SIDES 177

Traditional Hummus Recipe 177
Simple Sautéed Mustard Greens 178
Cauliflower-Spinach Purée 179
Fresh Okra with Tomatoes and Ginger 179
Sautéed Radishes with Radish Greens & Chives 181
Roasted Rainbow Carrots with Roasted Garlic and Lemon 183
Roasted Brussels Sprouts with Hazelnuts 185

THE HEALTH BENEFITS OF GOOD FATS 187

Nut "Mylk" Shake 191

Strawberry Cashew Milkshake ... 193
Chocolate Chip Macaroons ... 195
Dehydrated Herbed Flax Crackers with Lavender Buds ... 197
Curried Almond Pate ... 199
Falafel with Tzatziki Sauce ... 201

SUPERFOODS & SMOOTHIES ... 203

Protein Powders ... 204
Blueberry Açai ... 207
Orange Boost ... 207
Green Goddess Smoothie ... 209
Beets and Berries ... 209
Raspberry Kisses ... 211
Mint Madness ... 211
Mango-Coconut Smoothie ... 213
The Palms ... 213
Coconut Coolada ... 215
Hydrating Smoothie ... 215

BREAKFAST IDEAS ... 216

Chocolate Sesame Energy Bites ... 219
Pumpkin Pie Spread ... 221
Chocolate Chia Pudding ... 223
Pitaya Bowl ... 225
Coconut Bowl ... 225
Avo Toast ... 227
Tofu Scramble with Asparagus and Basil ... 229

MEATLESS MEALS ... 230

PLATE SHIFTING ... 230
WHY GO MEATLESS? ... 230
Tempeh Reuben ... 233
Vegan Mac-n-Cheez ... 235
Vegan Lasagna with Spinach, Mushroom, and Zucchini ... 237
Chayote and Kabocha Tacos with Jicama Slaw & Pepita Cream ... 239
Zucchini Spirals with Cool Red Pepper Marinara ... 241
Zucchini Noodles with Basil Pesto ... 243

DRESSINGS   245

Buttermilk Ranch Dressing   246
Meyer Lemon Vinaigrette   247
Miso Peanut Ginger Dressing   247
Japanese Style Ginger Dressing   248
Shallot Vinaigrette   248
Roasted Cherry Tomato Vinaigrette   249
Remoulade   249

FISHLESS FRIDAYS – SEA VEGGIES   250

Jackfruit Tacos with Cabbage Slaw and Coconut Lime Crema   253
Grilled Romaine with Caesar Dressing   255
Pad Thai Noodle Salad   257
Faux Salmon & Seaweed salad   259
Thai Soba Noodle Salad with Vegetables and Wakame   261
Vegan Crab Cakes with Remoulade   263

DIPS AND SAUCES   265

Delicious Guacamole   265
Fresh Tomato Salsa   265
Raw Vegan Cheddar Cheese   266
Coconut Lime Crema   266
Pepita Cream   267
Jicama Pico de Gallo   267
Chipotle Vegan Queso   268
Cashew Cream Cheese   269

SOUPS & STEWS   271

SOUPING   271
Spiced Pumpkin Soup with Toasted Pumpkin Seeds   273
Split Pea Soup   274
Oriental Sweet Potato and Carrot Soup   275
Tom Kha Gai with Tofu   277
Creamy Broccoli Leek Soup   279
Zucchini & Watercress Soup with Black Garlic   281
Traditional & Watermelon Gazpacho   283

Lithuanian Borscht Soup with Forager Cream 285
Ginger & Turmeric in Warm Coconut Milk 286
Vegan Southwest Soup with Cilantro Lime Crema 287

ELIXIRS AND TONICS 289

Loving Liver Elixir 289
Bragg's Alkaline Elixir 289

TONICS 291

Golden Sunshine Tonic 293
The Immune-Slayer Tonic 295
Cheery Cherry Tonic 297

DESSERTS 299

Banana Ice Cream with Chocolate Sauce 301
Raw Chocolate Mousse 303
Raspberry Mousse 305
Sweet and Tangy Baked Apples 307
Chocolate Almond Butter Cups 308

OPTIMAL DIGESTION THROUGH FOOD COMBINING 310

INDEX 315

REFERENCES 317

about me

*my story
is one of
finding
hope when
health
was lost*

Due to a strange and unexplained illness in 2011, I became intimately familiar with the slow progression of healing and the multitude of challenges faced with overcoming it.

Unable to find answers from traditional doctors about my condition, I turned to the Internet, where I found, among a plethora of confusing information, a local doctor familiar with my symptoms. After being sent away several times from traditional medical care, this particular doctor diagnosed my condition with a simple lab test. It didn't relieve me of my symptoms, but it helped shape my journey.

As I began to help myself by experimenting with a holistic means of healing, I realized my calling was to help others in ways I had so desperately sought. In order to see my plan to fruition, I enrolled as a student at the world-renowned Hippocrates Health Institute (HHI) in the summer of 2012. Hippocrates Health Institute is a holistic retreat, having built its reputation on healing individuals through diet and lifestyle. While at Hippocrates, I learned the true meaning of "health."

I arrived that summer determined to heal and to help others. The results were conclusive: I would never be confused about diet, dietary fads, or nutrition again.

I received my certification in August of 2012 as a Health Educator from the Hippocrates Health Institute in West Palm Beach, Florida, and hold a Master's Degree in Education from Manhattanville College. I currently write, speak, and work as a personal holistic chef specializing in detoxifying and healing foods.

What I created, I believe, is a strictly common-sense based program. There isn't some magic formula for health and wellness.

During my healing journey, I developed a motto: "without our health, we have nothing." I took that motto—and my personal experiences—and started Kitchen of Life, a business that melds my work as a teacher, my love of good food, and my educational background to help others.

My story is one of finding hope when health was lost.

My passion and expertise led to the creation of Kitchen of Life, a much-needed in-home service providing individuals the knowledge and tools to overcome the symptoms of chronic illness, injury, and disease...and for those simply wanting to eat healthier. I have found that the majority of my clients come to me with familiar stories, and by using the information and recipes contained here within, their symptoms subside, and their health improves.

I have used my Kitchen of Life program with clients since January 2013. My research and writings are based on the philosophy and teachings of the Hippocrates Health Institute. My recipes have come from a variety of sources, again based on my raw food training while at Hippocrates and tweaked by my incredibly talented colleagues.

My program was designed (and improved year after year) to take an individual eating a standard American diet and introduce them to the fundamentals of plant-based eating using a relaxed, comfortable, step-by-step process. Not all of my clients elected to progress to the raw and living foods lifestyle of the Hippocrates Health Institute, nor is it a requirement of the program. However, noticeable changes still took hold.

The Kitchen of Life program offers a unique approach to healthy eating, as well as minimizing the adverse effects of chronic or nagging health conditions. The method used stems from a practical and well-mapped program. The recipes have been created to appeal to the Americanized palette. It incorporates a desirable concept using decadent and gourmet flavors to create delicious and healthy meals. There are more than 100 recipes in the program meant for all levels offering a variety of flavors, textures, and ingredients. The food pairings are designed for both health and taste.

The stark difference between my work one-on-one with clients and this book is that I am not standing in the kitchen assisting you, so the recipe segment has been re-written to introduce you to each plant-based concept by offering helpful tips and suggestions in my absence. There are no marketing gimmicks, no scare tactics, no crazy formulas or dietary fads, just good old-fashioned (centuries-old) advice teeming with ways to eat healthier and smarter in our ever-changing world.

The recipes in this book are 100% plant-based, but you will also learn about how to shop smarter when it comes to purchasing meat, dairy, and seafood. As Americans, we rely heavily on animal products and by-products, so it makes sense for overall health and wellness to minimize your daily intake of conventional livestock and fish. A healthy, plant-based diet is designed to promote wellness by lessening the body burden and allowing the body to do what it needs...and that is work for you.

about kitchen of life

introduction

Much of our commercially grown food is no longer raised by mom and pop farms, nor by large companies either, but rather by enormous big-agricultural conglomerates, many of which now own some of the most notable organic companies (who have since sold out either due to competition or for monetary benefit). And with bigger multinational corporations means more government involvement. Why should that concern you? Well, it means that politics plays an integral role in how our food is grown.

Commercial technology is changing faster than a blink of an eye, as is our environment and lifestyle too. Many of these changes are celebrated, but with it comes a heavy burden. Modern-day living is taking its toll on our health. Our bodies are being inundated with more and more chemicals, toxins, and food additives, all the while negatively impacting our health.

Our industry standards, when it comes to commercial growing practices and raising livestock, is one of the most important sections in this book. Again, it's not necessarily what you're eating but how your food has been grown and raised. We've been led to believe that food is cheap but cheap food comes at a heavy price—our health.

The delicate ecosystem of our planet, down to our internal biological system, is out of whack.

There are many things we cannot control that impact our health. For instance, it's not possible to hold our breath for a lifetime to avoid breathing in polluted air, nor is it possible to change our genetic make-up. However, it *is* possible to control what we put into our mouths. And what we put into our mouths can have a huge impact on our health. The power of food is more powerful than you may realize.

The key to better health has become quite confusing with expert upon expert pumping out the 'right' way to become healthy, but it shouldn't be difficult to understand. You needn't be an expert in nutrition to know what is beneficial and what isn't.

We have been 'sold' how to eat rather than 'taught' how to eat. Once it is explained here and broken down, it feels a lot less complicated. What you will learn is how to shop smarter and wiser and learn how to purchase food that will work for you, your gut, *and* your health.

This book introduces you to the "why" behind plant-based. It also uncovers many of the modern-day methods that go into growing and raising our food. So many Americans are largely unaware of our food production, but as you continue to read, you will develop ways in which to shop and eat smarter to avoid poor industry standards.

While this program promotes plant-based whole foods, it is not a requirement to become a vegetarian or vegan. It's a lifestyle change without losing the lifestyle.

Trying to emphasize that health and nutrition are not found in a box is a hard concept for many to understand. Telling someone they are going to have to invest a lot more time into preparing meals is a tough pill for many to swallow. When I get a little pushback, I often say, "How much is your health worth, because without our health we have nothing?"

Information on how to get healthy is widely publicized, but no one really knows what's fact and what's fiction. We're marketed to death, literally.

We no longer grow our food from the source anymore. We buy mainly from companies who grow, produce, and sell our food. If you think about it, many of the natural, plant-based foods don't have much marketing appeal, so they don't get promoted and are often overlooked as an amazing food source. When they are noticed, they are usually sold as a supplement or 'the next best thing.'

Health and nutrition are found in the abundant colors of nature, but we are guided in our society to eat a different way. The goal of healthful eating is not to take food away, but to enlighten you to the idea that foods for optimal health are easily attainable and surprisingly tasty.

how to use this book

When reading along, making the recipes and creating meals is the first and most important step in your wellness journey. There is no magical formula for what to eat for optimal health. Food is not complicated, nor should it be. What is equally important is your view towards food. Do you live to eat or eat to live? Once you learn to eat to live, finding the right foods in nature's bounty will introduce you to what living *really* means.

utilize
sensible eating

Sensible eating makes sense. Many of us know the basics. Carbs can be good *and* bad, sugar is bad, caffeine is bad, alcohol is bad, and processed foods are bad too. If indulging, sure eat those things, but if we want to live healthfully, the easiest way to remember what makes us healthy is....*greens*. The key to better health is simple! It boils down to greens! The benefit to greens? All greens are anti-inflammatory.

There is nothing unhealthy or controversial about plant-based foods, spices, and herbs. But when eating beyond greens, learn to approach grains, meat, fish, and dairy with caution. Let the plants be your base as in "plant-based." Even that alone will have a huge impact on how you feel.

Is it any wonder why some of the largest animals on this planet live off of grass, and many of the fish species live off of sea vegetables? It's no mistake. The energy generated from the sun and the process of photosynthesis plays a significant role in the nutrients of our plants. Greens contain chlorophyll, one of life's most dependable health foods. It's the sustenance of life.

If we purchase a processed product, we know it's been manipulated and denatured. If we fill our plates with a majority of whole, plant-based foods, we are getting the best bioavailable nutrients. Eating as close to the source as possible means eating what Mother Nature provides. It's quite sensible, isn't it!

where to start?

During the initial stages of the program, there are a multitude of ways to begin the journey to a healthier lifestyle and body while simultaneously practicing with the recipes. The first and best way to transition away from a typical Standard American Diet is by taking these steps:

- Eat less or no dairy products, red meat, alcohol, coffee, tobacco, candies, soft drinks, pastries, and sweets (all junk foods)

- If you do consume animal products, make sure to buy pasture-raised eggs and wild-caught fish, while limiting poultry and domesticated red meat

- Eat 6 to 8 servings of vegetables and fruits per day—eat at least 50% raw

- Do not overcook! Only lightly cook your foods such as sautéed, steamed. Never boil. All nutrients are lost in boiling.

- Chew your foods a long time to stimulate enzymatic breakdown at the mouth to help with digestion

- Do not drink water during meals, but 30 minutes after

- Eat organic foods as much as possible

There are so many plant-based nutritional powerhouses that the list could go on and on, but for starters, this is a great way to begin and carry out each day!

Happy reading and Bon Appétit!

digestion and optimal health

Without optimal digestion, it's not possible to have optimal health, nor is it possible for your health to be optimal without a properly functioning digestive system. The two are truly symbiotic.

Diets generally focus on what to eat, and while that's all well and good, there's more to health than what we eat. The digestion/optimal health duo are intricately entwined because being healthy stems from not just what you eat but from what you absorb and assimilate. And to go a bit further, it's more about the *quality* of what you eat rather than *what you eat* that plays an integral role in digestion. A general understanding of how our digestive system works can go a long way in figuring out what to eat and how to eat for optimal health.

The beginning basics of digestion can give us a pretty good understanding of how our digestion works. And with a general understanding, we can make some pretty informed decisions. You see, eating for health or eating healthfully isn't complicated, nor should it be. Moreover, learning a few holistic tips about digestion can help pull it all together. If you're concerned it might seem elaborate, it won't be! Learning just a little bit about digestion will go a long way! You won't look at eating the same way again! I promise.

Digestion can be viewed from two different perspectives: a scientific, allopathic model (think your general practitioner) or from a holistic, alternative health model (think nature). The information presented hereafter stems from a traditional perspective, but the 'what, where, and why' comes from an alternative and "whole" perspective of what an optimal diet looks like. And there's no mistaking it; optimal digestion leads to optimal health.

How is that possible? Well, for starters, you can't control the air you breathe, and you can't help your genetic make-up, but what you can control is what you put in your body (including what goes on your skin). What you put inside your body can make you sick, and alternately, it can also make you well.

So, let's start by introducing digestion! Here are some common factors when it comes to poor digestion. I call them the obvious signs!

Signs of poor digestion:

- Food allergies
- Gas
- Bloating
- Fatigue after eating
- Abdominal pain
- Tooth decay or plaque
- Thrush
- Hot and cold sensitivities
- Constipation
- Nutritional deficiencies
- Acne
- Nausea
- Heartburn
- IBS (intermittent bouts of constipation/diarrhea)

And what usually causes poor digestion?

Poor digestion is usually a result of years of bad habits. It can be caused by a combination of things, but in some cases include:

- Low stomach acid
- Drinking any type of fluid during meals—including water!
- Certain pharmaceutical drugs like antibiotics
- Eating too much or too frequently
- Eating too many animal foods or processed foods
- Drinking or smoking

Now on the flip side, you can be eating the healthiest diet on the planet, but if your digestive tract does not absorb what you eat, your food is seriously *not* working for you. Health food or not, if you're not able to properly digest your food, you're not getting the benefit of what you're eating.

Before we get into discussing ways in which to improve digestion, we need to talk about enzymes and our digestive system. The two are instrumental in keeping our bodies healthy. Enzymes and the anatomy of the digestive system go hand in hand here, too! Let's understand how:

WHAT ARE ENZYMES?[1]

Before you learn how these helpful little guys work for you, you need to know what they are. Enzymes are complex proteins that *can help break down the foods we eat so the body can more easily absorb their nutrients.* Absorption, as you are keenly aware of at this point, is a key factor in optimal digestion and takes place with the fine hair-like villi in the small intestine. In order to adequately absorb the nutrients, the villi need to be in good working order, and our food needs to be completely broken down by the time it gets to that point. Think high acid for breakdown and the assistance of enzymes. These two words can help jumpstart the way you will begin to think differently about food!

Bodily enzymes, food enzymes, as well as chewing and stomach acid, assist in this process. When you think about it, we wouldn't be able to do much without a working digestive tract!

DIGESTIVE ENZYMES

Digestive enzymes have three main jobs. They are:

To digest proteins. These enzymes are called PROTEASE.

To digest carbohydrates. These enzymes are called AMYLASE.

To digest fat. These enzymes are called LIPASE.

If you're having trouble remembering the names of the food enzymes, don't worry—you're definitely not alone. A fun way to keep them straight is to think about the enzyme name and what it does. For instance, protease enzymes digest proteins. That's pretty easy, right? The words even *sound* the same!

But what about the other two? It all depends on how your brain works, but we like to think about it this way: What happens when someone gets liposuction? They suck the fat out. So, lipase enzymes digest fat. Then you're left with the carbohydrate digesting amylase enzymes. Simple!

FOOD ENZYMES

Food enzymes help with digestion instead of demanding that the body's digestive enzymes do all of the "dirty work." Enzymes are naturally present in the digestive tract, but the philosophy of Dr. Howell, author of *The Enzyme Concept*, suggests that we have a limited bodily supply. We need to do what we can to take care of and preserve these extremely important little workhorses instead of unwittingly burning them out!

Processed foods (you know, those highly tasty but chemically-laden denatured foods) are devoid of enzymes because they've been cooked out. To keep the body working properly, we need to make sure we don't stress the body out by requiring it to produce more enzymes. Eating enzyme depleted foods offer no benefit and also strain certain parts of the digestive system, namely the pancreas. Enzyme depleted foods are often referred to as "dead foods." Dead or denatured foods are generally cooked and/or processed in some way. Contrary to dead foods, nutrient-rich foods include raw fruits and vegetables (including raw fish, meats, dairy, and cheese) and fermented foods. Now, while cooked foods aren't completely stripped of their nutrients (with the exception of boiling), they *are* stripped of their enzymes that are necessary and beneficial to—you're on it—optimal digestion!

What can you do to avoid this drain? Well, cut out those chemical-ridden processed foods for starters! Consuming foods in their raw or living state ensures that we are using the highest amount of natural enzymes needed for digestion and not drawing from bodily reserves. Based on Dr. Howell's research, the philosophy is—once they're gone, they're gone.

If you feel that you struggle with digestion, there are multiple products on the market that promote digestion through the use of supplemental enzymes. If you feel your diet is lacking in high enzymatic raw and living foods, trying supplemental enzymes to assist with digestion may be an "optimal" choice.

WHY ARE ENZYMES SIGNIFICANT?

Our over-consumption of meat, fish, dairy, poultry, conventional produce, processed, and fast foods is, frankly, a detriment to our health!

Why? Much of our conventionally grown produce contains a significant amount of chemicals from pesticides and herbicides that have been grown in mineral-depleted soil. What is not widely known is that plants get their nutrients from the soil, not from the plant itself. In order to ensure our food source contains a high nutrient content and vital minerals that our bodies need in order to function, plants need to be grown in the highest quality soil. Additionally, the meats we consume have been raised on crowded feedlots, given less than optimal livestock feed while spending a lifetime on veterinary

medicine to keep infections down and growth rate up. Our modern-day food source is a very different type of food than from years past.

There is an ideal remedy (besides the obvious— consuming a lesser amount of those foods), and that would be to incorporate more organic, plant-based foods into our diet. Put down the hamburger and think about your body for a minute. Do you need that? Or is there something better out there? According to Dr. Howell, a body weakened by disease is a body in an enzyme-depleted state.

Dr. Brian Clement, director of the Hippocrates Health Institute in West Palm Beach, FL, author of numerous books on health, states that he (at HHI) has witnessed the reversal of disease due in significant part to the great energy that enzymes provide for a diseased body.

That's right—it's your enzymes at work!

He goes on to say that our ancestors consumed an enzyme-rich diet, and without question, it is the nutritional basis of human survival. Enzymes, he believes, are at the heart of physiological healing, which benefit brain waves, thereby stabilizing and enhancing emotions.

In Dr. Howell's words, "moving toward a healthier diet using enzyme-rich raw and living foods will stop the waste of enzyme energy." Think of it as making daily deposits into the enzyme account. Few withdrawals and large deposits are the keys to being richly supplied with the metabolic enzymes that are responsible for building, cleansing, and healing the body.

The most important thing to mention when discussing enzymes is their ultimate destruction when heated over 118 degrees, which supports the case for consuming foods in their raw state. Cooking leaves behind an enzyme-less food that makes up the bulk of the modern enzyme-deficient diet. In essence, those all-important enzymes just get cooked away! And while this is true, this, to a larger extent, pertains to the large amounts of processed foods that make up the bulk of the aisles in our modern-day grocery stores, convenience stores, and grab-and-go restaurants.

A HEALTHY DIGESTIVE SYSTEM

Here's a quick anatomy lesson for you. Our explanation is pretty simple, and definitely something you should know! When we think of optimal health, we need to think of it in terms of:

A) digestion, and

B) absorption.

Once you make sense of that, everything else comes together.

A SHORT LITTLE LESSON ON DIGESTION—IT'S EASY TO DIGEST

Digestion begins in the mouth. The role of the mouth is to chew food to begin breaking down the fibers so some of the vitamins and minerals can be released. Our saliva is made up of its own different enzymes, which begin digesting our food before it even gets to our stomach. In other words, the body is remarkably already producing enzymes for you!

Your saliva produces:

Amylase, which breaks starch into sugar

Lipase, which breaks down fat.

Once the food leaves the mouth, it goes down the esophagus and takes about 6 seconds to get into the stomach.

There, **protease** is released to digest proteins.

The enzymes naturally present in living foods also help to digest the nutrients and break them down into chemical substances. This is so they can pass through the lining of the digestive tract and enter the bloodstream.

The stomach is a highly acidic environment for the purpose of breaking down the food we eat. The stomach produces hydrochloric acid (HCL), which is necessary for the stomach to do its digestive work. All those antacids you're taking to suppress acidity works *against* your digestive system! Once you get to the end of this chapter, you'll understand how to take that very upset, highly acidic, and uncomfortable stomach (and belly bloat, belching, and discomfort) and turn it around *without* the use of antacids. Eliminating your tummy's misery through food is the best remedy—however, please understand that eliminating some of your favorite not-so-good-for-you, convenient, and satisfying foods may not be what you want to do. Still, it may be what's needed to heal your pain!

After tossing and turning in your stomach, the food now heads to the small intestine where most of the nutrients are absorbed. The digested "fiber-rich foods" from your nutrient-rich plant-based diet enter the small intestine where the plentiful nutrients are absorbed by the villi. Villi are tongue-shaped "hairs" designed to absorb nutrients and distribute them to the body's cells through the bloodstream (Remember this point: We want this area *oxygen-rich and alkaline*—we'll get to this in a bit).

The pancreas and liver also do their job at this stage. The pancreas produces enzymes that break down carbohydrates, fat, and protein, while the liver produces bile. Bile is stored in the gall bladder, and when you eat a meal, it goes into the intestine to mix with fat. This helps digest the fat in the foods.

The food is then passed along to the large intestine, which is about five feet long. Here, water and electrolytes are reabsorbed back into the bloodstream.

There are over 700 different types of bacteria located in the large intestine. The toxic waste from food is bound for swift elimination by the friendly lactobacillus family of bacteria present in the colon. The remaining fiber in the large intestine helps to dilute, bind, and deactivate many carcinogens (sea vegetables are especially good at this). Waste is eliminated from the body through daily bowel—at least daily! Better out than hanging out! As you can see, your digestive system plays one of the most important roles in keeping you healthy!

The glands and the major organs, including the brain, are affected most from a poorly functioning and toxic digestive system. A natural diet of plant-based foods helps to replenish the elements necessary for your body to function optimally and minimize acidic waste by-products. In simpler terms, eat the right foods, keep your enzymes in check, reduce waste by-products by eliminating frequently, and feel *better*.

This leads us to our next topic on a healthy system, pH! The chemistry that is going on within our body, too, is a symbiotic relationship—you are what you eat! And you're not fake, right? So, don't eat fake foods.

PH BASICS

pH (which stands for potential hydrogen) levels measure the acidity of a solution on a scale from 0 to 14. Lower numbers are more acidic; higher numbers are more alkaline. Why is this important to know? Because what you put into your mouth can affect your internal pH system. Your digestive tract is looking for foods that are more alkaline, and your external areas, more specifically the skin, seek a more acidic environment!

The body has its own natural ability to normalize acid production. Therefore it is constantly working to maintain neutral (pH 7) blood acid levels. The fluids and tissues do not stay in these fluctuating states of "too acidic" or "too alkaline" for very long because the body is always striving toward balance. That's why if you can give the body what it needs (hint: a diet consisting of foods on the alkaline side) instead of constantly allowing the body to work overtime drawing on its own reserves, you can give yourself some balance—just think of a balanced diet! Not too far one way or the other! Somewhere right in the middle is neutral, which would be around 7, but let's try to keep our body around 7.35. This is what holistic health professionals like to call "homeostasis" or a body in balance.

If you eat a highly acidic, enzymeless breakfast like a bagel with cream cheese, a side of bacon, and a cup of coffee, the system must counteract the acidity by drawing on reserves (like calcium) to neutralize the acidity level. Acidifying foods are generally meat, poultry, seafood, eggs, cheeses, and animal fats. Additionally, grains, legumes, sweets, alcohol, coffee, and soda produce acidic residues after digestion.[2] While the food tasted good going down, you've put a lot of strain on the body. What if we were to start our day off with lemon water, a green drink or smoothie, and a low-acid fruit like strawberries? You have given your body the opportunity to focus less on bailing you out of an acidic nightmare and more on easily digesting an alkaline and nutritious breakfast. Suppose you need to indulge, set aside a special day to have your excess. You can indulge a bit more on a weekend morning if you want to! Just don't do it every single day. Many health experts have asserted that

diet can play an essential role in maintaining a healthy body.[3]

UNDERSTANDING PH

As mentioned before, your body is always working to neutralize acids and maintain the proper pH in organs, tissues, and body fluids. To keep your engine running properly by giving it what it needs, in the form of alkalizing fruits and vegetables, it can more easily maintain the delicate acid/base balance.

Have you ever sat right next to a person that just reeked of body odor? Like, you almost couldn't stay there without pinching your nose? Although it could be a sign that the person didn't shower, it's more likely a sign that they're highly acidic! You can apply that same mindset to yourself, too, if you find yourself needing to re-apply your deodorant during a hot summer day, or needing possibly a second shower. You may re-evaluate your eating habits and start to shift your diet away from acid-forming foods and move more toward alkaline-forming foods.

WHAT ARE ALKALINE FOODS?

The quickest and easiest way to do this is to start by incorporating leafy green vegetables into your diet—and if you find it necessary to cook them, then try steaming rather than boiling or sautéing in oil. And, yes! This program focuses on plant-based—but we don't want to turn anyone away! The top seven alkaline foods are listed for you at the end of this chapter, including some scrumptious recipes for you to try at home that will start to turn the acidic burn, gas, bloat, sick feeling into a thing of the past!

A highly alkalizing diet can affect your overall well-being. It's true! I've witnessed it in others and experienced it myself! In today's Western diet, it's tremendously difficult to keep the body on the alkaline/neutral side because of the abundance of packaged and processed foods, meals heavily laden with meat and dairy, and the encouragement of eating refined grains and white sugars. Raw fruits and vegetables help balance the body's pH level and reduce acid accumulation that, over time, can deteriorate your health. Too much acidity creates too many de-oxygenated cells. That just means the cells are not receiving enough oxygen to repair themselves. Eating alkaline-rich foods provides an alkaline and oxygen-rich environment that our cells love! Keep in mind our cells receive oxygen from food, too, not just from the oxygen we breathe.

STRESS, PH, AND HEALTH

Imbalance and disease can set in when the body is not only dealing with too many acid-forming foods but from too much stress, as well. The body is quite extraordinary, and it can fairly easily handle stress-induced pH imbalance—except if you compound the problem by eating a cheeseburger, fries, and a soda for lunch! Then the body becomes so focused on the acidic food load that the build-up of carbon dioxide gets dealt with later—if at all. Then you just end up with an

acidic internal environment. And, if you've been paying attention, you know that too much acid inside is a bad thing. Finding the balance between too acidic and too alkaline can be a challenge in today's stressful, fast-paced, fast-food environment.

Most acid is formed by the metabolism of fats, carbohydrates, and protein. Fats break down into fatty acids, proteins into amino acids, and carbohydrates into carbonic acids. Acids are normally released as carbon dioxide when you exhale and as urine by the kidneys. However, a pH imbalance can also result from an underlying condition such as diabetes or starvation—besides just a large quantity of ingested poor quality foods.[4]

ACIDIFYING DIETS

A chronic acidifying diet depletes bones of minerals, a primary cause of osteoporosis. The body pulls calcium from bones to buffer acidic food residues. Think about that the next time someone tells you to "break a leg!"

As if that wasn't enough, irritation and inflammation from exposure to internal acids (not to be confused with the acidic environment the stomach needs to digest food) can spur ulcers and arthritis. An acidic environment can also lower the immune system, cause fatigue, and lower energy levels by slowing vital enzyme functions.

A balanced diet high in alkalizing fruits and vegetables and moderate in acidifying products will ensure a happy, healthy you.[5]

Need some guidance as to what is alkaline? Just remember it like this: Green and brightly colored vegetables are the primary sources of alkaline substances for the body! Eat foods with color! Pick from the family of reds, oranges, yellows, greens, blues, and purples. Now that is simple! It's like eating in Technicolor.

EATING FOR HEALTH. EATING FOR BALANCE.

Now that you know a little bit about alkaline and acidic foods, how do you do turn this over into meal planning? An easy way to accomplish this, without thinking too much about it, is to make fruits and vegetables the main part of each meal. Most fruits and vegetables are alkaline in nature; it is that simple. Some fruits, such as citrus, have an acidic pH outside of the body but leave an alkaline residue in the body after being consumed and broken down in the digestive tract. A prime example of this would be lemons. By its very nature, lemons are acidic. You know that if you've ever accidentally squirted lemon juice in your eye. Ouch! When metabolized in the body, lemons have an alkalizing effect. Mother Nature and all her talents—if we didn't know the science behind it, we'd say it was magic.

Eating the right foods is not the only way to maintain balance! Deep breathing also has a vital impact on the body's pH levels. Oxygen rids your body of stale, acidic carbon dioxide. How else do you get rid of it? Massage, meditation, and yoga are some prime CO2 reducing activities. Finding balance in the areas

of diet and lifestyle is critical to the body's overall health. Do the best you can for now. It just gets better with time.

OXYGEN AND SUGAR— HOW SWEET!

Sugar carries a pH of 7 and is generally harmless when ingested as nature intended. How's that? With proteins, vitamins, minerals, and fiber intact. Unfortunately, the Standard American Diet (otherwise aptly known as SAD) is heavily laden with refined sugars, which, in turn, wreak havoc on the metabolic process of the body. When refined sugar is digested, it no longer remains neutral at a pH of 7. This results in the formation of toxic by-products like pyruvic and lactic acids, to name a few. The acids interfere with the respiration of cells, inhibiting them from receiving sufficient oxygen to survive and function normally. In other words, sugar is highly acidic, promotes inflammation, and creates a deoxygenated internal environment. All these low to no sugar diets now make a whole lot of sense.

Want to know which foods boost the most alkalizing benefits? Scan through our top 7 super-alkaline foods list! The goal here is to make it nutritious *and* delicious!

TOP 7 SUPER ALKALINE FOODS

1. **SPINACH:** As with all green foods, spinach is rich in chlorophyll (we will discuss the health benefits of chlorophyll later. Sit tight!), a potent alkalizer, and blood builder. It's high in vitamin K, vitamin A, manganese, folate,

magnesium, iron, vitamin C, vitamin B2, calcium, potassium, vitamin E, and dietary fiber. Popeye had something going here. All leafy greens should be eaten in abundance, but spinach is great raw (or steamed). Spinach is easy to use in recipes and salads—and it's straight-up delicious. Baby spinach or fully-grown spinach is incredibly alkaline.

2. KALE: Kale is another leafy green that has gained much popularity lately. It's widely known for its cancer-fighting, cholesterol-lowering, antioxidant-rich, detoxifying properties. When prepared properly, it is absolutely delicious. Like spinach, it is massively high in vitamin K, vitamin A, and vitamin C and also has a huge chlorophyll content. Kale contains at least four glucosinolates, and as soon as you eat and digest kale, these glucosinolates are easily converted into cancer-fighting compounds. As if being a champ cancer fighter wasn't enough, kale is also quite amazing at lowering cholesterol.

3. CUCUMBER: Cucumber is most noted for its water content: 95%! This makes it an incredibly hydrating food and a great base for juices. It also contains superb amounts of antioxidants, including the super-important lignans. (Lignans are great at scavenging free radicals that play a role in aging and disease.) A strong history of research shows that cucumbers are connected with a reduced risk of cardiovascular disease as well as several cancer types, including breast, uterine, ovarian, and prostate. Cucumbers also contain the following alkaline minerals: calcium, iron, phosphorus, potassium, magnesium, selenium,

copper, manganese, iron, and zinc. And you thought cucumbers were only good for facials, think again!

4. BROCCOLI: Broccoli (and broccoli sprouts!) is a must. Broccoli has been proven over and over and over again to be incredibly powerful in inhibiting cancers, supporting the digestive system, the cardiovascular system, the detoxification processes in the body, and also supporting the skin, metabolism, and immune system. It's anti-inflammatory and provides ample antioxidants. It's a hugely alkaline, hugely nutritious food. Put it in salads, juices, smoothies, soups—anything! I prefer mine steamed and opt to send the stalk through the juicer.

5. AVOCADO: Avocados have a high-fat content—but think fats will make you fat? Not necessarily. These fats are good fats! Due to the high content of oleic acid (Omega 9), it can lower total cholesterol levels and raise levels of high-density lipoproteins (HDLs) while lowering low-density lipoproteins (LDLs), also known as the "bad" cholesterol. Oleic acid slows the development of heart disease and promotes the production of antioxidants. These beneficial omega oils also help speed metabolism. Avocados contain a wide range of other nutrients that have anti-inflammatory, heart health, cardiovascular health, anti-cancer, and blood sugar benefits. Containing key antioxidants such as alpha-carotene, beta-carotene, lutein, selenium, and more—it is a powerful, alkaline, nutrient-dense, and above all, delicious food. The creamy texture is just a bonus. Add it to soups and smoothies!

6. CELERY: Celery, like cucumber, is also very alkaline and has significantly high water content, so it is a great choice to use as a base in juices. Couple it with cucumbers! Celery is loaded with vitamin C, but two of its lesser-known nutrients are phthalides (which have been shown to lower blood pressure and cholesterol) and coumarins (which have been shown to inhibit several cancers). The beauty of vitamin C rich foods is that they help support the immune system, lessen inflammation, and also help support cardiovascular health. Crunch away, celery lovers!

7. CAPSICUM / BELL PEPPER / PEPPER: The antioxidant superpower, the red bell pepper is sweet, crunchy, loaded with moisture, and refreshingly delicious. You can use it in almost any meal. It is a great flavor enhancer and base for salad dressings and coatings for kale chips. Impressively beneficial to our health, red bell peppers contain 30 members of the carotenoid family, phytonutrients known to contain antioxidants, lower blood pressure, and prevent cancer. The only other food that is close to this is the tomato. Bell peppers are a good source of the more common antioxidants: vitamin C, vitamin A, and vitamin E. Did you know bell peppers contain twice as much vitamin C as oranges?[6] Bet you didn't "C" that one coming.

So, with all of this information, you ask, "where do I go from here?" Head on over to the Kale and Quinoa intro! Start by incorporating our kale and quinoa recipes to begin moving your body toward the alkaline side. Try at least one recipe before moving on to the next chapter! They're great for lunches and easy to take on the go! Also, try adding the foods above into your daily diet. Change doesn't happen overnight, nor should it! As we all know, change takes time. We want you to enjoy these changes; relish them. We want you to reap their rewards.

alkaline

EAT MORE RAW & FRESH

HIGH	MODERATE	MILD

HIGH

VEGETABLES

ARUGULA
ASIAN GREENS
ASPARAGUS
BARLEY GRASS
BEET GREENS
BROCCOLI
CELERY
CUCUMBER
ENDIVE
GINGER
KALE
KELP
KUDZU ROOT
LETTUCE
SEA VEGGIES
SPROUTS
SWEET POTATO
WATERCRESS
WHEATGRASS

DRINKS

HERBAL TEA
LEMON WATER
MINERAL WATER

OILS

COCONUT OIL

HERBS

CHIVES
PARSLEY
BASIL

FRUITS

CANTALOUPE
GRAPES
SWEET
KIWI
LEMON
LIME
MANGO
MELONS
PAPAYA
PEARS
PINEAPPLE
RAISINS
WATERMELON

SEEDS

FLAX SEEDS
PUMPKIN SEEDS

SPICES

CAYENNE PEPPER
CINNAMON
CORIANDER
CURRY
PEPPER
HIMALAYAN SALT

OTHER

BAKING SODA
BAKING POWDER
BEE POLLEN
PROBIOTIC CULTURES

MODERATE

VEGETABLES

ALFALFA
SPROUTS
ARROWROOT
AVOCADOS
BAMBOO
SHOOTS
BEANS
FRESH GREEN
BEET ROOT
BELL PEPPER
BROCCOLI
CABBAGE
CAROB
CARROTS
CAULIFLOWER
CELERY
CORN
SWEET + FRESH
DAIKON RADISH
GARLIC
GINGER
KHOLRABI
LETTUCE
LEAFY GREEN
PEAS
FRESH + SWEET
PARSNIP
POTATO W/SKIN
PUMPKIN
SWEET
SPINACH
SQUASH
SUMMER
TURNIP
ZUCCHINI

FRUITS

APPLES
SWEET / SOUR
APRICOTS
BANANAS
RIPE
BERRIES
CHERRIES
DATES + FIGS
FRESH
GOOSEBERRY
GRAPES
SOUR
GRAPEFRUIT
GUAVAS
NECTARINE
ORANGES
PEACHES
SWEET
PEARS
LESS SWEET
RASPBERRY
STRAWBERRY

HERBS

THYME
MINT
FENNEL

CONDIMENTS

APPLE CIDER VINEGAR
TAMARI
SEA SALT

MILD

VEGETABLES

ARTICHOKE
GLOBE / JERUSELUM
BRUSSEL SPROUTS
EGGPLANT
LEEKS
MUSHROOMS
OKRA
OLIVES
RIPE
ONIONS
RADISH
RHUBARB
SPIRULINA
TARO
TOMATOES
SWEET
WATER CHESTNUT

HERBS

AMARANTH

NUTS

ALMONDS
CHESTNUTS
DRY ROASTED

SEEDS

SESAME SEEDS
WHOLE

OTHER

GOATS MILK & WHEY- *RAW*
PICKLES
FERMENTED
SOY MILK & CHEESE

FRUITS

CHERRIES
COCONUT
FRESH

GRAINS

ESSENE BREAD
MILLET
OATS
QUINOA
SPROUTED GRAINS

SWEETENERS

HONEY *RAW*
BARLEY MALT
BRONNER
BROWN RICE SYRUP

CONDIMENTS

HORSERADISH
MAYONNAISE
HOMEMADE
NUTRITIONAL YEAST
SWEET BROWN RICE VINEGAR

PROTIENS

TEMPEH
MISO
SOY BEANS

OILS + FATS

AVOCADO OIL
FLAXSEED OIL
OLIVE OIL

acidic

EAT LESS FRIED & PROCESSED

NEUTRAL

VEGETABLES

MACA ROOT

NUTS

BRAZIL NUTS
CASHEWS
HAZELNUTS
MACADAMIA
PECANS
PISTACHIOS
WALNUTS

SEEDS

PUMPKIN SEED
SUNFLOWER

GRAINS

BARLEY
BRAN
BUCKWHEAT
CORNMEAL
RICE
UNREFINED
RYE
GRAIN
RYE BREAD
ORGANIC SPROUTED
SPELT

FATS + OILS

AVOCADO OIL
SESAME OIL

SPICES

MUSTARD SEED
NUTMEG

FRUITS

BLUEBERRIES
COCONUT
(DRY)
CRANBERRIES
PLUMS
PRUNES

LEGUMES

ADZUKI
GARBANZO
KIDNEY
LENTILS
MUNG
PINTO

PROTIENS

TOFU

SWEETENERS

MAPLE SYRUP
(UNPROCESSED)
MOLASSES
(UNSULPHERED ORGANIC)

OTHER

ALOE VERA
CACAO
CRACKERS
(UNREFINED RYE)
POPCORN
(PLAIN)

MODERATE

VEGETABLES

POTATOES
WITHOUT SKIN

GRAINS

OATS
RICE
BASAMATI
BROWN RICE
WHEAT GERM

BREADS

BREADS
REFINED
CORN BREADS
RICE BREADS
WHEAT BREAD
SPROUTED ORGANIC

PROTIENS

EGG WHOLE
COOKED HARD
FISH
SHELLFISH
SEITAN

SWEETENERS

MAPLE SYRUP
PROCESSED
MOLASSES
SULPHURED

CONDIMENTS

KETCHUP
MAYONNAISE
SOY SAUCE
COMMERCIAL

FATS + OILS

VEGETABLE OIL

FRUITS

APPLES
APRICOT
BANANAS
GREEN
BLACKBERRY
GUAVA
MANGO
PAPAYA

NUTS

PEANUTS

DRINKS

FRUIT JUICES
W/SUGAR
WINE

DAIRY

CHEESES
SHARP
YOGURT
SWEETENED

OTHER

CEREALS
REFINED
CIGARETTE
ROLL YOUR OWN
CREAM
OF WHEAT
UNREFINED
PASTA
WHOLE GRAIN
PASTRY
WHOLE GRAIN
PICKLES
COMMERCIAL
TAPIOCA
WHOLE
WHEAT FOODS

HIGH

PROTIENS

BEEF
CHICKEN
DEER
GOAT
LAMB
PORK
RABBIT
TURKEY

DAIRY

CHEESE
PASTEURIZED
MILK
PASTEURIZED

BREADS

WHEAT
WHITE

GRAINS

RICE – WHITE

CONDIMENTS

TABLE SALT
REFINED & IODIZED
VINEGAR
WHITE PROCESSED

DRINKS

ALCOHOL
BEER
BLACK TEA
COFFEE
LIQUOR
SOFT DRINKS
CARBONATED/FIZZY

SWEETENERS

ARTIFICIAL
SWEETNERS
MOLASSES
SULPHURED
SUGAR
WHITE / BROWN

OTHER

CAKE
W/WHITE FLOUR
CHOCOLATE
CIGARETTES
TAILOR MADE
CUSTARD
W/WHITE SUGAR
FLOUR
WHEAT / WHITE
JAMS / JELLIES
PASTA
WHITE
PASTRIES
W/WHITE FLOUR
PROCESSED
FOODS
SEMOLINA

DRUGS

ASPIRIN
MEDICINAL
PSYCHEDELIC

CHEMICALS

HERBICIDES
PESTICIDES

become a champion grocery shopper

It's nearly impossible to write a holistic health education program that discusses the benefits of high-quality foods yet ignores the controversy surrounding the health impact of genetically modified organisms (GMOs). I say that because GMOs are found in significant numbers in a location often frequented; the grocery store. GMOs can be found lurking in packaged products or mixed in with fresh vegetables in the produce section of the grocery store. What's troubling is that they are often camouflaged and sold under the false pretense of being "all-natural." If you're familiar with GMOs, you may be able to recognize some of them, but would you be able to find every single one? They're more common than you think.

Processed products have and continue to make up the bulk of grocery store aisles. Approximately 80 percent of packaged foods are known to contain at least one genetically modified organism.[7] It'd be a daunting task to scroll through numerous processed products to find the offending culprit. Leaving products unmarked and without labels is convenient for the food industry but inconvenient for you. Without labeling, many consumers remain unwitting guinea pigs, as the long-term effects of GMOs are currently not known.

Outside the U.S., many countries, including the entire European Union, require GMO labeling. In total, there are 64.[8] Other countries use voluntary GMO labeling, while many more countries have plans to introduce some form of genetically modified labeling. Until recently, companies in the US were not required to label their products as containing genetically modified ingredients. It wasn't until President Obama enacted the National Bioengineered Food Disclosure Standard on July 29th, 2016, that companies were required to disclose such ingredients. It was nothing to write home about, as consumer advocates dubbed it the D.A.R.K Act (Deny Americans the Right to Know Act). Even with the recent regulations in place, have you seen a warning label on any of the food you have purchased? The current labeling laws in the US is nothing but a veiled attempt to disclose which foods contain GMOs. In order to understand the contents of your produce or packaged product, you'd have to be well... informed. And not to confuse matters, many more foods are coming to market that have some form of genetic modification but fall under the "no need to disclose" section of the DARK Act.

Real change stems from consumer demands, and, thankfully, the demand for GMO labeling is at an all-time high. Before 2016, a few of the bigger companies like Campbell's Soup, the candy company Mars, General Mills, Kellogg, and ConAgra were voluntarily labeling their products as "made without genetically modified organisms." This voluntary labeling was largely due to intense public pressure. And public pressure does have an impact!

THE REAL CONTROVERSY

The problem with GMOs stems from the very same companies that manufacture them. These companies, most notably Monsanto, wage campaigns maintaining their safety, while independent anti-GMO groups claim genetically engineered foods have adverse effects on our health and the environment. Who's to believe? It's a hotly debated topic with biotech companies sending scores of lobbyists to Washington to push for legislation that favors GMOs and smaller non-profits trying to prove their malfeasance. Companies who rely heavily on the use of GMO ingredients do not support labeling laws suggesting it gives a bad stigma to GMOs, yet conversely, they want to keep GMO ingredients disguised. If GMOs are safe to consume like the FDA would have you believe, then why not be transparent in labeling?

The often thorny and convoluted problem with GMOs affecting the American consumer isn't limited to fresh produce and packaged foods. GMOs can be found in scores of animal feed, including beef, poultry, pork and fish meal, biofuel, pharmaceuticals, supplements, and cotton (including tampons). The introduction of the first genetically modified animal, AquaBounty's AquaAdvantage® salmon, will make its arrival for sale in the state of Indiana by the summer of 2020.

While you may find yourself deliberately trying to avoid GMOs or products containing GMOs, the solution may not be so clear-cut. One of the unintended consequences of GMO farming is the continued threat of widespread proliferation in the environment due, in large part, to cross-contamination and polluted soils. The only surefire way to know if GMOs are in our food is to understand the current legislation and food labeling laws, requiring that we become astute consumers. But you don't have to become an investigator or researcher to be accurately informed. There are a few agencies and consumer groups that closely monitor the recent developments regarding GMOs by surveilling new and inadvertently contaminated genetically-engineered (GE) foods. It's perfectly acceptable to rely on them to be updated with currents trends and the latest happenings.

Following legislation may not be your thing, but keeping GMOs out of your diet may be, so a quick and easy way to avoid GMOs is to look for the USDA's certified organic white and green circular label on produce and packaged products. No matter where it was grown, if a product has the USDA Organic label on it, it wasn't produced with a GM seed.[9] To guarantee your processed food is without trace GMOs, look for a third-party verification label known as the non-GMO project. These are "must-haves" on your grocery shopping list!

WHY ARE GMOS OFTEN LINKED TO MONSANTO?

If you're unfamiliar with Monsanto, you shouldn't be. While its early history was relatively benign, Monsanto has become more notoriously known for its development and widespread use of the now-banned DDT, Agent Orange, PCBs, and the highly controversial rbGH (bovine growth hormone). What's rbGH? Think, 'Got Milk?'

WHAT IS A GENETICALLY MODIFIED ORGANISM?

In the early 1980s, Monsanto was looking toward transgenic modification of plants—

which is the controversial science behind GMOs. Genetically engineered food originates from Mother Nature, but through scientific manipulation, it becomes what people commonly refer to as "Frankenfoods."

In transgenic breeding, genes are taken from a particular species or bacteria that are completely unrelated and then transferred into plants.[10] If this is confusing, think mating a fish with an apple—two completely unrelated species. Genetic engineering creates a combination of plant, animal, bacteria, and virus genes that are not organically found in nature.[11]

Transgenic modification of Monsanto's corn and soy, for example, takes natural biological material—such as a soybean seed or corn kernel—which is then artificially mated (spliced) with an insecticide (most notably the Bt gene, bacillus thuringiensis). The mating of chemical with seed is facilitated through the use of either bacteria to deliver the new genetic material, or by shooting tiny DNA-coated metal pellets into the plant cells with a gene gun. The newly developed seed has been genetically altered to produce its own insecticide, the Bt toxin. When a bug takes a bite out of the plant, the Bt toxin splits open its stomach, ultimately killing it. But rest assured, it's safe to eat according to the biotech firms like Monsanto. Our own FDA gives it a stamp of approval.

THE BIRTH OF GMOS

Monsanto's genetically engineered (GE) seed was first successfully created in a lab back in

1983, but it wasn't until 1987 that Monsanto grew its first field crops. By 1996, Monsanto's GE foods had officially entered the grocery market without the knowledge or consent of the American people. Is it any coincidence that the rise in gut disorders markedly began to increase that very same year?[12]

Monsanto's first commercial cultivation of genetically engineered plants in 1996 had been modified to be tolerant to the herbicides glufosinate and glyphosate, both of which are manufactured by Monsanto. GE foods are hotly debated because their claim to fame is to eradicate world hunger by being able to grow crops that are virtually indestructible—free from pests, fungus, and weeds by being able to withstand the baths of chemical applications. GMOs are said to be resistant to virus damage (as in the Ringspot-virus-resistant genetically modified papaya currently grown in Hawaii) *and* can produce its own pesticide, the Bt toxin.

According to the FDA, USDA, and Monsanto, these foods are safe to eat. However, the only studies to date have been on animals, not humans.

LEGISLATIVE DECISIONS REGARDING GMOS

Decisions regarding the safety of GMOs do not come from independent government studies. Instead, the FDA requires that the *burden of proof* comes from Monsanto itself (which also means the studies Monsanto funds) or by the "independent" scientists who work at colleges and universities and who are also the recipients of large donations from Monsanto and its subsidiaries.

Granted, GMO legislation draws its conclusions from scientific research, but when push comes to shove, research can be manipulated and tainted—be it from lobbyists, from a shortened study, from a study lacking sufficient data, or even the abrupt cessation of studies due to a position of dissenting opinion.

When a company is pushing a product for profit, the results of those studies can often be biased in favor of the manufacturers, especially considering corporations not only sponsor a growing amount of research, they also frequently dictate the terms under which the studies are conducted. One could loosely say that Monsanto runs (or owns) the studies that prove that GMOs are safe. To further muddy the waters, several former biotech executives and lobbyists who sat on Monsanto's legal and advisory boards, and committees among many others, now work for the federal government, including the FDA. This agency ultimately concludes whether the food you eat is safe to consume.

MONSANTO'S NOT THE ONLY ONE

Two other seed companies collectively dominate the seed and GE seed market. They are Syngenta and Dow. These three conglomerates are rapidly buying up smaller seed companies and gaining control of entire food production systems, including educational research facilities. In June of 2018, Bayer purchased Monsanto and, in turn, (to avoid heading off potential antitrust concerns) divested their seed business to BASF, a German-based chemical company—the largest chemical company in the world. Farmers and farm groups are increasingly concerned due to a marked upturn in corporate concentration resulting in decreased competition. We lose our freedom to choose when only a few companies single-handedly control the food we eat.

ENVIRONMENTAL IMPLICATIONS OF GE FOODS

Initially, farmers were intrigued by GMO seeds due to promised higher harvest yields. It was also hyped as producing a more nutritious product even when grown in mineral-depleted soils, a result of heavy pesticide and herbicide baths along with monoculture farming.

But, these new practices—known as genetically engineered crops—are essentially making pests resistant to pesticides, creating "superbugs." Weeds are becoming resistant to weed killer requiring the use of *more* weed killer. Something has gone wrong with its science. But, as always, nothing is for free.

CROSS CONTAMINATION OF GMOS

The seeds developed by these particular companies threaten the very existence of original crops through natural wind/cross-pollination and new breeds. Pro-GMO proponents would say there is no cross-breeding from pollination, but do you believe them?

Organic farmers are held accountable to the national organic standard. They are expected to adhere to the policies and practices of organics to maintain their certification. Organic farmers also pay a large fee to be able to use the certified organic label – a label held revered by many consumers. To avoid organic and GMO crops flowering at the same time (which can cause cross-pollination), some farmers plant their seeds early or late in the growing season. Others harvest crops before flowering or sign cooperative agreements with neighboring farms to avoid planting GMO crops next to organic ones. Any certified organic operation found to use prohibited substances or GMOs may face enforcement actions, including loss of certification and financial penalties.[13]

Many farmers fear that Monsanto will sue them through inadvertent cross-pollination. Still, Monsanto insists it has never been, nor will it be their policy to exercise its patent rights where trace amounts of DNA from their patented seeds are present in farmer's fields as a result of inadvertent means.[14] Between 1997 and 2010, Monsanto brought 144 infringement lawsuits and settled another 700 cases without litigation.[15] With that kind of reputation, it's no wonder small organic farmers fear Monsanto.

THE SAFETY AND SCIENCE OF GMOS

A peer-reviewed article of Jeffrey Smith, founder of the Institute of Responsible Technology, published November 7, 2017, in the *International Journal of Human Nutrition and Functional Medicine*, concurred that

GMOs are likely taking a heavy toll on our health due to the microscopic chemicals that are still prevalent in the resultant food, contrary to pro-GMO beliefs. A survey of 3,256 people who avoided GMOs in their diet reported astonishing improvements in 28 health conditions, namely, gut health.[16,17]

THE POLITICS BEHIND GMOS

Let's be partial. Monsanto, politicians, companies, and scientists ask that we buy into the argument that GMOs are a better alternative to conventional seed. If you spend some time researching the GMO hotly contested debate, you will realize the enormity and scope of the GMO quandary and the profound impact Monsanto's agenda has had on the political, social, and environmental landscape, even around the globe. Politics aside, President Barack Obama in 2016 signed into law one of the only bills set forth for mandatory GMO labeling—the S.764 federal standard for food labeling—which, in an ironic twist, has been titled the National Bioengineered Disclosure Act. Disclosure can provide information necessary for a consumer to make an informed decision. In business, full disclosure specifically means telling the truth. Anything short of telling the truth becomes concealment, and depending on the industry, anything short of full disclosure can have legal consequences or financial penalties. Unfortunately, the people elected to congress sworn to represent us have been so corrupted by our political process from the huge sums of corporate money and the covert influence over studies done by reputable scientists. The "DARK Act" has been dubbed the Deny Americans the Right to Know Act by continuing to keep consumers in the dark about whether or not GE material is found in a certain food or food products. Many liken President Obama's actions to that of fulfilling the Monsanto Doctrine. The law has been a huge loss for consumers, especially Vermonters, by invalidating the GMO labeling laws that the state had passed in 2016.

The bill is viewed negatively by anti-GMO advocates because it does not clearly establish a uniform national standard for full disclosure of GE food ingredients and gives the USDA the right to determine how much of a product needs to be bioengineered before a label is created. It continues to keep consumers in the dark by allowing food companies to avoid the whole truth—full disclosure. The Act also blocks states from issuing their own mandatory labeling laws, such as the case with Vermont. It requires food manufacturers to use one of three different labels to inform consumers of the presence of GMOs in products.

Manufacturers can comply with the ruling by providing a label that includes a U.S. Department of Agriculture (USDA) symbol indicating the presence of GMOs, print a label using plain language, or add a scanner- or smartphone-readable QR code that links to ingredient information.[18] The Act also omits GE foods that have been processed, such as oils and sweeteners, because it removes the evidence of modifications. The other limitations of the Act include language that limits labeling to GE foods that "could not otherwise be obtained through conventional breeding or found in nature."[19]

IN CONCLUSION

Not enough independent, unbiased, longitudinal studies are being done to say whether or not GE foods have a long-term negative effect on human health. Without transparent labeling, people are largely unaware that they are consuming experimental foods. Has the safety of these new foods been tested long enough and without bias? Are the decisions made by the Food and Drug Administration and the Environmental Protection Agency enough to warrant an approved safety rating?

Until that is done, we should label GE foods and return to sustainable, organic growing practices. Despite all of the smoke and mirrors, there are many ways to avoid GE food. Thankfully there are tips, tricks, and shortcuts. Here's how:

Number #1 Look for the Non-GMO project label!

WHAT IS THE NON-GMO PROJECT?

The Non-GMO Project is an independent, nonprofit monitoring agency, which continually maintains an accurate list of non-GMO ingredients.

You can find their logo displayed on the front of processed food boxes scattered throughout grocery stores. For more information on their testing and verification of at-risk ingredients and processed foods, please see the Non-GMO Project standard online.

GMO CROPS IN PRODUCTION[20]

Agricultural products are segmented into two groups: (1) those that are high-risk of being GMO because they are currently in commercial production, and (2) those that have a monitored risk because suspected or known incidents of contamination have occurred or the crops have genetically modified relatives in commercial production with which cross-pollination (and consequently contamination) is possible.

HIGH-RISK CROPS[21]

(These crops are currently in commercial production; ingredients derived from these must be tested every time before use in Non-GMO Project Verified products (as of December 2011):

Alfalfa (first planting 2011)

Canola (approx. 90% of U.S. crop)

Corn (approx. 88% of U.S. crop in 2011)

Cotton (approx. 90% of U.S. crop in 2011)

Papaya (most of Hawaiian crop; approx. 988 acres)

Soy (approximately 94% of U.S. crop in 2011)

Sugar Beets (approx. 95% of U.S. crop in 2010)

Zucchini and Yellow Summer Squash (approximately 25,000 acres)

Artic Golden Apples (Gone to grocery markets in Midwest 2017)

Innate Russet Potatoes (Approved by FDA 2015)

ALSO high-risk: animal products (milk, meat, eggs, honey, etc.) because of contamination in feed.

MONITORED CROPS[22] (those for which suspected or known incidents of contamination have occurred, and those crops which have genetically modified relatives in commercial production with which cross-pollination is possible:

Beta vulgaris (e.g., chard, table beets)

Brassica napa (e.g., rutabaga, Siberian kale)

Brassica rapa (e.g., bok choy, mizuna, Chinese cabbage, turnip, rapini, tatsoi)

Cucurbita (acorn squash, delicata squash, patty pan)

Flax

Rice

COMMON INGREDIENTS DERIVED FROM GMO RISK CROPS[23]

Amino Acids, Aspartame, Ascorbic Acid, Sodium Ascorbate, Vitamin C, Citric Acid, Sodium Citrate, Ethanol, Flavorings ("natural" and "artificial"), High-Fructose Corn Syrup, Hydrolyzed Vegetable Protein, Lactic Acid, Maltodextrins, Molasses, Monosodium Glutamate, Sucrose, Textured Vegetable Protein (TVP), Xanthan Gum, Vitamins, Yeast Products.

Wheat: There is not currently, nor has there ever been, any genetically engineered wheat on the market. Of all "low-risk" crops, this is the one most commonly (and incorrectly) assumed to be GMO. It is a key commodity crop, and the biotech industry is pushing hard to bring GMO varieties to market. The Non-GMO Project closely watches all GMO developments.

WHY ORGANIC IS WORTH THE PRICE

I continually encourage clients to buy certified organic produce, which is sometimes met with apprehension and skepticism. Why? Because certified organic products are grossly misunderstood.

I commonly hear the arguments over the cost of organics and the legitimacy of certified organic labeling. Clients wonder if it is even worth buying into. As the program progresses, it becomes abundantly clear the significant differences between conventionally grown produce and organically grown produce.

The distinction of organic produce does not mean the *absence* of pesticides. In fact, organic produce can *contain* pesticides.

Organic residues on organic produce come from bio-pesticides (derived from plants), not from the application of synthetic pesticides (man-made chemicals).

I repeatedly get challenged about the negligible dangers of pesticides and the unnecessary cost of organic products. I hear quite often that the "dirty dozen" covers the basics. It doesn't. In fact, the *process* by which organic food is grown and where the seed has originated has considerably more to do with the advantages of buying organic than the absence of pesticides; a *lot* more.

It is important to note that pesticide application is a small slice of what it means to be "certified as organic." Buying organic is buying into the belief that organic farming practices are actually better for us and better for the environment. Conventional farming and organic farming practices are two entirely different species.

When buying organic is not an option, try buying produce at farmer's markets, buying in season, and avoiding imported produce from countries outside the US (too much time in transit).

The benefits of organic farming are plentiful. Organic farming practices do not allow the use of synthetic fertilizers, sewage sludge, irradiation, and genetic-engineered seeds in the food it plants and harvests. In order to call a farm "organic," it must be free from synthetic application for at least three years after the most recent use of prohibited material.

WHAT EXACTLY IS AN ORGANIC FARMING PRACTICE?

• Organic farming provides cover crops: Cover crops, also called green manure, suppress weeds, build healthy soil, and help control pests and diseases. Green manure crops are generally part of the pea family and can often provide the needed amount of nitrogen for crop production naturally. In conventional farming, this nitrogen is typically applied in chemical fertilizer form. Cover crops are easy to plant and require only basic care to thrive! They grow well in nearly every part of the country, needing little water as they retain a sufficient amount of moisture.

• Organic field crop rotation: Field crop rotation is exactly as the name suggests. It involves a rotating planting cycle (a centuries-old practice) that is utilized anywhere from two to four years. What that means is that the same section of land is not used to grow the same crop more than once in a specified period. Instead, crops that are very different will be planted in the same tract of land in the off-year or offseason. Crop rotation is vital because it replenishes the soil year over year. Doing so usually results in crop production that is far superior to what is achieved when planting the same crops (mono-culture farming) in the same location year after year. Conventional farming uses the practice of monoculture farming, which depletes the soil of necessary nutrients (also due in part to synthetic pesticide application).

• Organic Farming's irrigation practices: Organic farmers usually use drip irrigation vs.

large industrial sprinklers typically found in conventional farming. Drip irrigation offers closely spaced drip emitters, which creates a wet line down the lowered portion of the plant bed. This allows for both germination and irrigation of the crop and drastically reduces weed growth.[24] Since the crop can be spoon-fed water and organic nutrients as needed, and the plant itself remains dry, the crop is healthier and more resistant to insects and diseases. Organic farming does not allow the use of sewage sludge (bio-solids) in irrigation, as defined in 40 CFR part 503.[25]

• What are biosolids? This is going to be fun. Biosolids are solids, semi-solids, or a liquid residue generated during the treatment of domestic sewage (human waste) at a treatment facility. According to the USDA's webpage, "when sewage solids are treated and processed, these residuals can be recycled and applied as biosolids to improve and maintain productive soils and stimulate plant growth," which, if you haven't figured already, means that this water can be used for commercial irrigation. Unfortunately, however, these regulations test for only nine metals before irrigation, and *not* for any toxic chemicals[26] before this wastewater is sprayed on your conventional produce.

• In the U.S., sewage solids must be treated to meet EPA's Part 503 sewage sludge regulatory requirements if they are to be used in irrigation.[27] Bio-solids are not allowed for use in organic farming *but* allowed for use in conventional farming. Many U.S. consumers are largely unaware of the fact that sewage sludge is *often* used for fertilizer in conventional agriculture.

• Organic farming practices nourish the soil: Conventional farming practices generally "beef up" the plants through artificial and synthetic means; however, much of the conventional soil has been stripped of its nutrients due to repeat plantings of the same crop, also known as monoculture farming. Organic farming practices, on the other hand, naturally nourish the soil through cultivation practices of tillage, vermiculture, and organic fertilizer. Organic farming practices also use various techniques to build up minerals and healthy bacteria in the soil that were once lost due to monoculture farming and synthetic pesticide application.[28] The continuous removal of nutrients through conventional farming has left our soils depleted and lifeless. The mineral content of our produce, grains, and fruit has rapidly declined.[29] Although we are encouraged to eat fruits and vegetables, much of the conventionally-grown produce does not provide the nutrients our bodies need. Organic produce is higher in mineral and nutrient content than its conventional counterparts.

• Irradiation or ionizing radiation: Irradiating food involves the practice of emitting X-rays and electron beams into food.[30] It is in place by the government as a precautionary measure— to keep us safe from microorganisms. Its purported benefits include: prevention of foodborne illness, extended shelf-life due to destruction of organisms, pest control management on imported goods, delayed sprouting and ripening, and sterilization of food to eliminate the need to refrigerate. It has been 'likened' to canning vegetables and pasteurizing milk. These forms of ionizing radiation are also used in the treatment of cancer, and the FDA, the CDC, WHO, and the USDA claim irradiation is safe when used on our food. Organically grown produce is *not* allowed to be irradiated.

• Organic seeds are not bioengineered (GMO): Buying organic seed is important because it guarantees that your seeds are not treated with fungicides. It also means Certified Organic Seeds are harvested from certified organic crops. Organic seeds may be a hybrid (one related species mated with another related species through traditional breeding) or heirloom variety (never been altered in any way). In order to qualify for the USDA Organic certification, farmers must purchase organic seed only. If they cannot find organic seed, they are allowed to use conventional, *untreated* seed. All organic seed is non-GMO.

What to do or where to go next? Pick up your phone and download the non-GMO app by heading to the non-GMO project's website at www.nongmoproject.org. You'll begin to notice the logo (if you haven't already) on food products within your grocery store. Also, look for the USDA's widely recognized green circular organic food labels when shopping for produce. When grocery shopping, try to leave conventional produce and processed foods without the organic or non-GMO app label where they belong—on the shelf.

blood, the sustenance of life

Is blood that important to overall health and well-being? Wouldn't it be our brain, our liver, or our heart!? Well, let's find out.

Our blood is responsible for nourishing every organ and cell in our body. In a way, it is our transport system. Think about it this way. A trucking company can't transport goods without a truck. You can't get your precious cargo across the ocean without a ship! Blood is an important facilitator responsible for the delivery of nutrients and oxygen to the cells within the body. The blood is also responsible for the transport of metabolic waste products away from those same cells (remember the first chapter, acidic by-products?) so that they may be removed from the body via the excretory organs (skin, lungs, colon, kidneys, etc.). These cells are suspended in a liquid called blood plasma, and they contain hemoglobin, an iron-containing protein.

When we think of iron in food, we generally think of iron that comes from meat. The type of iron we consume from animal products is called heme iron, and the iron that comes from plants and beans is called non-heme iron. Simple enough, right?

Blood is responsible for picking up the oxygen from our lungs *and* nutrients in our gastrointestinal tract. Oxygen is contained within the nutrients! The blood then carries the nutrients to cells throughout the body for metabolism. It finalizes its trip by picking up other wastes, including carbon dioxide, and transports them to the lungs and excretory organs. It then starts the cycle all over again. It's "in with the good, out with the bad" all day long. The blood is like your freeway system. Plug it up, and you've got yourself a nasty traffic jam.

Oxygen, the driver in the car on the freeway, is vital to many body processes:

- It stimulates digestion
- It promotes clearer thinking (the brain uses 25% of the bodily oxygen supply)
- It offers protective oxygenation of the blood
- And it promotes better circulation of the blood, ultimately nourishing every cell of the body.

SCIENTIFICALLY SPEAKING...

The cells in your body need oxygen to carry out metabolic processes and produce enough energy to live and support your daily activities. Red blood cells, like the cars mentioned earlier, are responsible for picking up oxygen from your lungs, transporting it in your bloodstream, and delivering it to cells that need it. Talk about meals on wheels!

Red blood cells are a good indicator of health. To ensure you have the right number of healthy red blood cells and to keep oxygen levels in your blood as high as possible, you need iron and a variety of vitamins. The hemoglobin is exceptionally important as it is responsible for delivering oxygen to all of the cells. A low red blood cell count could mean anemia. It could also mean blood loss or malnutrition. Patients undergoing chemotherapy can experience a drop in red blood cell counts as well. A proper blood cell count is so important that health practitioners check for a complete blood cell count known as a CBC at every yearly physical. Your blood may be more important for optimal health than you may have suspected!

There's a little catch when it comes to plant-based forms of iron (non-heme)! It needs to be paired with Vitamin-C and Vitamin B-12 for the best absorption. Non-heme iron is easily absorbed by the body, but strict plant-based eaters may need to eat just a tad bit more of it. Iron is essential for proper immune function and helping the body to fight infections.[31] It can be found abundantly in legumes and leafy green vegetables.

It is worth mentioning that as an herbivore, supplementation of Vitamin B-12 is key. Vitamin B-12 is found abundantly in animal-based foods such as fish, yogurt, milk, chicken, beef, and shrimp... but that won't work if you eat a strict plant-based diet! So what's an herbivore to do? Supplementation is key, and you can supplement in one of two ways:

Incorporating plants like algae (spirulina), sea vegetables (kelp and dulse), or wheatgrass (juices) into your diet increases the amount of B-12 that you aren't getting via meat sources. While various algae, sea veggies, and wheatgrass contain some vitamin B-12, they do not contain enough to provide all the B-12 you need. *Only a fraction of the B12 is bioavailable.*

It's important to prevent your B-12 levels from dropping, so try eating foods that contain folic acid (*green leafy vegetables*) instead. The body needs both B-12 and folic acid to maintain adequate vitamin levels.

The best advice is: When in doubt, take a Vitamin B-12 supplement.[32] Sublingual is best!

If you're looking for a boost of oxygen in your blood, there are definitely other foods that increase oxygen levels! They are B-5, B-6, and Vitamin A (or the precursor to Vitamin A, which is beta-carotene). The body converts beta-carotene into Vitamin A in the intestines—again, the importance of digestion! It's not necessarily what you eat but what you absorb and assimilate!

Here are a few quick tidbits on where we can find a great source of Vitamin B-5 (AKA pantothenic acid), Vitamin B-6, and Vitamin A (& the precursor to A, beta-carotene).

VITAMIN B-5

These vitamins are in a wide range of foods, such as vegetables, nuts, and lentils. Vitamin B-5's main role is metabolizing carbohydrates, proteins, and fats and turning them into usable energy. You know that these are energy-packed foods, and this is your body's way of making use of that energy. Skimp out on these, and you could find yourself deficient in vitamin B-5. Remember, B-5 is important for making your body, well, work!

Vitamin B-5 has another serious task of secreting hormones, as it supports the adrenal glands. Think you might have a B-5 deficiency? Well, there are a couple of things to look out for. Low energy levels, general fatigue, and weakness might signal a need for more B-5. Arthritic symptoms and a tingling or burning in the feet or legs also might be another clue. Try to eat B-5 foods in their natural, raw form because B5 is easily lost in cooking and freezing.

B-5 is naturally present in leafy vegetables, mushrooms, organic corn, sweet potato, and a lesser amount in cauliflower, broccoli, and collard greens.[33] Try to avoid foods that put stress on your adrenal glands like caffeinated drinks and sports drinks. These are just "false" forms of energy. Try getting your energy boost with some energy-packed foods like carbs, proteins, and fats.

Next on our list is Vitamin B-6. Vitamin B-6 is an essential nutrient that helps create antibodies to fight infection, supports normal nerve function, helps to form red blood cells, and breaks down proteins in the body. It promotes the proper breakdown of sugars and starches and helps prevent the buildup of homocysteine in the blood—which can cause clotting or a narrowing and hardening of the arteries. And you don't want that!

Still not convinced? Deficiency of this nutrient can cause sores in the mouth, skin conditions, malaise, depression, and confusion. Because Vitamin B-6 is water-soluble, it cannot be stored in the fat cells of the body and needs constant replenishment. Certain vegetables like spinach, potatoes, green peas, yams, broccoli, asparagus and turnip greens, chickpeas, lentils, and wheat bran are all high in B-6, as well as bananas, avocados, and sunflower seeds.[34] (As if this list didn't seem tasty enough!)

And lastly, Vitamin-A. If you are deficient in Vitamin-A, it makes iron deficiency more severe. So if you have low blood oxygen levels, be sure to take in enough vitamin A. Vitamin A can *only be found* in animal products such as liver, beef, chicken, turkey, and dairy, especially butter and egg yolks or a supplement of cod liver oil. A family member to Vitamin-A is beta-carotene found in carrots, red bell peppers, sweet potatoes, spinach, mangoes, melon, and pumpkin—generally foods that are primarily orange in color. Beta-carotene, a family member through phytochemicals called carotenoids, is converted into Vitamin A by an enzyme in the intestine. Each individual differs in the amount that gets converted to Vitamin-A, so there's no telling *how much* gets converted. You may also supplement with Vitamin-A, but it is possible to get toxic doses of Vitamin-A from dietary supplements. Getting this vitamin from fruits and vegetables does not lead to symptoms of toxicity. Rule of thumb with Vitamin A: Keep it real.

DE-OXYGENATED CELLS

Remember, in Chapter 1, we covered alkalinity vs. acidity and keeping our body's pH balance in check? We also discussed that metabolic enzymes have the ability to repair. Well, we're going to build on that a bit more now as we dive into the topic of oxygenated cells. Our body continues to strive for balance or what we like to call "homeostasis." The primary goal of eating healthy and living a healthy lifestyle is to minimize the drain on the body's system. We do this by minimizing our assault on it.

Think about it—are you being as good to your body as you can be? We need to stop beating on our bodies and give them a chance to regenerate! How do we do that? By giving the body as much assistance and love in areas that we have control over. Your body will thank you.

As we move further into this information, we will continue to mention acidity. Remember, deoxygenation of cells pairs well with acidity. If we keep our body too acidic (from foods and bad dietary habits), the acidity in the body suffocates the cells necessary for "life." In this state, our cells cannot adequately take in nutrients and oxygen. Furthermore, an acidic environment compromises the cells' ability to efficiently expel toxins. After a prolonged period of time in an acidic condition, the body becomes susceptible to disease.

A body deprived of oxygen can cause circulatory problems, respiratory problems, and fatigue. Lack of oxygen can also cause psychological problems like short-term memory loss and even impaired judgment. By increasing the oxygen in your blood, not only are you more energetic and alert, you are helping your body remove harmful toxins.

It's interesting to note that new cells are constantly being formed as old ones die. They must be swept away to be expelled from the body, and the body does this by performing its own form of detoxification, naturally. The interesting part about the body creating new cells is how we can rebound from disease or nagging health issues. As time goes on, the more we help the body mend and repair through consuming nutrient-rich and highly oxygenated foods, the more we can see bodily changes take hold.

"Scientists have discovered that green juices increase the oxygenation of the body, purifies the blood and organs, aids in the metabolism of nutrients and counteract acids and toxins. Green juices are the superstars of the nutrition world." ~ David Sandoval, Founder, Green Kamut

WHEATGRASS AND CHLOROPHYLL

Chlorophyll

Many of the earth's largest and heaviest animals consume grass—and only grass—as their primary source of food. What is in that grass that is vital to the animal's existence? Besides the grass's numerous vitamins, minerals, and protein content, it contains a substance called chlorophyll. Chlorophyll is the green (or sometimes purple) pigment found in growing plants.

Years ago, Dr. Hans Fischer and a group of associates won a Nobel Prize for their work on red blood cells. During their research, they noticed that human blood, which carries oxygen to all our cells, is practically identical to chlorophyll on a molecular level. In the human body, red blood cells have the mineral element **iron** as its central nucleus. Most green plants, on the other hand, are characterized by chlorophyll, have **magnesium** as the cell nucleus. While this may seem coincidental, it is certainly worth considering as the life force supplied by plants, namely grasses, are high in both oxygen and chlorophyll. Chlorophyll is touted as being the best blood builder and oxygen-rich deodorizer.

Healthy cells love the oxygen that the aforementioned provides while decreasing the chance for unhealthy cells to live in a highly acidic environment. Many of the animal products (including dairy), processed and refined foods, and even synthetic chemicals can cause a highly acidic and deoxygenated environment in our blood and our cells. One of chlorophyll's more important functions is oxygenation of the bloodstream. It is found in both plant and vegetable sea life. The health benefits we obtain are immense. Chlorophyll can be found in leafy greens, wheatgrass juicing, vegetables, sprouts, nuts and seeds, grains, seaweeds, and especially green juices!

"Whole and unprocessed raw and living foods flood our bodies with chlorophyll, enzymes, vitamins, minerals, phytonutrients, fiber, and oxygen." ~ Ann Wigmore, founder of the Hippocrates Health Institute Wheatgrass

Ann Wigmore firmly believes that the fresh juice of young wheat plants is a storehouse of natural vitamins, minerals, chlorophyll, enzymes, and life energy. As the pioneer behind wheatgrass juicing, she declares that wheatgrass helps to nourish every cell of the body, while cleansing them of toxins. She goes on to explain that fifteen pounds of wheatgrass is equal in protein and overall nutritional value to three hundred and fifty pounds of ordinary garden vegetables.

Considering we wouldn't consume that much wheatgrass in one sitting, let's break those numbers down. If you consume the suggested amount of wheatgrass as 2-4 ounces daily, then that means you would be consuming equal in protein and nutrition 6 lbs. of ordinary garden vegetables daily. Not a bad idea!

Although maybe not the tastiest, using wheatgrass is the quickest and easiest way to become vitally healthy.

GLUTEN INTOLERANCE AND WHEATGRASS JUICING

Although wheatgrass comes from the same seed that is used to produce the wheat grain used to make flour, wheatgrass is harvested before the plant matures and produces grain, which means that the young wheatgrass blades (if processed correctly) do not contain wheat gluten. The only thing to watch for would be an errant seed still attached to the blade. Give the wheatgrass a vigorous wash, and any seeds will come loose.

THE NUTRIENT PROFILE OF WHEATGRASS

While I don't mean to bore you with the details on wheatgrass, it is necessary to mention some of them here. If wheatgrass is touted as a 'superfood,' then one should know what makes it so special. Take a look...but don't stop here! The next biggest superstar, chlorophyll, is featured next!

MINERALS IN WHEATGRASS

- Wheatgrass has about as much calcium as milk minus the acidity

- A fairly good source of iron

- Sodium, Potassium, Magnesium—electrolytes the body requires

- Excellent source of a wide variety of trace minerals like selenium and zinc.

- Eight essential amino acids, which the body can synthesize only from the proteins we eat.

Now, do you understand why wheatgrass is such a beneficial inclusion into the diet due to its nutritional value and its conversion into blood in the body? We didn't even get into some of the heroic stories of wheatgrass, but we're running out of space!

ABSCISIC ACID

A formidable anti-cancer agent, abscisic acid is a plant hormone closely related to Vitamin A. Small amounts of abscisic acid proved to be a great weapon against any form of cancer, and it's therefore considered to be an anti-cancer agent, according to Metropolitan State College of Denver. Sweet potato, flax, and wheatgrass are superior sources of abscisic acid in case you were wondering![35]

CHLOROPHYLL

The nutritional value of chlorophyll is endless! Chlorophyll is a vital part of healing, recovery, and repair.

The chlorophyll in wheatgrass has deodorizing properties, but don't clear out that personal hygiene cabinet just yet! One of the obvious ways of testing the effects of wheatgrass on bodily toxins is the noticeable absence of body odors. Remember that terrible question I asked you in the first chapter? Body odors, actually secretions from inside the body, begin to smell offensive after they react with bacteria on the skin. Showering alone doesn't fix this problem. However, in a matter of weeks, the secretions that caused the odor can be neutralized if you use wheatgrass juicing daily. Try it and see for yourself!

The enzymes, amino acids, and chlorophyll in wheatgrass juice contain anti-bacterial compounds that are especially good at destroying anaerobic bacteria that thrive in oxygen-poor blood and tissue. Certain infections, ulcers, and putrefaction (rotting due to bacteria) are caused in part by anaerobic bacteria that cannot live in the presence of oxygen or oxygen-producing agents such as chlorophyll.

Wheatgrass juice deactivates these anaerobic bacteria and promotes the regeneration of damaged areas.

Think we're full of hot air, here?

Lose the flatulence! Chlorophyll also eases the severity of chronic constipation and reduces the presence of gas. Letting go just got that much easier!

ENZYMES AND AGING - SUPEROXIDE DISMUTASE

In case you were wondering, one of the most important enzymes in wheatgrass is superoxide dismutase, and it's aptly named. It certainly does have superpowers!

Superoxide dismutase (SOD) is an enzyme found in cereal grasses, which plays a crucial role in wheatgrass' ability to fight aging.

Additionally, wheatgrass lessens the effects of radiation, acts as an anti-inflammatory compound, and may prevent cellular damage following heart attacks. Wheatgrass is a superior food source of SOD! SOD has been proven to protect us from cell damage due to superoxides (things that age every part of us), infections, aging, radiation, poisoning by chemical additives, bad air, recreational, and pharmaceutical drugs.

DNA REPAIR AND WHEATGRASS

WHEATGRASS AND FREE-RADICALS

This wildly overused and often misunderstood term 'free radical' has gained much popularity lately and for good reason! Free radicals are pretty nasty, and they're everywhere. In the air we breathe, in the water we drink, and in the food we eat. Their claim to fame is aging us, all of us—every bitty cell within us. Most of the time, we can't avoid them, but for the times that we can, let's do it! Free radicals are created within us by the consumption of processed and cooked fats in our diet and from the toxins in our environment. Free radicals tend to disrupt anything they get close to and can damage nearly every system in the body.

When free radicals damage cells, their remnants persist. These further disrupt health by inhibiting the flow of oxygen into cells. Free radicals are rebels without a cause.

Wheatgrass can effectively reduce and prevent free radicals because of its vitamin C, E, and carotene, which are *all* natural antioxidants. Cooking oils, butter, margarine, mayonnaise, and other free fats can age your body to the extent that you indulge in them and cannot rid your body of the excesses, and they love to sink their teeth into your fat cells.

There's a strong link between weight gain and toxicity. Weight loss occurs when the body becomes alkaline, and the cells begin to detoxify. Hint. Hint.

Vitamins A, C, and E are examples of natural antioxidants. Vitamin C not only prevents free radical formation but also prevents vitamins A and E from being destroyed. Wheatgrass juice contains about as much vitamin C per ounce as orange juice (seriously, and without all that sugar, too!) and more than most common vegetables. Again, Vitamin A is not found in wheatgrass juice or any other plant food, but its precursor carotene is. Carotene has not been found to be toxic in any amounts when consumed as a whole food source. Wheatgrass juice is a fabulous source of carotene and contains more carotene per pound than iceberg lettuce, tomatoes, and many other garden vegetables!

IN CONCLUSION

It's pretty apparent now that oxygenated blood, chlorophyll, and wheatgrass juicing is essential to a body in balance. As mentioned, chlorophyll has been shown to build red blood cells quickly, normalize blood pressure by dilating the blood vessels, helps to release carbon dioxide, distribute oxygen, promote higher metabolism, and stimulate enzyme systems. In addition, consuming chlorophyll from wheatgrass is a highly effective way to alkalize the blood.

Alkalinity reduces the level of acidity in the body, which can reduce the symptoms of many conditions, including arthritis, heart disease, high blood pressure, and insomnia, to name just a few.

Where to go from here? Head on over to the Cruciferous Vegetable intro section! Try some of these amazing foods in the recipe section and see if you notice a difference in how you feel! Don't forget to keep a kale and quinoa dish in your daily or almost daily diet. And begin to build from there. Keep it easy and simple by allowing your lunches to change first. Let the rest of your daily diet remain the same. Looking for a little more right now? Change up some of your side dishes at dinner! Head on over to the Detoxifying Sides section of the recipes. Many of those dishes are full of cruciferous vegetables as well.

From the Cruciferous section, move directly to the Juicing section to begin the juicing process. There you will find detailed information regarding juicers, how to juice, and what to juice and when! You will not feel left out in the cold. I promise! It's all spelled out clearly how to embark on this amazing process. Juicing should replace your morning beverage altogether. If not ready to let go of your norm, then begin with a morning juice and imbibe a little later on! These two sections, Cruciferous Vegetables and Juicing, will catapult you to the next phase of feeling fantastic!

phytochemicals, antioxidants and the controversy over soy

Antioxidants seem to steal the show these days, but there's a bigger, larger, more powerful plant compound that deserves some major street cred. It's called a phytochemical! Phytochemicals or phytonutrients are chemical compounds found naturally in plants that protect the plant against bacteria, viruses, and fungi. Phytochemicals help shield the buds of plants from predators and the elements of nature and pollution. But how does that translate into a benefit for me from a health perspective? Research is finding that the protective compounds of phytochemicals are passed along to us when we eat the plant. More than protect us from bacteria, viruses, and fungi, studies are showing that phytochemicals can prevent disease from developing by maintaining healthy cells. A big bonus? This applies to cancer prevention, as well! If it's potent enough to thwart the onset of cancer, then it most certainly can provide other health benefits as well!

According to WebMD, there are over 25,000 known phytochemicals and more that are yet to be discovered. Since there are so many, we are going to keep the types of phytochemicals to a minimum and focus on those that are researched extensively, not to mention the ones you might commonly hear or read about. We want to keep you knowledgeable and informed without feeling like, well...you're back in school! Here's a fairly simple way to understand the complexity of phytochemicals. The principal phytochemical association with a given food just by the color, smell, and type of food is known as polyphenols. Polyphenols are the largest subset of the phytochemical family. And from there, flavonoids are the largest of the polyphenol family. Not to worry! We explain it in simple detail. Just think of phytochemicals in comparison to a multigenerational chart!

A phytochemical's main purpose is to repair damage caused by aggressors, which in turn allow the plant to survive in hostile conditions. How that translates to us is it's just a matter of fighting hostile invaders within our blood cells! For instance, when grapes are grown on a vine and attacked by certain microorganisms, the plant secretes a large quantity of a substance that acts as a fungicide and counteracts the negative effects of that fungus. Plants cultivated naturally without the use of synthetic pesticides are more susceptible to attack and therefore contain *greater* quantities of self-defense molecules. Not a believer yet? Here's an interesting story. Take, for instance, the wine-growing practices of decades ago. Grapes grown for wine were one the most heavily sprayed crops (and some still are).

Most winemakers used chemical fertilizers and potent chemical fungicides and insecticides even when problems didn't exist. It was commonly used as a preventative measure. The pesticide baths created a slurry of chemicals that remained in the ground creating a depleted, lifeless soil. Some pests had even mutated to withstand the chemical baths, and fungal overgrowth was common. Many orchards were entirely wiped out! For the past 15-20 years, many winegrowers have turned back to sustainable, biodiverse

organic farming practices. Their categorical efforts have since created a nutrient-dense soil replete with beneficial bacteria. This new crop is now stronger, healthier, and better for us and the environment. It just shows that farming practices using the power of Mother Nature yields life back to the soil and, in turn, the plant.

Phytochemicals aren't discussed as much as antioxidants, which is unfortunate as they offer significant health benefits by incorporating them into our diet. In discussing phytochemicals, it's important to differentiate essential vs. non-essential nutrients. Phytochemicals aren't necessary for keeping you alive, unlike vitamins, minerals, proteins, carbohydrates, or fats. While they aren't responsible for keeping you alive, they **are** responsible for keeping you healthy. When you eat or drink foods that contain phytochemicals, you may potentially be consuming hundreds if not thousands of different phytochemicals. The compounds isolated from these foods have shown that a large number of them interfere with the sequence of events that trigger the birth of a tumor (however, many of the phytonutrients showing the **highest levels of cancer prevention** activity are present only in a very few specific foods, which are listed later on). While there are no recommended dietary allowances for phytochemicals, they are a vital part of a healthy dietary regimen.

POLYPHENOLS - THE LARGEST FAMILY OF PHYTOCHEMICALS

As we mentioned earlier, polyphenols are the largest class of phytochemicals. Flavonoids are the largest of the polyphenol family—don't panic. You'll see many of them listed over and over again. Within the family of phytochemicals, you will typically find mentioned: antioxidants, flavonoids, flavones, isoflavones, catechins, anthocyanins, isothiocyanates, carotenoids, allyl sulfides, and polyphenols.

The chapter categorizes more of the highly publicized phytochemicals. While these aren't all of them, please know many of these foods can be found in more than one category. You don't need to memorize them or be a scientist to understand. Just keep telling yourself, "fruits and veggies; fruits and veggies." And if you're thinking, "Gosh! The list is so long! How can I eat all of those foods in one sitting!?" Well, eating *all* of them in one day isn't necessary! Eat these foods whenever you can, but definitely don't avoid them! Try to make sure they become a part of your *weekly* diet! It's not possible to eat them all in one day!

Think of a rainbow being your food options, and you're mouth being the pot of gold at the end. In order to eat as many phytonutrients as possible, eat a variety of colors on the rainbow spectrum. Eat vegetables during every eating occasion (food in natural colors only) and fill half your plate of them! Yes, half! Eat more veggies than fruit, but make sure you vary your fruit choices as well.

Want to go a step further and maximize your anti-cancer potential? Focus heavily on these foods: tomatoes, cabbage, green tea, red bell peppers, turmeric, soybeans (organic fermented products like tempeh), garlic, and grapes.

And don't forget to eliminate the bad ones! You know which ones I'm talking about!

Since we mentioned the word cancer, I'd like to go a little more into detail on some very specific phytochemicals. They're worth spending a little extra time on:

• Allium (plant sulfurs), contained in the onions and garlic family, has been widely studied for its potential to reduce cholesterol levels and protect against heart disease. Studies show that people who eat garlic have lower levels of LDL cholesterol (the "bad" form of cholesterol) than people who do not eat garlic.[36] Garlic is also a great blood cleanser and has been touted for centuries as having antibacterial and antifungal properties. To get the most out of the alliums, it's best to eat them raw. While there are over 500 species within the allium family, you will mostly recognize them as leeks, scallions (green onions), red, white, and yellow onions, shallots, garlic, and chives.

• Ellagic acid found in many berries may prevent healthy cells from turning cancerous. It may also protect your noggin as it ages!

• Flavonoids are a part of a phytochemical family called polyphenols. This is the largest of all the polyphenol families. More than 4,000 different flavonoids belong here. You'll find flavonoids in cranberries, onions, broccoli, kale, celery, soybeans, tomatoes, eggplant, cherries, apples, cranberries, and tea. Red wine and grape juice contain a high level of phenolic flavonoids. Studies have shown that flavonoids can fight heart disease, slow cancer tumor growth, prevent blood clots, reduce inflammation, and act as antioxidants.[37]

• Indoles are found in the cruciferous vegetables, including broccoli, cabbage, Brussels sprouts, cauliflower, kale, bok choy, and turnips. Their primary benefit appears to be in protecting against certain forms of cancers. They may counteract carcinogens (cancer-causing agents) in the body, and they may play a role in blocking the growth of new prostate and breast cancer cells.[38]

• Isoflavones (or phytoestrogens) are a type of flavonoid similar to the female hormone estrogen. They are found primarily in soy, but also in grains, berries, seeds, and certain vegetables (such as chickpeas). Like estrogen, isoflavones can improve bone density and lower cholesterol levels, as well as reduce some of the symptoms of menopause. They may also protect against hormone-driven forms of cancer, such as prostate and breast cancer.[39]

While all of these families play an important role in maintaining a healthy, body of particular importance when detoxifying the body would be the consumption of those foods found in the Indole and Allium family.

HOW TO INCREASE YOUR INTAKE OF PHYTOCHEMICALS

It's real easy. Start by eating the colors of the rainbow! In need of pointers? Here they are:

• Be liberal with spices and herbs when cooking. Buy fresh or high quality organic. Include into your homemade dishes: basil, oregano, parsley, sage, thyme, turmeric, garlic, and ginger. Don't forget your curries, cumin, coriander, and dried chilies.

• Keep frozen veggies on hand, just in case you don't have fresh.

• Eat the white part of citrus fruits (despite being bitter!) as they contain the most amount of phytonutrients.

• Drink green tea instead of coffee.

• Make a nut mix with organic dried superfood fruits like goji, noni, and cranberry and sweeten with morsels of dark chocolate.

• Familiarize yourself with ancient cereal grains.

• Experiment with fermented soy products like Nama Shoyu, tempeh, and miso.

• Put into practice meatless Mondays.

While all these suggestions are very helpful in making you aware of how to increase the disease-fighting chemicals of phytonutrients, the majority of Americans eat less than two cups of vegetables per day and only one cup of fruit per day. In order to maximize the intake phytochemicals, it is NOT advised to get them through supplementation. The high dosage of isolated phytochemicals may have unexpected effects. Plant foods contribute 100% of phytochemicals to the human diet, so the recommendation is to fill half your plate with plant foods each time you eat.

ANTIOXIDANTS

Everywhere you turn these days, we hear about antioxidants and better health. But what is an antioxidant, and what do antioxidants do for us?

(Here's a little known fact. Phytochemicals have the ability to act like antioxidants, but antioxidants AREN'T phytochemicals).

Antioxidants are substances that inhibit the oxidation process (think rust!) within our bodies. The antioxidants act as the body's WD-40 by lubricating it and keeping it running! Antioxidants thwart the damaging effect of free radicals (the aggressors causing the rusting of our cells). Confused still? Think of it in these terms "free"—out of control, at liberty, without obstacles, and "radical"—extreme, drastic. And what do these free radicals feel at liberty to do? Wreak havoc on your body's cells—by basically "rusting" them out!

Before we think we can completely rid ourselves of these negative influences, it's important to note that, unfortunately, free radicals are just a part of everyday living and breathing. It can occur even when doing something good for yourself, like exercising. Free radicals are also naturally formed within the body when your body converts food into energy. Your body can also be exposed to free radicals from a variety of environmental

sources, such as cigarette smoke, smog, and sunlight. Free radicals go through the drastic measure of destroying healthy cells, which is termed oxidative stress, which in turn *changes* the DNA (*Hello*, that means trouble's on the horizon!). Oxidative stress is thought to play a role in a variety of diseases, including cancer, cardiovascular diseases, diabetes, Alzheimer's disease, Parkinson's disease, and eye diseases such as cataracts and age-related macular degeneration.[40] Free radicals and its by-product, oxidative stress, are sabotaging you of being the "best that you can be." While there are some factors we can change, others we cannot. What's the solution? The antioxidant potential!

Did you know that the body has its own inner mechanisms for fighting free radicals? It's not simple, but we'll make it sound simple...through glutathione production originated in the liver, but that begins to diminish around age 20 (Darn that thing called aging!), so in order to assist the body, it is best to consume antioxidants.

Now, it's important to make a distinction. Antioxidants are not anticancer, but remember in the earlier section, we said phytochemicals are anticancer and can also double as antioxidants. Here's how to differentiate the two:

Phytochemicals can target a variety of things going on in the body, including the chemical process involved in tumor growth or the proliferation of cancer cells. Phytochemicals—and most notably polyphenols—can search and destroy free radicals.

Antioxidants, on the other hand, fight the harmful effects of free radicals, including waste products from the air we breathe, the processed food we eat, and the environmental toxins we are exposed to. Antioxidants prevent or delay some types of cell damage and can be found in many foods.

Given the option to be on the antioxidant team or the phytochemical team, I think I may be going with phytochemicals for sure! But wait, antioxidants sound pretty impressive too!

Below you will find a list of antioxidants brought to you by the National Institute of Health:

Beta-carotene enhances white blood cells in the immune system and helps protect the lining of the mucosal membranes in the body. We hear it again; beta-carotene is the precursor to the formation of Vitamin A, which occurs in the intestines. Beta-carotene gives foods their yellow, orange, and red color. Foods high in beta carotene are squash, carrots, red bell peppers, cantaloupe, apricots, tomatoes, sweet potatoes and spinach, and broccoli (the green chlorophyll happens to mask the orange color).

Lutein is the deep yellow pigment found in the leaves of plants. Foods high in lutein include kale, spinach, dandelion greens, paprika, cayenne, turnip greens, mustard greens, watercress, swiss chard, radicchio, and collards.

Lycopene is one of the major carotenoids that give foods their red, yellow, and orange pigment present in tomatoes and many berries and fruit. Foods high in lycopene are watermelon, guavas, tomatoes, papaya, grapefruit, sweet red peppers, asparagus, red/purple cabbage, mango, and carrots.

Selenium is an essential trace element found in certain foods. However, plants do not manufacture minerals—they absorb them from the soil. There has been a significant amount of interest in the role of selenium and cancer prevention, heart disease, immune function, and thyroid health. Again, supplementation is more detrimental than the need for this mineral. Foods high in selenium include brazil nuts, sunflower seeds, and mushrooms.

Vitamin A - beneficial for vision, bone growth, reproduction, cell functions, and immune system. Vitamin A is converted in the body through the intake of beta-carotene. For a list of foods high in beta-carotene, see above. Vitamin-A foods can only be found in animal products, including dairy, as well as fish.

Vitamin C captures free radicals and neutralizes them. Foods highest in Vitamin C are yellow bell peppers, chili peppers, kale, broccoli, papaya, strawberries, kiwi, pineapple, Brussels sprouts, and mango. Hey, where's the o.j.? Try the former instead!

Vitamin E breaks the chain reaction of free radicals in a membrane. Foods highest in Vitamin E include tofu, spinach, almonds, sunflower seeds, avocados, olive oil, broccoli, swiss chard, hazelnuts, mustard greens, and squash and pumpkin.

High doses of direct antioxidant supplements may be linked to adverse health effects. Again, the recommendation is to consume antioxidants through food instead of through a pill.

SOY – THE CONTROVERSIAL BEAN?

Gosh. Is there something *wrong* with soy? It's a fantastic protein replacement for meat, right? Well, not exactly. Above we state that the isoflavones found in soy prevent cancer, and now we're cautioning you about soy? Why the contradiction!? Well, the reason is fairly simple. There's much processing that is done to soy that *is* bad for you. There are specific types of soy that are *better* for you. So, what we're doing is uncovering the fine print on soy. Again, we want to keep it simple, so we are going to try and make it less complicated—less complicated means we can't give you all the minute details, just the silky on soy. Read on soy lovers.

Long ago, in Ancient China, soybeans were grown as a cover crop plowed under the soil between food crops as a means of fertilization. Initially, the Chinese ate small quantities of fermented soy foods, but not the bean itself. The first foods made from soybeans were products of fermentation as in miso and soy sauce, then followed by the discovery of tofu preparation thousands of years later. Naturally found in soy are high levels of phytic acid, which may block the body from absorbing minerals like calcium, magnesium, zinc, and iron as well. To counteract the phytic acid, the process of

fermentation helps to neutralize the phytic acid and instead ends up producing a healthy probiotic effect. Fermented soy is the easiest form of soy for your body to digest and absorb nutrients. This includes again: miso, tempeh, and Nama Shoyu.

There are substantial benefits to soy, which include isoflavones, a sub-class of polyphenols, considered noteworthy to the fight on cancer, especially breast cancer. The flip side to that is if you already have cancer, particularly the estrogen-sensitive type, those same isoflavones could further promote the growth of a tumor. The confusion again? Studies show that the slowing of cancer progression is dependent upon several factors, namely the age of onset of the introduction of soy. It seems that soy consumption at an early age, before puberty, might better reflect the anticancer effect of soy.

In contrast, consumption at a later age could potentially promote the growth of certain types of cancers. Also, keep in mind the types of soy that are with and without benefit. Please understand that the medical community is at great odds over the benefits of soy and soy isoflavones. If we go based on the philosophy of the Hippocrates Health Institute, Director Brian Clement, Ph.D., N.D. adamantly states "no soy" for women with breast cancer. More on that in a moment.

THE HIGHLY PROCESSED SOYBEAN

Soybeans are crops that have been hybridized over many, many years. Altering the proteins of a crop can alter the nutritional components. In this case, hybridized soy is almost impossible to digest, often giving individuals extreme discomfort and further compromising the benefits of those cancer-attacking isoflavonoids. Typically the American diet relies heavily on highly processed, genetically engineered soy. A majority of the American soy crop used by the food industry includes processing the bean to use in salad dressings, cooking oils, emulsifiers (soy lecithin), breads, crackers and cereals, prepared foods, non-dairy creamers, and as a primary feed source for livestock and farm-raised fish. It is also used for infant formula, protein bars, protein drinks, milk substitutes, and tofu, etc. Soy is also a US commodity crop second to corn. In other words, we produce a LOT of it. Furthermore, as of 2019, 94% of the soy cultivated in the US is grown as genetically modified.[41]

The more soy is consumed in processed form, the worse it is for you. This includes faux meats, treats, and snacks and salad dressings made with soy or soybean oil. Processed soy is highly acidic to the body and can be mucous forming. Furthermore, much of the soy milk manufactured today is made from isolated soy proteins combined with other artificial ingredients and a significant amount of sugar, which compromises any benefits one would receive from the isoflavones. The proteins used have long been subjected to processing before being added to our diet that any anticancer properties associated with soybeans have long since disappeared.

As mentioned earlier, consuming phytochemicals in supplement form can be a cause for concern. As with the case of isoflavones, supplements can be as high as 100 milligrams per tablet, whereas daily consumption of isoflavones in an Asian diet consists of 25-60 milligrams. Asia has the lowest rates of breast cancer in women.[42] Again, the best way to consume phytochemicals is in their original form, not by way of a pill.

What's recommended when it comes to soy:

• consume organic fermented soy like miso, Nama Shoyu, and tempeh

• avoid all soy (isoflavone) supplements

• avoid all processed GM soy found in all of the products mentioned above

• avoid consuming CAFO meats (meat not certified as **organic, grass-fed, or pasture-raised**), including farm-raised fish whose main diet consists of GM corn and soy (especially tilapia)

• if you have breast, ovarian or uterine cancer or a history of estrogen-dependent cancer in your family, consult with your physician regarding his/her recommendation on the consumption of soy as we are not a replacement for medical advice.

Where to go from here? Head to our phytochemical section of the recipe book under Colors of the Rainbow! You will also learn about food preparation when it comes to beans and legumes, which also includes a small amount of soy. Here you will want to make some of these meals for dinner. Not ready for a meatless meal just yet? No problem, follow the recipe as is, and add your favorite meat on top, keeping with the whole plant "based" philosophy! But first, be sure to spend some time in the kitchen gadget and small appliance section to get you on your way to home-based healthy cooking.

omega oils 3, 6, 9 and saturated fats

Fats have gotten a bad rap despite their necessary role in healthy brain and bodily functions.

Why? Information about fats can be misleading and is presented to the public with a general statement that all fats are equal. It's a big fat lie! They are not!

Not all fat is bad (though too much of a good thing can still be bad, so watch your amounts of the good fats, too!). Our bodies need a certain amount of fat to function properly as they contain essential nutrients our bodies require. Fats also contribute to cushioning our vital internal organs. We just don't want excess cushioning.

Fat is necessary for the transport of fat-soluble nutrients like Vitamins A, D, E, and K. Healthy fats provide us with gorgeous locks of hair and supple skin—and if consumed responsibly, fat can also help us lose weight!

In today's on-the-run, faced-paced environment, fat is almost unavoidable. But which fats should we avoid? You may be surprised!

TRANS-FATS

America is the land of processed foods and the creator of the convenient meal. It is called mainstream America, and we are all a part of it. With cheap and quick food readily accessible, overconsumption has become the norm. The culprit in all that processed food? Trans fats.

Trans fats are found mainly in processed food items. Trans fat is a manufactured fat. It cannot be found in nature. Trans-fat's origins began as either a mono- or polyunsaturated fat. Through an industrial process called hydrogenation, the fat is structurally changed. It starts out as a natural fat, and through the chemical alteration process, the result is something entirely unnatural and unrecognized by the body. If the majority of your food is coming from the pantry in decorative and colorful packages, then you may be eating a lot of this stuff.

Trans-fats have an unnatural melting point, which allows it to sit at room temperature in a solid form. What was once oil at room temperature is now solid. Manufacturers see this as a big benefit because the hydrogenation of oils increases the shelf life of foods. Food with a longer shelf life saves the food companies money because these foods can be stored at room temperature for longer periods during shipping and storage. Consumers also love this advantage because these foods can last for months if not years in the pantry. I hope you're starting to wonder if this is real food?

No amount of trans fat is healthy. Why? Trans fat raises the LDL (bad) cholesterol in the body, the one that clogs the arteries. Unfortunately for us, that means the possibility of an increase in heart disease. Heart disease just happens to be the leading cause of death in the United States. So, with overconsumption of processed foods combined with the leading cause of death being heart disease and an obesity epidemic at large, could there be a correlation?

Today we know that trans fats have also been implicated in stroke, diabetes, and other chronic conditions. Eating trans fat also reduces the normal healthy responsiveness of the cells that line the blood vessels. In animal studies, eating trans fat also promotes obesity and resistance to insulin, the precursor to diabetes. When in doubt, steer clear of what industry is selling. Try to rely on Mother Nature instead.

Not sure where you'd find trans fats? Here is a potential list of offending culprits: certain brands of pizza dough and frozen pizzas, canned frosting, crackers, potato and corn chips, pies, meat pies (like chicken pot pie) and sausage rolls, non-dairy creamers, bakery products, certain kinds of margarine and vegetable oils and certain varieties of microwave popcorn. The best way to spot them? Look at the ingredients. If the ingredients show partially hydrogenated oils, you have found yourself a trans fat!

Moving on to repair the reputation of saturated fats.

SATURATED FATS

Saturated fat is a type of fat that comes mainly from animal sources of food, including meat and dairy. Other sources of saturated fat include palm oil and coconut oil. According to the Mayo Clinic, the problem associated with saturated fat comes from its very make-up. Saturated fat raises total blood cholesterol, which causes a build-up in the heart and arteries, increasing the risk of cardiovascular disease.

There's a new paradigm shift, however, regarding the demonization of saturated fats. A study published in 2010 by the American Journal of Clinical Nutrition pooled together

21 unique studies that included 248,000 people over a period of 14 years and found no relationship between intake of saturated fat and the incidence of heart disease or stroke. What the authors did find was that the 11,000 of whom who developed cardiovascular disease consumed a diet rich in trans fats from processed foods. A diet of saturated fat was replaced with a higher intake of carbohydrates (particularly refined), which can exacerbate insulin resistance and obesity, increase triglycerides and small LDL particles and reduce beneficial cholesterol.[43] In other words, a diet high in sugar (the breakdown of the refined carbohydrates in those very same processed foods) and dangerous trans fats is what the authors felt contributed to a risk of heart disease.

Saturated fat, once vilified by the American Heart Association, does everything from enhancing the immune system to protect the liver from toxins. Saturated fat is needed for optimal brain health. At least 50 percent of our cell membranes are made up of saturated fatty acids. So the skinny on saturated fat is it's not that bad after all.

Proponents of this new study argue that the studies since the 1950s have not differentiated between saturated and trans fats. Based on Dr. Mercola, here are some of the many benefits to saturated fat consumption:

- provides a concentrated source of energy

- provides the building blocks for cell membranes

- builds a variety of hormones

- slows absorption of meals

- acts as a carrier for fat-soluble Vitamins A, D, E, and K

- needed for the conversion of beta-carotene to Vitamin A

- needed for mineral absorption

- fuel for the heart

- source of fuel for energy expenditure

- antiviral agent (caprylic acid)

- antifungal agents (lauric acid)

- lowers bad and raises good cholesterol

- prevents cancer (butyric acid)

Please know that organizations such as the American Heart Association still encourage us to consume tasteless and useless vegetable oils, including margarine and packaged and processed foods with refined carbohydrates. Those foods negate the real benefit of fat consumption. The AHA also claimed that certain oils, as well as low-fat cuisine loaded with refined carbohydrates, would protect us from heart disease but subjected us to heart disease over the years instead. The final verdict on saturated fat is still being deliberated. More and more research is pointing to processed foods and not saturated fat as a contributing factor to an increased risk of cardiovascular disease.[44]

HEALTH BENEFITS OF POLY & MONOUNSATURATED FATS

Polyunsaturated fats have a different chemical make-up than trans fats and saturated fats. Polyunsaturated fat is responsible for the liquid consistency. Polyunsaturated fats consist of both omega-6 and omega-3 fatty acids.

Monounsaturated oils are generally liquid at room temperature but turn slightly solid when chilled, much like olive oil. Omega-9, a monounsaturated fat, can be found in avocados, olive oil, non-GMO canola oil, nuts, and seeds.

Since the body does not produce omega-3s, 6s, and 9s, they must be consumed through diet. They are considered essential fatty acids. Each type of fat creates different actions within the body.

• Omega-9 is oleic acid and is a monounsaturated fat

• Omega-6 is linoleic acid (LA) and is a polyunsaturated fat

• Omega-3 is alpha-linoleic acid (ALA), also a polyunsaturated fat

Each omega oil has a unique property to it, and we'll discuss a little bit about what each one does. The body takes the molecule from plant-based sources of omega-3s and converts **ALA** into **(EPA)** eicosapentaenoic and **(DHA)** docosahexaenoic acid. **EPA** is believed to play a role in the prevention of cardiovascular disease, while **DHA** is necessary for proper brain and nerve development.

Plant-based omega-3s and marine life omega-3s, it's important to note, are technically not the same omega-3s, although they are often lumped together. Like I mentioned above, plant-based sources of omega-3s contain a rich source of ALA, which is the body then converts into DHA and EPA. Much like the body's conversion of beta-carotene into Vitamin A, ALA conversion into EPA and DHA is similar. ALA is the precursor to EPA and DHA.

How much does the body convert? Well, there aren't any guarantees. Why? Because again, we rely on the functionality of an enzyme within our bodies to do the conversion. Some say as low as 1%, but it is also dependent on whether the body has adequate levels of vitamins and minerals.[45] So does that mean eating plant-based sources is nothing but a futile attempt to reap the benefits of omega-3s? Hold on! No! Vegans and strict vegetarians can get DHA and EPA directly from seaweed and algae sources while nom-nomming on plant-based rich dietary sources of omega-3s. Where do I find them, you ask? You will find an abundance of ALA based omega-3s in:

flaxseeds, walnuts, hemp seeds, soybeans, walnuts, soybeans, hemp seeds, chia seeds, flax seeds, pumpkin seeds, walnuts, and primrose oil and some dark green leafy vegetables. (Yes, you can actually find omega-3 oils in greens!). Plant-based direct sources of DHA and EPA include blue-green algae, chlorella, and seaweed.

THE OMEGA-3/OMEGA-6 CONNECTION

Many Americans are learning how important omega-3s are to heart health and for reducing inflammation, but why are we so down on omega-6s? We need omega-6s. They help with inflammation, and we need inflammation when tissues within our bodies are damaged. White blood cells flock to this damaged tissue and release a series of chemicals—one being blood clotting. But when the inflammation is on overdrive, too many inflammatory markers are present such as the pain signal of histamine, leading to redness and swelling and, ultimately, chronic pain.

Remember, omega oils are essential oils. Since our body doesn't make them, we need to consume them through diet. If the consumption of these oils is unbalanced, we end up with too much inflammation. And too much inflammation leads to disease.

Why have we been consuming too many omega-6s? Well, the American processed food diet pumps out a disproportionately high ratio of omega-6 to omega-3 to the tune of 20:1. In seeking a healthy balance, experts site anywhere from 4:1 or as low as 1:1 omega-6s to omega-3s. The culprits of high omega-6s include corn oil, safflower oil, sunflower oil, and canola oil. Other foods rating significantly high on the scale include meat and eggs, but more about why in later chapters.

The American Heart Association, although preferring mono and polyunsaturated fat over saturated fat, suggests limiting it to 25-35% of daily intake and no more.

DEFICIENCY SYMPTOMS OF OMEGA-3S

Symptoms of omega-3 deficiency can be vague and often misdiagnosed as some other health condition. Deficiency symptoms often include fatigue, dry or itchy skin, brittle hair and nails, constipation, frequent colds, depression, poor concentration, lack of physical endurance, or joint pain.[46] To maximize the benefits omega-3s offer, it is important to get a sufficient amount of vitamin B6, vitamin B3, vitamin C, magnesium, and zinc.

COOKING AND STORAGE OF OMEGA-3S

Polyunsaturated oils, including omega-3 fats, are easily damaged by heat, light, and oxygen. This is important for several reasons. When exposed to the elements, the oil becomes rancid, and the nutritional quantity is deeply diminished. Still, more importantly, the oxidation of these oils produces free radicals, which play a role in a host of degenerative diseases.

For example, an intact flax seed poses no issue. But when the outer shell is pressed to release its oil, the oil itself is no longer with protection. How do we keep it protected? By using a dark-colored bottle with a tight lid and storing in the refrigerator. This also means that omega-3s should not be used for cooking because, again, the heat alters the delicate chemical make-up. A better choice to use omega-3 oils would be for use in salads. Grapeseed oil and coconut oil can tolerate high heat and are a better choice for cooking.

TIPS TO INCORPORATE OMEGA-3S INTO THE EXISTING DIET

- Use olive oil, hemp, walnut, flax, avocado oil as a primary source of fat in oils

- Sprinkle flaxseed over breakfast cereals

- Use cereals like Q'ia, which include buckwheat, chia, and hemp

- Dehydrate or purchase flax crackers

- Use cracked chia in smoothies and desserts

- Consume walnuts

- Eat avocados

- Eat romaine lettuce, sesame seeds or sesame tahini, mustard seeds, tofu, spinach, collard greens, kale, soybeans, summer squash, turnip greens, winter squash, Brussels sprouts, raspberries, miso, green beans, and strawberries

- Increasing your intake of omega-3s through plant-based foods and minimize your intake of omega-6 oils by eliminating processed foods and oils. Reducing your intake of omega-6s may significantly reduce the risk of inflammatory ailments. A relief for many!

A QUICK ASIDE ABOUT FISH OIL SUPPLEMENTATION

When doctors recommend to their patients or make blanket statements about the benefits of omega-3s through fish oil supplements, the general public is relatively unaware that the fish oil pill they are consuming contains the omega-3s fatty acids not because of the fish but because of the marine algae and sea life they consumed. Interestingly enough, the foundation for algae oil is derived from sustainably sourced microalgae. The original source of marine omega-3s is a great alternative to fish oil for vegans, vegetarians, and anyone whose preference is to avoid fish.

WHAT'S WRONG WITH FISH OR KRILL SUPPLEMENTATION?

The problems associated with fish oil supplements are tied to the contaminants within the fish at harvesting and the rancidity of the oils once they are extracted from the fish. During fish oil processing, the fish are usually minced, then the oil is extracted by way of heat and chemical solvents. This process is an invitation for carcinogens and free radicals, which are left as by-products in the pills.

Mainstream medical practitioners recommend 300-400mg per day of fish oil supplements, which is twenty times or more what the average person needs. One study from the Fred Hutchinson Cancer Research Center in Seattle, Washington, published online July 10, 2013, in the Journal of the National

Cancer Institute, had looked at blood levels of omega-3s and determined that there was a link between high blood levels of omega-3 fatty acids and prostate cancer. They claim that the consumption of fatty fish and fish-oil supplements are linked to a 71% increase in risk.[47] Dr. Brian Clement of the Hippocrates Health Institute writes in his book, *Killer Fish*, that using fish oil supplementation is a misguided attempt to correct essential fatty acid deficiencies in mainstream diets, which are based on processed foods. Changing the diet, minimizing inflammatory omega-6s (letting go of processed foods and conventional meats), and incorporating omega-3s is a worthwhile attempt with zero risks, he claims.

LET'S TAKE A CLOSER LOOK AT SOME OMEGA-3 SUPERSTARS

- Spirulina—a therapeutic type of blue-green algae. Spirulina is rich in protein and contains all the essential amino acids, making it a complete protein as well.

- Chlorella—often sold in tablet or liquid form it can reduce cholesterol, high blood pressure and can enhance the immune system

- Spinach—contains high levels of antioxidants, vitamins, and other nutrients in addition to omega-3s.

- English walnuts—are known to contain higher concentrations of omega-3 fatty acids than any other type of nuts and might be expected to lower cardiovascular risk.

The traditional thought on plant-based omegas vs. fish omegas is that the omega oils produced by fish are a superior version of plant-based omegas, but we can provide ourselves a balance. If the EPA and DHA concern you, then finding a reputable supplement company like Nordic Naturals or E3Live would be a good place to inquire about marine sources of omega-3s, but don't devalue the benefits that mother nature plays when it comes to consuming plant-based omega-3 foods.

How would I prepare omega-3s? It's quite simple. Head over to our recipes in the Health Benefits of Fats section. There you'll find some interesting and unique ways to prepare omega-3 fats! Incorporate these recipes sporadically throughout the day. You'll find smoothies, side dishes, and some amazing snacks to further your quest for all things healthy—the honest form of healthy!

superfoods

Superfoods are everywhere these days: in almost every grocery store, online, and even paired with non-healthy foods. Not surprisingly, Dr. Oz, dubbed America's doctor, is a big proponent of them.

How often have *you* seen or heard of superfoods?

Companies touting superfood products is nothing short of a marketing ploy to encourage you to buy their product. Why? Because they know you're concerned about your health. More often than not, processed products touted as a "superfood" product usually contains just one superfood. Do your due diligence! Turn the label around and read the fine print to ensure there aren't ingredients that work against your health like genetically modified or hydrogenated oils, food additives, or fillers.

Let's move on to find out what a true superfood is!

SUPERFOODS—DEFINED

By definition, a superfood is an organically grown raw food that is exceptionally nutritious, easily digestible, and contains proportionately higher quantities of nutrients than other foods. It's relatively easy to understand what a superfood is, but with vague wording, it encourages manufacturers to jump on the latest health trend and lure you into their web of deception. A product that contains one superfood by no means makes it a super product. Since there are no labeling laws or any specific percentages to render a product a 'superfood,' anything is game. What if the superfood product contains ingredients that work *against* your health like sweeteners, gluten, and soy? This, again, is where marketing can be somewhat misleading, potentially counterproductive, and disruptive to your health goals.

In order to be a true superfood, a food must contain the following attributes:

- vitamins, minerals, proteins, and fatty acids

- antioxidants and phytochemicals that strengthen the body and immune system

- non-addictive

Cacao is touted as being a superfood, but it contains caffeine. Therefore it is considered addictive. It's not that super if you become addicted to it, which is why cacao is not found on our list.

Heed caution, however, when buying into superfood labels as they are without any regulatory oversight. All sorts of experts, health gurus, nutrition authors, industry promoters, and talk show hosts use the term 'superfood.' Some foods that are included on superfood lists may indeed be bad for you if you have certain health conditions, even if they are good for everyone else. The biggest concern would be for those with compromised immune systems and allergies.

Superfoods have the characteristics to assist in the prevention and elimination of disease and premature aging. They are meant to help with efficient elimination and promote the presence of healthy intestinal flora.[48] Superfoods are an excellent, permanent daily dietary choice. No food, however, no matter how "super," can stand alone or replace a complete and well-rounded diet.

The top ten superfoods listed here are the superfoods promoted by the Hippocrates Health Institute of West Palm Beach, Florida. In existence since 1956, the dietary methods and food served at Hippocrates has not changed since its inception. The foods mentioned today are not new and have been around for centuries.

TOP 10 SUPERFOODS (AS PROMOTED BY HIPPOCRATES HEALTH INSTITUTE)

1. Wheatgrass

2. Blue-green algae, spirulina, chlorella

3. Sea vegetables

4. Aloe vera

5. Coconut

6. Açai and goji

7. Maca root

8. Bee pollen

9. Hemp seed

10. Chinese herbal mushrooms

1. WHEATGRASS

Earlier reading detailed this amazing superfood because it certainly needs to be in the spotlight! It's the number one pick because it contains all of the characteristics a superfood should have, including vitamins, minerals, chlorophyll, enzymes, phytochemicals, antioxidants, amino acids, abscisic acid, and superoxide dismutase. Remember, there is some controversy over whether or not wheatgrass contains gluten, so it gets a little dicey. Wheatgrass is a baby blade that has not matured into seed; therefore, it remains gluten-free. However, when running wheatgrass through a juicer, make sure none of the seeds are attached to the wheatgrass blade. This is when contamination from gluten could occur.

2. THE ALGAE FAMILY

Blue-green algae, spirulina, and chlorella are one of the richest sources of chlorophyll. Chlorophyll is most known for its antibacterial, anti-fungal, anti-inflammatory, and blood-building benefits. Algae has the highest amount of chlorophyll, surprisingly surpassing wheatgrass.

Chlorophyll content[49] (per 10 g):

- AFA blue-green algae (300mg)

- spirulina (115mg)

- chlorella (280 mg)

- barley grass (149mg)

- wheatgrass (55mg)

Blue-Green Algae

What is blue-green algae, you ask? It's a form of cyanobacteria that structurally resembles bacteria; however, unlike other bacteria, cyanobacteria contain chlorophyll. One of the amazing benefits of blue-green algae is that it utilizes energy from the sun and, in turn, releases oxygen. The action of this light-driven photosynthesis produces not only oxygen but other health benefits, as well. Contained within blue-green algae are more than 65 vitamins, minerals, amino acids, and essential fatty acids, which is readily absorbed by the body. Blue-green algae are wild harvested and sold in either pill or liquid form.

Special precautions and warnings: Blue-green algae products must be certified free of contaminants, such as liver-damaging substances called microcystins, toxic metals, and harmful bacteria, and then they are considered possibly safe for most people. Paradoxically, recent research has identified—BMAA—a neurotoxin responsible for ALS, Parkinson's disease, and Alzheimer's, which can be found in other sources such as the roots of the cycad plants in Guam, in the accumulation of fish and shellfish of South Florida waters and in blue-green algae.[50] And as always, consult your physician before embarking on a dietary change. For more information regarding the testing of algae-free of microcystins and other contaminants, please visit or contact www.e3live.com.

Spirulina

Spirulina is one of Earth's oldest inhabitants. It grows naturally on every continent, especially in mineral-rich lakes near volcanoes. Since it came into vogue in the 1960s as a health food, scientists have studied its extremely high protein count. Spirulina contains a significant amount of iron, vitamin A and boasts 60% digestible proteins. A traditional steak is 22% protein, so this shows spirulina in an amazing vegan protein source. Spirulina is also high in vitamin B-12, vitamin E, omega-3, and omega-6 fatty acids and calcium. Good vegan sources of B-12 are virtually rare, so spirulina is indispensable when it comes to a plant-based diet. Spirulina is also a concentrated source of beta-carotene, boasting fifteen times as much vitamin A as carrots.[51] Spirulina is full of magnesium-rich chlorophyll. Consuming spirulina in powdered form is best, although the drying and packing of spirulina decreases its beta-carotene levels. Be aware that the FDA does not regulate spirulina for safety, so approach spirulina with caution.

Chlorella

Chlorella is a green alga that grows in freshwater. Although the algae grow naturally in fresh water, chlorella destined for human consumption is generally cultivated in large, fresh mineral water pools under direct sunlight.[52] The outer cell wall of chlorella has a low digestibility, which requires opening to digest its nutrients.[53] The broken cell version will have a higher absorption rate than the unbroken cell. Chlorella can typically be found in tablet or liquid form.

Special precautions when consuming chlorella: Chlorella may cause an allergic reaction, including asthma and other breathing problems. It can cause the skin to become extra sensitive to the sun. It can contain iodine; therefore, heed caution if faced with an iodine allergy or sensitivity. Always consult with a physician before using supplements or supplementation.

3. SEA VEGETABLES: KELP, DULSE, NORI, ARAME, SEA LETTUCE, WAKAME, BLADDERWRACK, IRISH MOSS

When I first embarked on my health journey, I had no idea the benefits of consuming sea veggies, let alone the multitude of them. Sea vegetables are one of the richest plant sources of minerals found in the ocean. They offer a variety of unique phytonutrients and antioxidants, are an excellent source of vitamin K, B-folate, magnesium, iron and calcium, and the B-vitamins riboflavin and pantothenic acid. Not enough? Try measurable amounts of antioxidant vitamins C and E. Many health benefits stemming from the consumption of sea vegetables include improved metabolism, removal of heavy metals and toxins from the body, and cleansing of the digestive tract, lymphatic system, blood, and kidneys. With that record, they've definitely earned their spot on this list!

For those concerned about contaminants of sea vegetables like that found with fish, sea veggies contain glycoprotein, which is a coating that protects the sea vegetables from pollution.[54] Certified organic sea veggies can be found almost anywhere. If you're like me, I like to purchase dry goods off of the Internet if I can't find locally. Try www.seaveg.com for Maine coast sea veggies.

Special precautions when consuming sea vegetables: Sea vegetables are more commonly associated with adverse reactions than other foods due in part to shellfish allergies.

4. ALOE VERA

Aloe Vera is the very few foods that contain vitamin B-12, making it a great choice for those on a strictly plant-based diet.[55] The aloe vera plant is high in vitamin C, antioxidants, fiber, amino acids, enzymes, steroids, and the mineral germanium, which supports the immune system. It also contains the minerals valium, magnesium, zinc, selenium, and chromium. Aloe Vera contains glyconutrients that assist in cell-to-cell communication, a purported benefit to the immune system.[56] The best way to consume aloe vera internally is in the form of juice, which can be bought at a health food store ready to drink. Aloe vera juice provides relief for a variety of digestive problems, including constipation, heartburn, and stomach aches. It has been shown to alleviate the burning pain associated with ulcers.[57]

Aloe vera's many benefits include:[58]

• cuts and dissolves mucous in the intestines allowing for better nutrient absorption

• boasts oxygen increasing levels in the blood

• eases inflammation and soothes arthritis pain

• contains antioxidants that protect the body from oxidative stress

• prevents the formation of kidney stones

• slightly raises the alkalinity levels in the blood

• assist with the healing from damage caused by ulcers, IBS, Crohn's disease

• assists with lowering high blood pressure

• promotes glutathione production in the liver[59]

• stabilizes blood sugar levels[60]

• prevents and assists with intestinal candida overgrowth

• and #1 on my list, hydrates the skin and accelerates skin repair

5. COCONUT: MEAT, WATER, OIL, AND MILK

Inside young Thai coconuts, the white tender, pliable soft fruit called the meat. The meat of brown and green coconuts is not tender but rather tough and chewy. Regardless of consistency, all coconut meat contains lauric acid, which helps fight bacteria from intestinal parasites and wards off countless infections.[61] Eating coconut meat helps fight gas, constipation, ulcers, and other digestive ailments.[62] Coconut also supports thyroid function and can help prevent goiter because it naturally contains iodine.[63]

Coconut water is the clear, and sometimes pink, liquid that pools inside coconuts. It's touted as nature's sports drink rivaling those brand name icons due to the significant amount of potassium it provides. Potassium is the mineral lost in sweat. Coconut water provides twice as much potassium as one banana; however, it also costs twice as much! On a budget? Bananas will work just fine. Coconut water, as with all electrolytes, helps the kidney and bladder to maintain proper functioning.

Coconut oil also comes from the meat of the coconut. It contains a type of heart-healthy fat called medium-chain triglycerides, which are metabolized differently than fats from other oils.[64] Most of the fat in coconut oil is saturated, but as was shared in the last segment, not all fat robs you of good health. Coconut oil can raise your good HDL cholesterol and provide antioxidants.[65] Pay close attention, however—not all coconut oils are created equal. When wanting to get the best health benefits, be sure to purchase unrefined, organic, first cold-pressed virgin coconut oil. It has serious drawbacks when processed, refined, and hydrogenated. The lauric acid is lost during processing and can clog arteries and decrease heart health.[66]

Coconut milk is also produced from the fatty meat of the coconut. What's remarkable about this superfood is that 50% of the fatty acids in coconut come from lauric acid, an antiviral and antibacterial agent, which is adept at fighting off infection. Being that coconut is a healthy omega-9 fat, it is great for skin rejuvenation and prevents wrinkles.[67]

6. AÇAÍ, GOJI AND NONI BERRIES

Açaí

The açaí berry is an inch-long, reddish-purple fruit and originates from the açai palm tree, which is native to Central and South America.

Research performed on the açai berry has focused on possible antioxidant activity due to the plethora of phytochemicals it contains.

Açai berries contain:

- essential fatty acids

- antioxidants

- sterols (which reduce cholesterol)

- 19 amino acids

- fiber

- minerals

A sustainable brand of packaged açaí can be found under the name Sambazon. The company engages in fair trade practices, and as stated on their website, their Fair Trade certification helps them to raise the standard of living for Açaí family farmers. The company invests 5% of fruit purchases directly back into local communities, and in turn, has been able to build schools, a library, a sports center, renovate healthcare centers, thus improving literacy and access to healthcare. Sambazon products can also be found on www.amazon.com if unable to find in your local store.

Goji

The goji berry has been used in Asian medicine for centuries as a healing plant. Asians have used goji berries to treat many common health problems like diabetes, high blood pressure, fever, and age-related eye problems.[68]

What can we find eating a handful of goji berries?[69]

• more beta-carotene than carrots and zeaxanthin (an antioxidant which protects the eyes)

• B-complex vitamins

• 500 times more vitamin C than oranges

• Vitamin E, a rare find in fruits

• excellent source of selenium (thyroid health) and germanium

• 21 trace minerals (the body requires 52)

• linoleic acid

• polysaccharides which strengthen the immune system

• 18 amino acids (including the eight essential ones)

• protects cellular DNA[70]

If hard to find in your local grocery store, you can always try to locate goji berries at this site www.extremehealthusa.com.

Noni

The noni berry made its way to this superfood list due to its phytochemicals, antioxidants, polysaccharides, flavonoids, fatty acids, and catechins. It boasts 17 different amino acids.[71] What else does the noni berry have to offer?

Noni berries may provide:

• protection against tobacco smoke-induced DNA damage

• normal homocysteine levels

• lowered systemic inflammation

• improved joint health

• increased physical endurance

• increased immune activity

• aid in weight management

• maintain bone health in women

• maintain normal blood pressure

• improve gum health

To get the most benefits from the noni berry, it is often consumed as either a juice from dried powder, as an extract or tea. The dried powder can be mixed with yogurts, smoothies, juices, or nut milk. The Polynesian peoples used the noni berry widely as a dye and to treat wounds, inflammation, infections, and other ailments.

Want to purchase noni? You can find dried powders most anywhere online, but the most potent of the noni berries comes from French Polynesian berries. One such brand containing French Polynesian berries is Tahitian Noni®.

7. MACA ROOT

Maca is a root plant consumed as a food as it has a malt flavor, but its claim to fame is for its purported health benefits. Maca is known for its ability to increase stamina, energy, and sexual function. It has been touted as an aphrodisiac and as a way to improve sexual performance and fertility.[72] Maca's beneficial attributes include fighting off anemia, chronic fatigue, depression, poor memory, stress/tension, energy, stamina, and athletic performance. It has been known to relieve symptoms of menopause, PMS, and can balance the endocrine system, hormones, and thyroid function.[73]

What's it got?[74]
• high mineral content (calcium, potassium, iron, magnesium, phosphorus, and zinc)

• sterols

• vitamins B1, B2, C, E

• 19 amino acids

• essential fatty acids

• phytonutrients

• fiber

• carbohydrates

It is either taken as a pill or as a powdered maca root. Its rich malt flavor is an added boost to soups and smoothies.

Special precautions and warnings: There is a risk of allergic reaction to using maca root. These can range from skin rashes to hives. Maca also contains high levels of iodine.

8. BEE POLLEN

Bee pollen is considered by some to be a vegan food product as the pollen is considered a waste product; the bees have not collected it for their own purpose. The question remains, however, whether humans have exploited the bees to obtain the pollen balls.

Bee pollen contains vitamins, minerals, carbohydrates, lipids (fats), and up to 40% protein. It boasts 22 amino acids and more than 90 nutrients.[75] It comes from the pollen that collects on the bodies of bees. Bee pollen may also contain bee saliva.

Special precaution and warnings: Bee pollen contains trace amounts of the plant material that may trigger allergies. Those taking warfarin, a blood thinner, may want to check with their doctor before taking bee pollen.

9. HEMP SEEDS

Hemp nuts or hemp seeds nuts are the shelled inner portions of the hemp seed. Hemp seed for food consumption is not the same as the leaf, which is used for marijuana and contains the psychoactive drug THC. Hemp is an eco-friendly plant used to make anything from paper and protein powder to building materials, bedding, and clothing.

Hemp offers a myriad of benefits, one being that it is a complete protein. Hemp nuts are approximately 33-35% protein. A mere two tablespoons of hemp nuts contain 11g of protein! Another big plus is its near-perfect ratio of omega-6 to omega-3, with that ratio being 4:1. Hemp also contains omega-9s.[76]

What else do they provide us with? Hemp nuts are a good source of iron and also contain significant levels of the antioxidant vitamin E. They contain both oil and chlorophyll, which is extremely nourishing and detoxifying to the body.

Chlorophyll's presence in a nut is unusual in that it is typically found in blatantly green foods.

10. MUSHROOMS

Reishi

The reishi mushroom is a shiny little fungus, which grows on rotten wood. For 2,000 years, the Chinese have used reishi in medicine because of its presumed health benefits and absence of side-effects.[77] The mushrooms are generally cultivated and harvested in elixir or capsule form. Here are the health benefits of reishi:[78]

- immune system support

- cancer prevention

- lowers blood pressure

- lowers cholesterol

- blood sugar regulation

- speeds relief from cold sores and herpes

- has antiviral benefits

- radiation damage protection

Special Precaution and Warnings: Reishi mushrooms may interact with high blood pressure medications and may not be the best supplement for those with very low blood pressure.

Also, discuss with your doctor if you are using anti-coagulant or anti-platelet drugs such as aspirin, NSAIDs, Warfarin, Heparin.

They may also interfere with blood pressure medications.

Cordyceps

Cordyceps is a parasitic fungus, indigenous to China that attacks moth caterpillars. Cordyceps has been used in traditional Asian medicine for centuries.[79] According to the Memorial Sloan Kettering Cancer Center's laboratory studies, cordyceps contain anti-diabetic, anti-tumor, and radioactive properties, and one human study showed improved kidney function.

The nutrition found in cordyceps includes protein, carbohydrates, sterols, oils, vitamin B1, B2, B12, E, and K. When harvested from the wild, it is considered to be a superior product.[80]

Cordyceps purported benefits include:[81]

- improving energy and performance

- increases oxygen in the blood

- assists with Hepatitis B

- has antibiotic properties

- improves liver and kidney function

Special Precaution and Warnings: Medications that decrease the immune system interact with cordyceps. Those who are pregnant should not take cordyceps.

Chaga

Chaga mushrooms are hard much like wood. Chaga contains numerous B vitamins, flavonoids, phenols, minerals & enzymes. It is disproportionately high in pantothenic acid, which is needed by the adrenal glands...think energy. It also contains riboflavin and niacin.

Chaga's most potent ingredient is a substance also found in high quantities in wheatgrass. That enzyme is called SOD, superoxide dismutase. This enzyme halts oxidation, which is responsible for oxidizing and damaging tissues, resulting in aging. Chaga, like many other mushrooms, are rich in beta-glucans, which have immunomodulating activities.[82] In laboratory studies, Chaga demonstrates anti-cancer activity due to its beta-glucans, and anti-inflammatory, antiviral and immune-stimulating properties.

Special Precautions and Warnings: Consuming Chaga could magnify the effects of anticoagulant medications such as aspirin and warfarin, which could raise the risk of bruising and bleeding, which is similar to the precaution when taking reishi. Chaga can also interact with

diabetes medication like insulin causing blood sugar levels that fall too low.[83]

Where to buy? Found in powdered, capsule, and liquid form, these mushrooms can be found at www.hostdefense.com.

So while you might find other superfoods not mentioned here in various articles, supplements, on the TV, and from friends, you are now better equipped to differentiate between a true superfood and an imposter!

Are you looking to embark on your superfood journey through recipes? Head on over to our Superfood and Smoothie section. Don't forget to read the all-important intro, which gives a thorough explanation of how to assemble all of these amazing and wonderful beauties that mother nature has provided! And don't stop with smoothies. Move straight into Breakfast Ideas, where you'll continue on your whole foods, alkalizing, detoxifying, healthy fats guided tour.

I bet you'll begin to see your days start to take shape with all that you have been exposed to! Getting started with wheatgrass and a morning juice, an amazing superfood smoothie or a new breakfast idea, a healthy cruciferous lunch with an amazing side, and an easy-to-make snack to hold you off from crashing late afternoon. Changing one's diet a day at a time is a surefire way to make sure it clicks and sticks! Changing one's lifestyle doesn't need to be difficult, but it surely takes time to adjust to new ways of doing things. Out with the old and in with the new! I hope you are starting to take notice of the new you!

where's the beef?

I vividly remember the idyllic pictures of rural farms in America's heartland from my childhood. Clear visions of vast landscapes with cows grazing in green pastures, giant bales of hay neatly arranged in diagonal patterns on freshly cut grass, rows of cornfields with silk tops blowing wistfully in the wind, a pastoral red barn off in the distance dwarfed by skyscraper-sized silos. It's an apt description of the dairy farm near where I grew up in Massachusetts in the late seventies and early eighties. Is this what you envision, too? The egg and meat packages of today certainly depict that view, but things aren't always as they seem.

THEN AND NOW

Unlike today, farms of the 19th and early 20th century were run by families. As a general rule, farmers would pass down their farms from generation to generation instead of selling out to larger companies, a common occurrence in today's agricultural climate.

FARMS AT THE TURN OF THE 20TH CENTURY

Within every early farm contained a veritable ecosystem. Farmers grew their own feed for their livestock and threshed harvest seeds by hand. From one growing season to the next, farmers had the customary tradition to use the best ears of corn or the best heads of wheat to use for plantings the following year. To protect and replace the soil's nutrients, farmers rotated their crops from year to year. Cattle and livestock roamed and grazed on the natural grassland only to come in for supplemental feedings and water.[84] Horses, instead of machinery, plowed and tilled the dirt. The hay fields were cut, dried, and stored to use as feed for the horses and livestock and the straw for their bedding.[85] Each person and animal on the farm had an important role to fill.

FARMS OF THE 1930S

A change in farming practices was already taking place in the 1930s. The use of tractors and combines, which mechanically remove seeds from the heads of grain, became commonplace. Farmers also began to implement the planting of hybrid seeds through natural selection. The objective of hybridization was to grow a heartier plant to resist the harsh conditions of Mother Nature. Nothing about this was unnatural, merely practical.

A pinnacle turning point occurred during the 1930s, however, that changed farming in the U.S. forever. The global economic slowdown due to the Great Depression and one of the worst droughts in America's history were a catalyst to this change. There were no longer buyers to support the crops or the animals the farmers produced. Further compounding this issue, the drought made it virtually impossible to plant and harvest in the first place. Due to these ill-fated events, livestock prices drastically dropped to cataclysmic levels. As a result, many farmers could no longer maintain their farms. Many farmers ended up walking away, becoming migrant farmworkers on the west coast.[86]

With the unintended consequence of this decline came government intervention. To improve this dire situation, the government designed programs to maximize output and stabilize pricing. This intervention, called the Agricultural Adjustment Act of 1933, artificially reduced the supply of commodities like livestock and crops. The government paid farmers to plant less of certain crops or to abstain from planting altogether and the most draconian of them all—destroy millions of livestock across the nation and name it "emergency livestock reductions."[87]

Because the federal buy-out saved farmers from bankruptcy, farmers felt compelled to sell their herds. Critics of this deal complained that millions of animals were being killed while many Americans were going hungry.[88] In the end, however, it was a big win for the American farmer but a misfortune for the majority of Americans.

These events eventually set the stage for the government's repeated intervention into U.S. farming practices. The approach of supporting farm prices by reducing supplies through government subsidies and price control practices remains on-going.

FARMS OF THE 1940S

In the 1940s, the widespread use of veterinary medicine in livestock became standard practice. The development of streptomycin, an antibiotic that eradicated bovine tuberculosis, a problematic farm disease that would wipe out entire herds of cattle and other animals, did away with limiting the number of animals in a flock or herd. Farmers could add more livestock to the same amount of square footage of containment space.

The promising use of antibiotics in cattle also helped defeat mastitis, a painful infection of the udder in dairy cows. With the continued use of antibiotics, farmers and researchers were finding that animals were not only healthier, but they also grew faster on the same amount of feed.[89] With its marked success, antibiotics were added to the feed of all animals in the herd, whether they were sick or not.

CRAMPED CONDITIONS ON THE HORIZON

The introduction of antibiotics created a new phenomenon of hog and poultry confinement facilities and huge feedlots for cattle. The bucolic setting of family farms was now solely left for history books.

With the success of technological advances—better feed, better medicine, and better machinery—the productivity of livestock began to increase, and so did the demand for meat from consumers.[90]

FARMS OF THE 1950S AND 1960S

Ironically, with the emergence of better technology, the 50s and 60s saw a decline in the number of farmers. What once was a conglomeration of small farms had now shifted to a limited number of large corporations. Large corporate entities began to dominate the nation's animal production system using confined containment systems. Fewer operations were raising more animals.

Also, during this pivotal period, there was an explosion in government-supported agricultural research.[91] Around 1950, spending on agricultural research increased exponentially. Research grants doubled from under $500 billion in 1950 to over $1 trillion in 1963. Research spending reached $1.5 trillion in 1972 and to over $2.5 trillion by 1990 (numbers adjusted to inflation).[92] How did all of this research change the way we farm in the U.S.?[93]

FARMING BASICS VS. MONOCULTURE FARMING

During the 19th and into the 20th century, farmers needed a generalized knowledge of how to prepare a seedbed best, how to apply manure for nutrients, how to cultivate weeds, and how to harvest. Farmers needed to know how to feed animals, collect their products (like eggs or cream), butcher them, and preserve meat—most of this knowledge applied to a variety of crops and livestock.[94] In the last half of the 20th century, researchers were developing means to create superior crops and improve pesticide application. Researchers were also rewarding farmers for specialized, one-crop farming called monoculture farming, a widespread practice used by big agriculture.[95]

THE CASE FOR MONOCULTURE FARMING

Demographers during the 1950s were predicting a population explosion resulting in famine. The answer to this impending doom seemed to be through government-supported agriculture research, which encouraged and rewarded farmers for specializing in one crop or one type of livestock and calling for mass cultivation.[96]

Another significant impact in the farming industry during this time was the discovery of DNA in 1953, which helped to create a new breed of crops, most notably genetically engineered foods or GMOs. Farming was leaving its humble beginnings behind for a more scientific, industrial process. The farmers who had survived and thrived during periods of uncertainty were now forced to apply scientific methods to growing commodities.[97]

By 1961, the world's total meat supply amounted to 71 million tons. By 2007, it had increased to 284 million tons, according to the U.N. Food and Agriculture Organization. Per capita consumption of meat doubled worldwide from 1961 to 2007. Since the turn of the 20th century, our consumption of milk, milk products, and meat have risen 50%, and chicken consumption has risen 280%.[98] According to a New York Times article written on January 27, 2008, the author Mark Bittman states that Americans eat about eight ounces of meat daily, about two times the global average. At only about 5% of the world's population, we slaughter nearly 10 billion animals yearly, which is more than 15% of the world's total.

The demand for more beef, pork, chicken, and other meats means that countless animals were switched to grain feed and living under duress in confined spaces. And more meat means a corresponding increase in demand for feed, namely corn and soy.[99]

BEHIND THE SCENES

Half of the pork produced in the US and three-quarters of the chickens raised today are in enclosed, pre-fabricated confinement buildings. The animals may never see the sun until they're loaded on to semi-trailer trucks for transport to the nearby slaughterhouse.[100] Cattle, being larger animals, live in massive, crowded feedlots. The meat we buy at the grocery store no longer comes from farms but rather from factories.[101]

TODAY'S FARM— IMPRISONMENT

Very few people today understand how or where their food is grown or produced. If you were to ask, they'd say from farms. Farm from the 20s? The 30s? The 40s? Farms of today are vastly different from a century ago. Because they are run as an industry, most of us are largely unaware of their "practices." Most of today's livestock lives its life on an industrialized "concentrated animal feeding operation" (CAFO). They're technically farms but with an industrialized bent, a place remiss with compassion or humane treatment. It is nothing but a disguised attempt to put a fancy name to a deplorable, inhumane, and morbidly sad way to raise livestock. Animals are so crowded and confined; they have nowhere to move. Chickens peck away at each other until death, pigs chew off other pigs' tails, and cattle walk in manure about a foot to two deep. Farming has undoubtedly changed with the help, support, and encouragement of the federal government.

FACTORY FARMED ANIMALS

By their very nature, cows have a digestive organ called the rumen, which dutifully digests the cellulose of grass while creating proteins. To live off of grass, cows need more land, and more land means the need for more money. In today's big-ag environment, farming practices boil down to cost. Slow down growth, expand unnecessary costs, and companies lose money. Feeding cows corn is an intentional way to make them grow bigger and fatter as rapidly and cheaply as possible. This is the kind of production companies strive for because costs are affected by efficiency and expediency.

Factory farmed animals are much higher in fat than pasture-raised animals because they get little or no exercise and eat a diet of milled grains, including genetically modified corn and soybeans. Factory farmed livestock are subject to vast quantities of chemicals, artificial hormones, and antibiotics to sustain their unnatural diets and environment.

On a feedlot, thousands of cows are packed into one farm. Some feedlots can contain 100,000 cattle with virtually no space between them. They live in an unhealthy and flagitious environment. Their feed demand is so astronomical that it needs to be purchased from huge agri-business firms and hauled in. To prevent the outbreak of disease on these cramped lots, the animal feed contains antibiotics as well as growth hormones and scores of veterinary medicine to prevent illness.[102]

Typically there are 2,000 cows per acre instead of the usual two for pasture. With this many animals in one space, it reduces the need for bedding while reducing production costs. However, it creates new problems in disposing of manure.[103] Urine and waste collect and drift downstream into what is called capture lagoons, which are vast open-air pits, sometimes as large as six to seven acres.[104][105] Once manure is stored in open-air lagoons, it is periodically pumped out to be sprayed on fields surrounding the farm, allegedly to be used as fertilizer. Manure is often mishandled and overapplied to fields, which causes it to run-off polluting rivers and streams and leaching into groundwater. Open cesspools containing human waste is illegal, so why are the rules for agriculture different?[106]

WHY THE NEED FOR HORMONES IN LIVESTOCK?

American cattle raised for slaughter today are injected with hormones to make them grow faster and to enhance beef production. Growth stimulants are used to offset the high feed prices for cattle. Often hormone implants will give at least a 10 to 1 return on cost, a big boon to farmers, but what's the trickle-down effect?

Today there are several natural hormones approved for use in cattle. Three of the natural hormones include estradiol, progesterone, and testosterone. Some of the more commonly used synthetic hormones are:

• Zeranol—a mycotoxin (mold) derived from fungi and may be found as a contaminant in fungus-infected crops. Zeranol is a growth promoter in livestock, including beef cattle in the US. It is not approved for use in the European Union

- Trenbolone—Another growth promoter. Studies of trenbolone are currently at odds in debating if trenbolone has carcinogenic properties. It's banned for use in humans, and one study shows it does not break down when excreted and can be found in water[107]

- Melengestrol—Melengetrol is a feed additive and is not injected but added to cattle feed

FINISHING FEED

In an article in the Wall Street Journal, Monday, August 19, 2013, author Jesse Newman and Kelsey Gee report that manufacturer Merck & Co. would temporarily suspend the sales of Zilmax, a feed additive used only a few short weeks before slaughter in cattle. The drug had been widely used in the industry to promote weight gain by stimulating the growth of lean muscle and not fat.

The suspension? Tyson, one of the world's largest meat producers, voluntarily withheld sales of animals fed Zilmax due to strange behaviors in the cattle upon arriving for slaughter. The article reports that cattle walking down the truck ramp enroute to the slaughterhouse exhibited unusual signs of distress: walking stiffly, having trouble moving, sitting in dog-like positions, and walking down the ramp tippy-toed. Zilmax is a supplement designed to add weight. Zilmax was used in roughly 70% of cattle sold to slaughterhouses.

All this demand means that we, as consumers, have exchanged a plant-based diet for a meat-based diet. What has changed?

WHY THE PUSH FOR ANIMAL PROTEIN?

The push for meat stems from the body's need for protein. Amino acids are proteins and used by the body to rebuild tissue proteins. Since our body doesn't make amino acids, it's "essential" we get them from food. There are eight essential amino acids that we must get from certain foods. Foods containing eight or nine amino acids are considered a complete protein, but various food proteins are said to be of different quality.

Proteins of the highest quality are those that provide the exact right amount of protein to synthesize new tissue proteins efficiently. High-quality proteins are considered meat, milk, and eggs. Lower quality proteins come from a plethora of plants, but as a group, they contain the necessary combination of amino acids. Many plant-based foods contain the right quantity of eight essential amino acids, but they are harder to come by in the American diet. Much to people's surprise, pea and sunflower are a complete protein.

WHAT IS THE SIGNIFICANCE OF HIGH-QUALITY PROTEIN?

High quality is often portrayed in the media as the best type of protein, which leads to a belief system that we must eat meat at every meal. Animal meat is viewed as high quality, which is factually true, but it also leads to the false sense that "high quality" equals "high health," to which it does not. A diet heavily reliant on meat is a highly acidic diet, and a highly acidic diet, in turn, leads to poor health.

Americans are led to believe that vegans and vegetarians are often weak or sick. If vegans or vegetarians rely heavily on processed foods, faux meats and consume a significant amount of dairy, then yes, that could be considered true. Instead, consuming a variety of plant-based foods, including beans, legumes, and a multitude of colorful produce, one can meticulously organize a healthy daily intake of nutrients to avoid getting sick. The word vegan connotates a diet without animal products. A plant-based diet is one that connotates the majority of the foods one eats comes from plants, including those who claim to be raw vegan or high raw (living foods). A vegan may consume processed foods while a raw foodist, living foodist, or a plant-based, whole foodist does not.

Meat is omnipresent in our country and easily accessible. What this means is that in our processed, fast-food world, it is quite possible to be missing nutrients from our diet if we don't embrace a diet replete with foods from nature.

Many consumers are largely unaware of what would be a good meat substitute. Try these high protein plant foods:

- Almond
- Lentils
- Sesame
- Mung BeanSprouts
- Rye
- Soybeans

- Sunflower Seeds
- Chia
- Buckwheat (does not contain wheat)
- Walnuts
- Amaranth

Want a complete protein? Try these foods:

- Spirulina
- Pea Sprouts
- Quinoa
- Sunflower Sprouts
- Hemp Seeds
- Wheatgrass

SO WHAT'S YOUR BEEF WITH BEEF?

Well, it's not only about beef. It's about all meat. While the American Heart Association has vilified domestically raised beef due to its saturated fat content and cholesterol, a widely *unknown* fact is that chicken and pork contain a significant amount of cholesterol as well. Meat is generally highly acidic and promotes inflammation, especially red meat. Chicken is also high in cholesterol (especially the dark meat) and high in saturated fat. Since we eat our meat cooked, the natural digestive enzymes found in abundance in raw or fermented meat is killed off. The digestion of meat proteins takes an arduous toll on our digestive system to break down the proteins. High protein meat diets, like the famed Keto diet, can induce ketosis, a state of hyperacidity that is dangerous to the body. Keto done right with ample greens can be beneficial, but again, much of a traditional American Keto diet contains a significant amount of animal proteins.

Toxic substances called ketones are formed as a result of the overconsumption of proteins and can damage the kidneys. Intensely high-protein diets may also bring on gout, increase cholesterol and triglyceride levels, stress the heart, may damage the liver, cause constipation due to the excessive use of fiber-poor animal foods, wash minerals and vitamins out of the body and increase the risk of certain types of cancer. T. Colin Campbell, the author of *The China Study,* states that the lower the percentage of consumption of animal-based foods, the greater the health benefits. According to Campbell, he states it is not unreasonable to assume that the optimum percentage of animal-based products is zero.[108]

Proteins and starches from seeds, nuts, and some grains are an excellent option for ease of digestibility, which provides good nutrition for the human body. Quinoa, an alkaline-forming food, contains high amounts of readily digestible protein and starch, making it a great addition to the diet. Brown rice is another option and remains neutral on the pH scale.

CAN WE LIVE ON PLANTS ALONE?

Proponents of a plant food diet believe that man's natural body physiology is not designed to eat or digest meat. It starts with the teeth and structure of the jaw. An animal such as a canine has an elongated jaw with sharp teeth. The jaw moves up and down to strip meat into pieces. A human's mouth has flattened molars and only four incisors. Our jaw moves in a masticating fashion, a movement which is generally used to chew vegetables.

The digestive system of an animal is short, which allows for swift elimination—the colon of a human spans over 20 feet with curves and pockets. The meat consumed sits in our digestive system for three days and upwards of 10 days, depending on the efficacy of elimination. Furthermore, meat and animal products (such as milk, yogurt, cheese) are all highly mucous forming.[109]

Since a human's digestive system is much longer than that of other meat-eating animals, the meat creates a putrefied or fermenting effect when it sits too long inside our colon. Due to the long transit time in humans and weaker stomach acid than carnivores, meat is not thoroughly digested upon leaving the stomach, thus causing undigested proteins to enter the small intestines while setting off a large mucous reaction within the whole digestive tract.[110] The body does this as a means to protect itself from the half-digested proteins. We may also encounter this in the mucosal linings in the ears, nose, and throat. Since our digestive tract is designed to consume vegetables, fruits, seeds, and nuts, it is a common recommendation for optimal digestive health to consume mostly plant-based foods. One of the best ways to cut mucous in the digestive tract is to consume one ounce of whole aloe vera juice before bed nightly.

IF I DON'T EAT MEAT, WHERE WILL I GET MY IRON FROM?

If one increases the consumption of plant-based foods, it is fairly easy to consume more iron. These plant-based foods offer the most amount of iron:

- Lentils
- Mung Bean
- Sprouts
- Sesame Seeds
- Almonds
- Beets
- Parsley
- Sunflower Seeds

Additionally, more consumption of dietary fiber from whole foods and beans provides for better elimination. When trying to obtain iron from plant-based foods, the absorption is best when consumed with vitamin C, which is discussed at length in Chapter 3.[111][112]

How to prepare meals without meat, fish, or dairy! This section probably becomes the most challenging of all ideas and concepts thus far. We, as Americans, are tied to our belief that meat must be a part of our daily diet. Not just one time a day but as many as three times a day. Sometimes it's just because plants don't appear to be all that satisfying or plant-based foods taste too "healthy." If you have played around with recipes, started juicing, and have been exploring with more plant-based, whole foods, this section may be a little easier to transition to.

I always like to start with the concept of Meatless Mondays, but there's more on that in the Meatless Meals section of the recipes, so make sure to spend some time there. The recipes that begin the meatless meals section showcase more comfort foods that offer deeply rich and satisfying flavors that can appeal to any palette. The soups in the Souping section are another amazing addition to your meatless meal repertoire. Not completely meatless, that's fine, but the beauty is it's all dairy-free. That is a ginormous step in improving one's health. For me, the Souping section is probably my most favorite of all the sections. Soups are hearty and flavorful, easy to make, assemble, and tote to work or play. Soups can also replace meals or be a part of a nourishing fast. So why not start today? Go ahead! Give it a try. If not today, then make it a Monday!

dairy farms and the 'got milk' campaign

Industrial farms like we discussed at the beginning of this chapter use several methods for increasing milk production in dairy cows, including selective breeding, grain-based diets (instead of grass), and exposing cows to longer periods of artificial light instead of pasture. Another more common and controversial way to induce greater milk production is to inject dairy cows with a growth hormone called rBGH (recombinant bovine growth hormone).

RBGH is a genetically engineered artificial growth hormone. Developed and manufactured under the brand names Posalic® by Monsanto Corporation, rBGH has been controversial from the start. Cows forced to produce unnaturally high quantities of milk have the potential for malnourishment because they lose more nutrients through their milk than they ingest in their feed. It causes them to become highly susceptible to disease. Milk

from rBGH-treated cows contains higher levels of IGF-1 (Insulin Growth Factor-1). IGF-1 has been linked to colon and breast cancer.[113]

Despite mounting evidence and pressure from the public, huge multinational agricultural companies are dropping their use of milk from rBGH treated dairy cows. The FDA stubbornly continues to assure consumers that rBGH is safe for cows and humans.[114]

DAIRY, MUCOUS, ALLERGIES, AND ASTHMA. WHAT'S THE CONNECTION?

After drinking milk, does your throat contain mucous, does your nose run, or do your ears clog? The body's formation of mucous is its attempt to protect itself from matter that can damage its delicate mucosal lining. Mucous can grow inside the intestines and line the mucosal walls, which problematically inhibits the proper absorption of nutrients. While mucous is beneficial in that it does not allow particles to exit the colon, it can provide a breeding ground for unfriendly bacteria, fungi, and parasites. An unhealthy condition in the colon can contribute to health conditions and disease.[115]

Ordinarily, the body can remove the mucous when the mucous forming source is removed from the diet.[116] Being that milk is highly acidic to the body, the body's response to neutralizing the pH of the blood is to release alkaline mineral reserves such as calcium. Where does the body get its calcium from? The bones, of course.

The body will always try to remain in a healthy pH state and will attempt to counteract the rise in pH levels due to the consumption of the milk (and other highly acidic foods).

Consuming a diet of either 100% alkaline-forming vegan food, or up to 70% alkaline-forming, 30% of acid-forming plant-based foods is suitable for good human health.

CALCIUM ONLY COMES FROM MILK, RIGHT?

An 8-ounce serving of low-fat 1% milk contains 290 mg of calcium.[117] People typically do not realize that many green vegetables are calcium powerhouses. Several servings of vegetables per day provide as much calcium, if not more, than a glass of milk. For example:

- A cup of broccoli has 94 mg.
- A cup of collard greens boasts almost 350 mg of calcium—more than a cup of milk.
- Turnip greens are also impressive, with 249 mg per cup.
- Kale and okra both have around 179 mg per cup.
- If you enjoy cabbage, a cup of bok choy has 158 mg.[118]

Additional sources of calcium come from beans, nuts, and seeds, though not as much as vegetables.

- Almonds boast 188 mg for a half cup. Trading in your peanut butter for almond butter will give you 86 mg in two tbsp.
- Sesame tahini has 128 mg in two tablespoons.
- The average one-cup serving of sprouted legumes has about 90 mg. of calcium in addition to being packed with protein and fiber.

Wondering where to get your calcium now that you might give up milk? Here's a list that will help you get all the calcium you need:

Almonds	Collards
Dulse	Kelp (1093 mg)
Kale	Mustard Greens
Parsley	Sesame Seeds (1160 mg)
Turnip Greens	Watercress

In general, almost all fresh fruits and vegetables do not cause mucous and are the perfect food for human consumption. This is due to their ease of digestibility, mineral makeup, and lack of anything toxic or damaging to the body. Steaming or baking vegetables also maintains their non-mucous forming qualities.[119]

CALCIUM AND ITS HELPER, VITAMIN D

Rice, soy, or almond milk sold on shelves is often fortified with vitamin D. Many name brands contain the same amount of calcium and vitamin D as cow's milk.

Natural sources of Vitamin D are shiitake mushrooms, which provide approximately 4% of the daily recommended allowance. Another natural source of vitamin D comes from the sun. The best hours to achieve vitamin D from the sun without damage occurs before 9 am and after 4 pm without the use of sunblock.

Transitioning diets should take time and research. It is not expected that you would drop meat overnight, although some do. To better understand what you may be purchasing in the grocery store, here is a list of how your meat has been raised *and* fed.

USDA'S LABELING OF LIVESTOCK[120]

Companies must abide by these labels and are inspected as such. This should also take much confusion out of purchasing meat and animal-based products in the store.

• All-Natural: As required by USDA, meat, poultry, and egg products labeled as "natural" must be minimally processed and contain no artificial ingredients.

• The natural label does not include any standards regarding farm practices and only applies to the processing of meat and egg products. There are no standards or regulations for the labeling of natural food products if they do not contain meat or eggs.

• Cage-Free: This label indicates that the flock was able to freely roam a building, room, or enclosed area with unlimited access to food and fresh water during their production cycle.

• Free-Range: This label indicates that the flock was provided shelter in a building, room, or area with unlimited access to food, fresh water, and continuous access to the outdoors during their production cycle. The outdoor area may or may not be fenced or covered with netting-like material. The USDA regulates this label.

• Pasture-raised: Due to the number of variables involved in pasture-raised agricultural systems, the USDA has not developed a federal definition for pasture-raised products.

• Grass-fed: Grass-fed animals receive a majority of their nutrients from grass throughout their life, while organic animals' pasture diet may be supplemented with grain. (Consumers take note, the grass-fed label does not limit the use of antibiotics, hormones, or pesticides. Meat products may be labeled as grass-fed organic.)

• Humane: Multiple labeling programs make claims that animals were treated humanely during the production cycle, but the verification of these claims varies widely. These labeling programs are not regulated under a single USDA definition.

No added hormones or a similar label that includes "Raised without Hormones" is misleading as federal regulations have never permitted hormones or steroids in poultry, pork, or goat.

Here we are again—moving right along, empowering you to make the right choices that work for you as an individual or part of a family or on a dietary journey. Now that you have a clear vision of milk and its alternatives, head on over to the Dressings and also Dips and Sauces section of recipes. There you will find an array of dressings, dips, and sauces that are sure to fill your fancy while leaving out all of the gunk! One of my favorite dressings of all times is Buttermilk Ranch, and here it is, unmistakably delicious. It'll be hard to tell it's made without animal products!

eating fish?
there's a catch!

The dilemma many consumers face when finding an alternative to red meat is, "what protein source is better for me?" We have fallen for the argument that fish and chicken is the better alternative to red meat. We believe the experts when they insist that chicken has less cholesterol than domesticated red meat and that we must get our inflammation-reducing omega-3s from fish, namely salmon.[121] The information you've been given is mostly true, but there's a 'catch.'

We've become entangled in a web of fragmented health information that touts the benefits of omega-3s while simultaneously vilifying saturated fats. We have come to realize that the widely publicized and controversial saturated fats from meat are not good for us and that omega-3 fats from fish are highly regarded. We've been told omega-3s can lower the chance of heart attack, makes babies smarter, ward off dementia and stroke in the elderly, and even guard against dry-eye syndrome.[122] No wonder we're seeking more of it. The best way to get omega-3s? In fish form, of course. But don't run to the fish counter just yet. Let's take a look at what the studies don't mention.

STRIKING A BALANCE

We have been told to eat fish as few as one time per week and up to as much as three times per week in order to get our recommended amount of omega-3s.[123] Americans are also encouraged to supplement with fish oil pills to account for the shortfall of good fats in our diet, especially those who do not eat seafood.[124] The supplements might be necessary if we consume highly processed foods coupled with a heavy meat protein diet. However, we are programmed to believe that pills are a quick fix and a viable solution to our health maladies instead of making dietary changes. Taking omega-3 supplements is merely one solution to take your inflammatory omega-6 riddled diet and to swing the pendulum back over to the anti-inflammatory side. But what if we chose instead to eat a multitude of plant-based sources of omega-3s and limited our consumption of fish or fish-based supplements?

For best absorption when consuming plant-based sources of omega-3s, pair with iron. Do that, and you're surely on your way to a well-balanced diet.[125]

Not all direct sources of EPA and DHA come strictly come from fish. However, sea and freshwater marine plants do! Algal oil, for instance, is an omega-3 oil made from certain types of marine algae and great for plantarians! According to WebMD, algal oil has been used safely for several years in studies and is also added to infant formula and pharmaceuticals. It differs from plant-based sources of omega-3s in that it is a direct source of EPA and DHA, much like fish oil, but should not be confused with blue-green algae, brown algae, chlorella, or seaweed.[126]

AVOIDING THE FAT AND CHOLESTEROL

Consumers are sadly misled when they believe that fish offers us one exceptional benefit - omega-3 fats. What we aren't told or made aware of is that fish and seafood generally contain excessive amounts of *both* fat and cholesterol.

People often mistakenly defend their healthy diet by stating, "I only eat fish and chicken" because this is what we have been deceived into believing. You have been convinced that by consuming fish and chicken, you are limiting not only saturated fat but cholesterol, too, while markedly increasing your omega-3 intake. What you may not realize is that many fish, including shark, catfish, swordfish, and sea trout contain almost one-third fat, while salmon and orange roughy contain over 50% fat. If cholesterol is a concern for you, prawns (shrimp) have double that of beef and a 3-ounce serving of salmon contains 74 milligrams of cholesterol, about the same as a comparable serving of T-bone steak or chicken.[127]

AQUATIC LIFE CONTAMINATED

What else aren't we being told? Animal-based sources of fat are still fat, and what lurks in fat? Toxins. In fact, pregnant women are advised not to consume any of the larger fatty fish like tuna, swordfish, and shark due to its mercury content. The reason for that is due to the toxins being stored in the fish's fat from bioaccumulation, which is the build-up of toxins from larger fish consuming smaller fish.

Contaminants continue to pollute our aquatic systems through the air, water, and bio-accumulation. Many of these contaminants are uncontainable due to the atmosphere's movement of air, wind, and rain. These aquatic pollutants can have originated from pesticides, fungicides, herbicides, heavy metals (such as mercury), flame retardants, PFC's (water and stain-repellents, which can be found on pizza boxes and the slick coating inside microwavable popcorn bags), and POP's (persistent organic pollutants, which include the formally banned DDT, Polychlorinated biphenyls [PCBs] and dioxins).[128]

BIO-ACCUMULATION

Pollutants love fat. As pollutants accumulate over time, the older and larger fish, such as swordfish, tuna, and shark, carry around toxins from ingesting smaller sea animals such as krill and shrimp. The pollutants bio-magnify up the food chain from the smaller fish to the larger fish residing in fat cells. When we consume these very same fish, the toxins are then released into our own delicate systems.

THE ENDOCRINE SYSTEM AND POLLUTANTS

The endocrine system is responsible for almost every cell, organ, and function in your body. It is equally important as the liver's job to remove toxins and the heart's job to pump blood. The endocrine system consists of a network of glands that make hormones to help cells (think blood) communicate with each other. If that communication network gets disrupted, bodily functions can start to go haywire. You might have problems with puberty (like we see with young girls entering puberty as early as six), getting pregnant, or managing stress. You might gain weight for no reason, have brittle bones, or lack vitality or stamina because too much sugar remains in your blood instead of entering cells to be used for energy. Having

a healthy endocrine system is essential for moods, growth and development, metabolism, organs, and reproduction.[129]

If the role of the immune system is to protect the body against foreign invaders and infection such as bacteria/viruses/fungus by mounting an immune response to attack and eliminate them from your body, could it be possible that endocrine disruptors are the cause of inflammation found in auto-immune diseases?[130] Is it plausible to say that endocrine disruptors could possibly be the cause of auto-immune diseases?

WHAT ARE ENDOCRINE DISRUPTORS?

Endocrine disruptors are just that. They disrupt the developmental, reproductive, brain, and immune systems in humans. They are foreign invaders that interfere with the endocrine system by mimicking natural hormones. Endocrine disruptors are found in everyday items, including food and beverages, pesticides, toys, cosmetics, creams (including sunscreen), and prescription drugs, all by-products of chemical industries. Contact with endocrine disruptors can occur on a daily basis through the food we eat, the air we breathe, the products we apply to our skin, and even the purified water we drink.

XENOESTROGENS

Xenoestrogens are one example of endocrine disruptors. Xenoestrogens act like estrogens, but more disturbingly, they mimic the effects of natural estrogens in the body. Xenoestrogens significantly affect males, regardless of species, because males are more sensitive to estrogenic influences. Even small changes in the body's normal endocrine system can cause significant developmental and biological effects.[131] Xenoestrogens love to attach themselves to testosterone with the goal of making it diminish completely. Scientists are now finding evidence of increasing abnormalities among boys, particularly large increases in the number of genital deformities among newborns.[132]

The most common endocrine disruptors are:

• Mercury: Most everyone is aware of the mercury content of some larger, fattier fish like tuna, swordfish, shark, and southern tilefish. One of the largest sources of mercury contaminants comes from burning coal. The EPA estimated in 1998, U.S. coal-fired plants emit about 50 tons of mercury a year into the atmosphere.[133]

Once up in smoke, mercury meanders around the globe, landing indiscriminately. Mercury residues that fall on the water are eaten by bacteria, which undergoes a chemical reaction resulting in a very toxic form of mercury called methyl-mercury. The body has the ability to excrete inorganic mercury, the kind found in old-style thermometers, but methyl-mercury binds very tightly to muscle tissue, which becomes more problematic for that reason.[134] With each step up the food chain, the amount of methyl mercury grows.[135] Tiny plankton that float on the upper part of the ocean are first affected by mercury. The plankton is then eaten by smaller fish that are then eaten by medium-size fish, which are then eaten by larger fish, amplifying the methyl-mercury until it has permanently attached itself inside of us after we consume those very same fish. At this point, it becomes very difficult to eliminate.[136]

• PCBs: Polychlorinated biphenyls, when absorbed, persist in fat tissues. PCBs have been known to cause cancer, and some of these compounds can cause neurotoxicity and endocrine disruption in humans. PCBs can suppress the immune system, alter thyroid and reproductive function, and increase the risk of developing cardiovascular and liver disease and diabetes.[137] The highest levels of PCBs are found in rock sole.

Shockingly, General Electric dumped an estimated 1.3 million pounds of different types of PCBs into the Hudson River in upstate New York from 1946 until 1997, when PCBs were finally banned.[138] PCBs can also be found elsewhere all over the world.

• Dioxins: The dioxin family boasts about 50 or so individual family members living for decades in our environment. Dioxins are formed either during high-temperature treatment of waste-water or through industrial processes of chemical agents. Dioxins travel without restriction through the air. Once in the environment, dioxins disrupt the function of the endocrine and immune systems. Dioxins are also found abundantly in beef, pork, chicken, and almost all animal-based foods that contain fat. The greatest amount, surprisingly, is found in farm-raised salmon.

• PBDEs: PBDE's are omnipresent in today's flame-retardant world. If you think about it, what you are touching, sitting on, sleeping on, or wearing is most likely flame-retardant. Flame retardant is such a pervasive chemical that an entire chapter could be devoted to it. Flame retardants are heavily pushed by the same industry that manufactures these chemicals, and many organizations are trying to ban flame retardants. The National Fire Protection Association claims firefighters who tend to fires riddled with PBDE experience sudden cardiac deaths, accounting for 42% of the on-duty deaths in the last five years, and several studies have indicated that firefighters have an increased risk of several cancers compared to the general population.[139] PBDEs disrupt the delicate balance of the human thyroid gland and the brain, resulting in behavioral changes and hyperactivity. In children, PBDEs are associated with developmental problems and lowered IQ. A primary animal source of ingested PBDEs? Fish and shellfish. Where one finds PBDE's the most? Breast milk.

• *BMAA: Remember the recent and heavily promoted social media ice-bucket challenge for ALS? Research is linking BMAA to the rise in ALS and other neurological diseases. Research is suggesting that this new toxin, called beta-methylamino-L-alanine, is produced by cyanobacteria, a common component in the diet of lake and ocean creatures. BMAA becomes a neurotoxin in the brain and becomes a trigger for neurological diseases, in particular, Alzheimer's, Parkinson's, and ALS. The reason for algal blooms? Increasing temperatures and contamination by sewage and agricultural chemical run-off in both fresh and salt waters. Where to find fish with high amounts of BMAA? In the state of Florida, the highest levels of BMAA contaminated fish are found predominantly in largemouth bass, pink shrimp, and blue crabs. Lower but still significant amounts were found in oysters and mussels.

• Toxaphene: Banned for all uses in the U.S. in 1986, toxaphene had been widely used on cotton and soybean crops in the midwestern U.S. and even around the globe. The highest level of toxaphene and DDE (a breakdown of DDT) was found in sockeye salmon. Both chemicals are well-documented endocrine disruptors.[140]

There are many other toxins found in the bodies of fish and shellfish, but these are the more commonly known potent, cancer-causing, and endocrine-disrupting agents.

PHARMACEUTICAL DRUGS IN FISH?

Unfortunately, fish have become the unintended recipients of pharmaceutical drugs that evade wastewater treatment filters. Municipal wastewater facilities do not have the technology nor the funds to appropriately eliminate the drugs coming through them. Many drugs that evade filtration include drugs that treat depression, psychiatric disorders, high blood pressure, allergies, cholesterol, and a wide range of other chemicals coming from personal hygiene and care products. Many, if not all, of these drug residues persist in discharged wastewater from these wastewater treatment facilities.

Fish that live downstream from wastewater treatment facilities are constantly inundated with wastewater that has not been completely purified, contaminating the fish living in the local water bodies, which should be rendered unfit to eat.[141] Treated wastewaters are also used for other purposes beyond what the EPA claims as "sustaining aquatic life." Treated wastewater is also used for irrigating crops, as mentioned in an earlier chapter, and for drinking water, which we will discuss in a subsequent chapter.

CHEMICAL SUNSCREENS

What would we do without our beloved sunscreen? It allows us to sit out in the sun for hours on end without burning! Doctors and dermatologists insist we use it to prevent skin damage, premature aging, and even cancer. This chemical that has afforded us many summertime freedoms now comes with a hefty price tag. Oxybenzone, the principal-agent in sunscreen, is a documented hormone disruptor. In 2005 oxybenzone was found in the bodies of 97% of the 2,500 US residents whose blood had been tested at random. Once in lakes, rivers, or oceans, oxybenzone settles into sediment and gets absorbed by small fish as they feed. The small fish are then eaten by the bigger fish. We then eat the fish, and hence the xenoestrogen cycle begins.

According to Brian Clement, author of *Killer Fish*, "The impact of chemicals found unnaturally in our waterways contributes to the disturbing alteration of fish hormones such as gonadal inter-sex fish, altered sex ratios, reduced gonad size, and disrupted ovarian and testicular tissue changes, which is consistent with exposure to estrogenic wastewater contaminants."[142] What does that all mean? It means that young boys and girls are at the most risk. As human actions continue to warp natural ecosystems, we will continue to see and feel firsthand the rapid demise of what nature intended.

Looking past local municipalities, the global demand for fish continues to diminish our oceans of fish. Overfishing and habitat destruction has left some species as a low at 1% of their original populations, according to federal data.[143] With the destruction of waterways through overfishing and pollution, consuming fish has become more so a matter of ethical implications rather than pollution alone.

AQUATIC LIFE - LIFE ON THE FARM - FARM RAISED FISH

Many consumers falsely believe that farm-raised fish are healthier than wild-caught fish because of the high levels of contaminants found in our oceans. Aquaculture (known as aqua farming or farm-raised fish) involves raising fish under controlled conditions. In an aqua system, both the environment and feed quality are regulated, so the assumption is that there will be less chance of contamination from toxins. What most people do not realize is that the level of contamination in farm-raised fish is due to the very practice itself. Farm-raised fish is the aquatic version of a concentrated animal feeding operation or CAFO. There are also many examples of man-made contaminants found at high levels in farmed fish due to the fishmeal and fish oil that the fish are fed while they are penned up. (The same fishmeal that is fed to fish is also fed to chickens and pigs.)

The species predominately raised on fish farms are salmon, bigeye tuna, carp, tilapia, catfish, and cod. Much of farmed raised salmon contains more contaminants than wild-caught salmon. The FDA has established tolerance levels of many contaminants for commercially sold fish – and what is shocking are the allowable amounts. For a detailed list of contaminants, go to https://www.fda.gov/media/80258/download.

The difficulty in determining the levels of toxicology is the impact of one or more combined chemicals resulting in a greater health effect, called synergistic properties. Or when a person eats fish exposed to two or more industrial toxins, the effects could be additive (each toxin adds to the health impacts of the other).

In nature, there are no controls in place regarding feed, contaminants, supply, etc. Not to suggest that wild-caught is any less toxic, but the belief that farm-raised is healthier is a misguided concept.

TILAPIA – CHEAP FISH AT A CHEAP PRICE

Tilapia is a cheap fish and is becoming an appealing staple in the diets of people with restrictive grocery budgets. Tilapia is easy to produce in large quantities on fish farms and develops well off of inexpensive GMO corn-based feeds. Tilapia contains very low levels of omega-3s due to its diet of omega-6 rich corn (tilapia is generally a marine plant eater, which would give it a higher omega-3 ratio). With an already disproportionate ratio of omega-6s to omega-3s in the Standard American Diet (SAD), consuming tilapia (and its plant-based counterpart, the catfish) further contributes to a chemical-ridden, nutritionally void, and inflammatory diet typical of Americans.

Additionally, overcrowding is the norm in fish pens, and with it comes the rapid proliferation and spread of viruses and bacteria. Let's not forget the problematic sea lice, too, which is then treated with anti-parasitic medication.

BUY LOCAL?

When it comes to fish, buying local may not be the best for your health. When in doubt, check your state's local advisory. The Department of Health issues fish consumption advisories in cooperation with the state Department of Environmental Protection.

Nationally, the U.S. Environmental Protection Agency (EPA) maintains a website that posts fish advisories with fish contamination alerts to consumers. To find this information, go to water.epa.gov and search for "fish consumption advisories."

Can't live without fish? We have some amazing alternatives for you in the Meatless Meals Part

Two section called Sea Veggies! They are sea plants and provide an incredible amount of health benefits with less of the contaminants found in a variety of aquatic life. Spend some time exploring. I think you'll be surprised by the information and more pleasantly surprised by their flavors! Again, make it a Meatless Monday or a Fishless Friday! Unfortunately, however, if you have a seafood or shellfish allergy, the seaweeds presented may not be an option for you. That doesn't mean you can't find an amazing alternative or just plan to omit altogether.

the "all-natural" chicken

Ah! The life of a chicken, living luxuriously in the red henhouse, dining all day long on seedlings in the thick green grasses of the sprawling farmland coming in at night only to be protected from wildlife. If only life on a farm could be this serene.

THE HAPPY LIFE OF HENS!

Hens naturally produce omega-3 rich eggs that actually come from the protein chickens consume, mainly bugs and insects from the ground. Chickens are not vegetarian like the manufacturers boldly claim on their packaging. Chicken are omnivorous. Chickens' natural diet includes bugs, ants, worms, grasshoppers, and fly larvae—larvae that come straight out of cow dung! If your chickens are high in omega-3s from being raised off of flax meal, you know they spent a good majority of their life indoors! Being that chickens are omnivorous, they also eat vegetation. They peck for seedling through grass, eat herbs, and even clover. Chickens will consume about 30% of their calories from grasses alone. Both the vegetation and insects provide the chickens with a naturally high omega-3 content.

Another little known fact? During the winter, when penned, chickens will eat the internal organs of vermin. They find freshly shot groundhog, opossum, and raccoon a delicacy. Worse yet, they'll eat each other—think "hen-pecked." During winter months, chickens can be supplemented with fresh road kill, earthworms, comfrey, milk, and whey and fermented green forage. Furthermore, they like to dig deep into their bedding to find bugs and other organisms invisible even to the human eye. Not the sweet, docile little bird you envisioned? Of course not! Industrial farming raises them in an entirely different way. Here's how conventional factory-farmed chickens are raised.

TODAY'S FACTORY FARMED CHICKEN

CAFO's aren't what we envision when we think of raising chickens. Due to agricultural changes in the US over the past 25 years, CAFO's have become the norm and have an unfortunate impact on both animal and human health. The US is the largest producer of broiler chickens with over 600 factory broiler farms in Alabama alone. The world raises and slaughters around 40 billion chickens per year.[144] CAFO chickens are raised in inhumane long windowless "houses," which are inaccessible to anyone outside the industry.[145] These so-called large-scale commercial farms account for 82% of overall broiler production.[146]

The new large-scale, cage-free, or free-range "all vegetarian fed" organic chicken is grossly undernourished. If the chickens did have access to insects, the store packaging would lose its feel-good label with the potential to turn ill-informed consumers away. Here is what your "free-range, all-vegetarian fed" chicken means: No access to pasture, little to no access to the outdoors, and worst of all, continuous confinement.

In keeping broiler chickens "pristine and pure"—essentially sanitized, we consume a weaker, paler, "nothing-natural" chicken. The nutrient profile of chickens and eggs raised in this environment are nutritionally inferior to birds with access to bugs and meat scraps. An all-vegetarian diet contains mainly corn and soy, another unnatural part of an omnivore's diet.

LIFE ON THE FACTORY FARM

It is difficult to control the problems faced with raising thousands of chickens in one chicken barn, 500 feet long, 40 feet wide, and windowless—chickens overcrowded, lame, limping, or possibly even dead, living without natural sunlight.

Chickens raised in these crowded, unsanitary farming conditions contract the very illnesses and infections that chicken producers are using antibiotics to protect against. While many companies are advertising "antibiotic-free," many still use them. With a nutritionally devoid diet and the continued use of feed additives and antibiotics, the chickens deceptively look healthier with larger, more succulent breasts. They are anything but "natural," as the label suggests.[147]

WHY THE BIG FARMS (CAFOS)?

With the changes seen in agricultural farming over the decades and the push towards monoculture farming comes with it another change: The farmer no longer has control of his farm, nor his livestock. What he does have, however, are the risks and responsibilities for the operation and maintenance of the chicken houses, including raising the birds and disposing of their waste.

How did this happen? The farmer entered into a contract with a multinational company to save his family farm. The deal he signed leaves him beholden to the practices of billion-dollar agribusiness companies such as Tyson Foods, Gold Kist, and Perdue Farms. These firms technically own the birds and provide the feed. They also provide the set pace of the input and output for production, paying the farmer for the realized weight gain of the birds. In this setting, the farmer has lost his negotiating power. He rendered himself powerless yet allowed himself to be squeezed in the middle. He essentially became a chicken factory worker rather than a poultry farmer.

POULTRY FEED

Mass producers of poultry are certainly leery of disease, which might bring about the destruction of their entire flock. The new "all vegetarian fed" chickens put to rest the worry over latent animal diseases found years ago in poultry feed. The antibiotics used currently in production contain compounds that can cause health problems in humans, according to Dr. Partha Basu, an associate professor in the Department of Chemistry and Biochemistry at Duquesne University.[148] The feed additives contain an antibiotic arsenic compound known as roxarsone, used since the 1960s, which makes the chickens healthier in terms of bigger breasts and pinker skin. The use of roxarsone in poultry feed has become common practice to help protect the chickens from illnesses and infections, namely parasites. Its ability to plump and beautify the breasts is a major area of concern. The studies that Dr. Basu conducted show a correlation between the stimulation and growth in the chicken carrying

over into the cells in our bodies when we eat chickens fed roxarsone.[149] The concern? Abnormal and overproduction of cell growth, called angiogenesis, which studies show can lead to cancer. What many people are unaware of is that the use of steroid growth hormones in poultry is prohibited by the FDA, but we still face other dilemmas associated with feed additives.

Poultry litter is the agricultural term for poultry waste. If chickens are consuming arsenic and other chemicals in their poultry feed, it is sure to exit as waste. Contaminants from poultry litter include ammonia, nitrates, pathogens, antibiotics, hormones, and heavy metals. When metabolized by the chickens, these compounds break down and cause arsenic to be passed through the chickens. The arsenic, a known carcinogen, then leaches into surface and groundwater. The large-scale feeding operations generate more waste than sewer systems of small towns can handle. Contaminants from the excess litter become a burden for nearby water sources, including drinking wells. Furthermore, consumers unwittingly purchase "all-natural" contaminated poultry litter sold as fertilizer for family flowers and gardens. The toxic feed given to CAFO chickens becomes a disastrous and pervasive ecological and health problem.

WHAT CHICKEN DO I BUY THEN?

When you are able to locate a pasture-raised, all-natural grown chicken, you are going to be quite surprised. The bird is significantly smaller compared to its conventional counterpart. Its skin is somewhat grayish in color with a pimpled texture from feather plucking. The meat is generally darker than the all-American yellow-pink breast we have become accustomed to seeing.

Two of the best alternatives to conventionally raised chickens:

• Certified organic free-range: This particular bird most likely lives in a row house, but there are windows that allow fresh air and sunlight. The floor is cleaned with a disinfectant prior to a new batch of chicks arriving. (The standard is sweeping only.) The feed is certified organic, which means no genetically-engineered products were given to the mother during any part of the chicks' life. The feed may not contain antibiotics or growth hormones. The chicken may or may not have access to the outdoors.

• Pasture-Raised: This is the most "natural" of all the chickens. The chickens either have access to the outdoors, and the indoor home is again a row house, or the chickens primarily live outside and have a hen house provided for perching. Their food comes naturally from the ground or is given as a supplement. The feed generally is not certified as organic, but a quick online inquiry or phone call will be able to tell you what is and is not in the chicken's feed.

Not sure what to ask when you call? Here's a list of things to inquire:

Are the chickens supplemented with:

- Flax Meal
- Fermented Green Forage
- Vermin
- Earthworms
- Fishmeal
- Proper Bedding for Microbial Food
- Milk, Comfrey, or Whey
- Grass, Herbs, or Clover

What would we do without eggs for desserts!? Pies, pastries, cakes, puddings, oh my! There's an easy fix! Head on over to the Dessert section of the recipe book and learn a few and exciting new ways to make desserts without the use of butter, milk, or eggs. You surely will not be disappointed. I promise you that!

water

These days pretty much everyone is dutifully aware of the need to remain hydrated. The best-touted source of hydration comes from water—rightfully so! Water has become one of the most popular drinks, which is why we see most Americans carrying with them various forms of bottled water everywhere we go!

Why the emphasis on water? Well, water is considered a necessary nutrient your body needs due to loss from sweat, evaporation, urine, and stools. Water also maintains the balance of bodily fluids. Since our body is comprised mostly of water, about 60%, to be exact, we need to replenish these fluids. Fluids help with digestion, transportation and absorption of nutrients, blood circulation, creation of saliva, and maintenance of body temperature. It also lubricates and cushions joints, protects sensitive tissues, and gets rid of waste through urination, perspiration, and bowel movements. Without the minerals and electrolytes from hydration, we would, unfortunately, die.

The eight glasses per day guideline is merely a guideline. Want to know how to personalize water consumption for you? The calculation calls for half your body weight in ounces. Are you having a caffeinated or alcoholic drink? Tack on an additional 16 ounces of water for each! What does that work out to be for you?

The information about water consumption has been so widely publicized, but what we don't hear about very much is from where? While our body needs water and lots of it, certain water sources enhance our health, and others could possibly undermine it.

We'll start with the most readily available source: tap water.

TAP WATER

What is tap water?

Tap water is one of the many success stories of the developed world and one of the many modern-day conveniences we enjoy. It flows freely from our faucets, shower-heads, outside spigots, and disappears down our toilets. Tap water is subject to stringent federal safety regulations at both the state and local levels. Tap water safety and testing results are made available to the public.

Generally, from lakes or rivers (surface water) or underground (aquifers), tap water is pumped into a treatment facility where it undergoes several purification processes. First off, it enters through a filtration system to remove debris. At this point, it is also treated to kill off any bacteria and viruses that could otherwise make you sick. The water is then remedied with an acid or a base to bring it to a neutral pH of 7. Because tap water is not naturally "clean" to drink, it requires further treatment with chemicals and several other filtration processes.

What is tap water treated with?

Water treatment facilities treat water destined for homes and businesses through the widespread use of disinfectants, with the most common being chlorine. Some municipalities are using newer technology such as ultra-violet (UV) irradiation to accomplish what disinfectants can do. All this disinfecting does not come without a price, however. Let's take a closer look.

While tap water disinfection is necessary for controlling waterborne disease, the chemicals used to eliminate disease, in turn, form harmful cancer-causing byproducts in the treated water. These byproducts occur when disinfectants come in contact with organic pollution from agriculture or urban and sprawl runoff. For example, chlorine introduced into the water supply reacts with other naturally occurring elements to form toxins called trihalomethanes (THMs), which then enter our bodies.[150] THMs have been linked to a wide range of human health maladies ranging from asthma and eczema to bladder cancer and heart disease.[151] So, by eliminating one problem, the microbes, another is caused. The government does not test by-products from synergistic chlorine reactions, so there is no limit set on these particular contaminants. The by-products are the ones of particular concern.

Jane Houlihan, EWG's Research Director, states, "Dirty water going into the treatment plant means water contaminated with chlorination byproducts coming out of your tap. The solution is to clean up our lakes, rivers, and streams, not just bombard our water supplies with chlorine."[152]

Between 2004 and 2009, water suppliers across the U.S. detected 316 contaminants in water supplied to the public. The list of detected contaminants includes:[153]

• 97 agricultural pollutants, including pesticides and chemicals from fertilizer- and manure-laden runoff;

• 204 industrial chemicals from factory discharges and consumer products;

• 86 contaminants linked to sprawl and urban areas or from polluted runoff and wastewater treatment plants;

- Forty-two pollutants that are byproducts of the water treatment processes or that leach from pipes and storage tanks.[154]

Many commonly detected contaminants have been found at concentrations exceeding mandatory federal drinking water standards.

Don't pass on tap water just yet. As we move further into this chapter, there are a few purification filters that can easily turn your dirty tap water into a clean and pure form of drinking water.

BOTTLED WATER

In addition to being an environmental nightmare from pollution to the cost of fossil fuels to produce and transport, bottled water is not safer than tap water, as one would believe.

What most people are unaware of is that 25 to 30 percent of bottled water comes straight from municipal tap water systems, despite the picturesque scenes on the labels that imply otherwise.[155] Need an example? Think Dasani or Aquafina.

Some municipal water sources destined for fancy plastic packaging may go through additional filtering, but there are no federal mandates that require any extra precautionary measures. The Natural Resources Defense Council (NRDC) has researched bottled water extensively and found that bottled water is "subject to less rigorous testing and purity standards than those that apply to city tap water."[156]

Furthermore, bottled water is not required to be tested as frequently as tap water for bacteria and chemical contaminants.

The U.S. Food and Drug Administration bottled water rules allow for some contamination by E. coli or fecal coliform, which are in direct contrast to EPA's tap water regulations that prohibit any such contamination.[157]

The NRDC also found that there are no requirements for bottled water to be disinfected or tested for parasites such as cryptosporidium or giardia, again unlike the more stringent EPA rules regulating tap water.[158] Cryptosporidium infiltrates the water supply by way of animal and human sewage. The eggs of the parasite hatch inside the intestinal tract and cause severe diarrhea, cramps, vomiting, fever, and in certain cases, death. With very loose bottled water regulations, it leaves open the possibility that we could become sickened by bottled water. How much is that bottle worth to you now?

Not the water but the packaging? Recent studies have shown that chemicals called phthalates (from plastics), which are known endocrine disruptors, can leach into bottled water over time. Although there are regulatory standards limiting phthalates in tap water, there are no legal limits for phthalates in bottled water—the bottled water industry waged a successful campaign opposing the FDA proposal to set a legal limit for these chemicals.[159]

The FDA requires that companies test for:

- bacterial contamination in water only once per week,

- only four empty bottles once every three months for bacterial contamination, and

- chemical, physical, or radiological contaminants once per year.

To determine if bottled water is just tap water, check the bottle label and even the cap. If it says "from a municipal source" or "from a community water system," this means it's derived from tap water. You're paying for free water packed into a disposable plastic bottle. Not only does it have environmental implications, but it can also negatively impact your health. There are solutions to the public water supply/disposable bottled water conundrum. Not all bottled waters are created equal, which we discuss later on.

REVERSE OSMOSIS WATER FILTRATION SYSTEMS

Benefits of Reverse Osmosis Water Filter Systems

The best reason to use a reverse osmosis system, also known as an RO system, is the purity of the water produced. These systems remove many harmful contaminants from the water or greatly reduce their number. Just a few of the many pollutants they remove include microbial cysts, bacteria, sodium, sulfate, nitrate, iron, mercury, lead, phosphate, nickel, fluoride, chlorine, chloroform, cyanide, and barium.

To put it into perspective, the best whole house water systems leave the water with less than 1,000 parts per million of dissolved solids, which is very good. Reverse osmosis (RO) water filter systems leave the water with less than 100 PPM, significantly much less.[160]

The one drawback to RO water is its thorough purification. Due to the extraordinary process of removing all pollutants and contaminants, it also removes all of the electrolytes rendering it "dead" water. An easy and relatively inexpensive way to remedy that is to replenish the water with mineral drops. I personally use ConcenTrace® Mineral Drops, minerals taken from Salt Lake, Utah. Our family bottles the water again in inexpensive gallon glass jugs and store in the refrigerator. ConcenTrace® is an all-natural, pH-balancing trace mineral product with over 72 trace minerals. For perfect water from your water distiller, reverse osmosis, or purification system—add 20 to 40 drops per gallon of pure distilled water or 1-3 drops to your glass. ConcenTrace® adds a complete, balanced spectrum of low sodium minerals and trace minerals.

Another big benefit to RO water is that it pours directly from a specialized faucet at your kitchen sink. It sits in a holding tank until used, so it's not possible to pour gallons upon gallons at one time, but it is possible to have on hand healthy drinking water without purchasing water housed in plastic bottles. Over the long term, RO water is the most cost-effective.

DISTILLED WATER

Distillation is the process in which water is boiled until it changes to steam and evaporated. When the steam cools down and condenses back into a liquid form, the result is called distilled water. Distilled water is free of dissolved minerals or contaminants and contains a pH level of 7. Because of this, it has the special property of being able to actively absorb toxic substances from the body and eliminate them.[161]

Drinking distilled water for purposes other than detoxifying is highly controversial among health gurus and notable physicians. Some believe that it helps flush away excess minerals and toxins from the body, only those in the bloodstream, not found in the organs. Others believe distilled water leaches essential minerals from the body and could leave teeth and bones vulnerable to damage.[162]

Dr. Mercola, a notable and leading health expert, emphasizes that fasting using distilled water can be dangerous because of the rapid loss of electrolytes (sodium, potassium, chloride) and trace minerals like magnesium, deficiencies of which can cause heartbeat irregularities and high blood pressure. He also believes cooking foods in distilled water pulls the minerals out of them and lowers their nutrient value.[163] Whether you agree or disagree with his argument, purchasing distilled water is an option as it is relatively cheap by comparison, and one could add minerals and electrolytes like potassium, calcium, and sodium back in by using ConcenTrace®.

SPRING WATER

Bottled spring water tastes good and is deemed safe, but it too may come from a contaminated source. Contaminants come from the ground as the water passes over the rock, which include acid rain, ground contaminants, toxins from factories and farms, and a wide variety of potentially harmful bacteria.

Municipal springs are tested periodically, and if you purchase from one, you can find the testing information from the spring's website. Many bottled spring waters do not cite their source except for Poland Springs, which cites six springs. Poland Springs is one of the very few bottled water companies that will offer the results of water testing. Just as a side note, Poland Springs also sanitizes the spring water with UV rays, so it is unclear just how much of the delicate balance of the water is disrupted.

WELL WATER

Well water is probably one of the most flavorful waters used as drinking water due in part to its mineral content. As many as 15 percent of Americans rely on their own private water supplies, but these independent systems are not subject to EPA standards. Because the EPA does not regulate private wells, however, some state and local governments set rules to protect users of these wells. Unlike public drinking water systems, households with wells must take special precautions, which tend to be costly, to ensure the protection and maintenance of their drinking water supplies.

If you own and drink from a well, you should have the well tested at least yearly.

What Might be Lurking in your Private Well Water?

Microorganisms: Bacteria, viruses, parasites, and other microorganisms. Some of these organisms can cause a variety of illnesses.

Radon: Radon is a gas that is a natural product of the breakdown of uranium in the soil — can also pose a threat. Radon is most dangerous when inhaled and contributes to lung cancer, while radon is less dangerous when consumed in water, but still remains a risk to health due to a higher risk of stomach cancer.

Nitrates and Nitrites: Although high nitrate levels are usually due to human activities (see below), they may be found naturally in groundwater. Drinking large amounts of nitrates and nitrites is particularly threatening to infants (for example, when mixed in formula).

Fluoride: In excessive quantities has been known to cause damage to bone tissue.

Septic tanks: The wastewater from septic tank leach fields can move into groundwater.

Industrial Products and Wastes: Many harmful chemicals are used freely in local business and industry. They can become drinking water pollutants if not managed or disposed of properly.[164]

In order to know for certain the contaminants that may or may not be in your well, conducting periodic is suggested. Check for well water testing companies in your area through a simple web search.

ARTESIAN WATER

Artesian water comes from (you guessed it) an artesian well. An artesian well comes from a source deep in the earth. The water found in these wells has been compressed between layers of rocks. This means that bacteria, acid rain, and other toxins can't penetrate the rock and contaminate the water as easily as found with spring water. The resultant water contains only minerals.

An artesian well must be drilled. After drilling, a pipe is installed, so when the water is pumped out, it doesn't come into contact with any potential contaminants.

There are many minerals and electrolytes found naturally in artesian water. The electrolytes potassium and sodium keep the body's chemistry balanced. Other minerals and electrolytes include:

Bicarbonate: Bicarbonate is an electrolyte that balances the blood's pH. Without the right level of bicarbonate in the body, the blood will become acidic.

Calcium: Calcium is a mineral that keeps the bones strong, the nerve functioning properly, and helps with muscle growth and tone. Too much of a good thing is no longer good, as is the case with calcium.

Silica: Silica is another mineral that the body requires. Without enough silica, the joints could become problematic. The silica that is naturally found in artesian water is what gives it its taste and body.[165]

Looking for the perfect artesian well water to drink? Find out if your area drills artesian wells.

SHOWERING IN TAP WATER?

For many Americans, although not all, showering is a daily event. For some, multiple showers are the norm. We talk a lot about the water we drink, but there needs to be some thought given to what we are putting *on* our bodies. Just remember that what goes on our bodies eventually ends up *in* our bodies. If it becomes soaked up by the skin, it bypasses the liver and enters directly into the bloodstream. If you're like most people and take hot showers, those delicate little pores open up due to the warmth of the water and let in whatever is present. When in the shower, not only is the skin absorbing the chemicals, but the lungs are inhaling them as well. Scientists have warned of the risks of showering in chemically treated city water.

Tap water on the skin.

When showering in tap water daily, the chemicals in the treated water changes the skin's natural pH balance (as do most conventional cleansers on the market). The normal, slightly-acidic pH of the skin helps to protect against bacterial infections, including staph, MRSA, and even acne. The more alkaline the pH level created by frequent showering is a better environment for bacteria to grow. It also strips away the skin's natural oils. Good-bye hydration and glowing skin!

Want to eliminate the problems associated with showering in tap water? Try a good quality shower head filter that balances the pH level, removes the chlorine along with other harmful chemicals. Showering in filtered water is better for your hair and skin, but the cosmetic benefits are just a minor consideration to your overall health.

If you want to do everything that you can for the health of your respiratory system and that of your whole body, the advice is to stop showering in chlorine. When the chlorine in publicly treated facilities is heated, chloroform gas and THMs form. Chloroform, a known carcinogen, "may be released to the air as a result of its formation in the chlorination of drinking water, wastewater and swimming pools. The major effect of acute (short-term) inhalation exposure to chloroform is central nervous system depression. Chronic (long-term) exposure to chloroform by inhalation in humans has resulted in effects on the liver. Chloroform has been shown to be carcinogenic in animals after oral exposure, resulting in an increase in kidney and liver tumors. The EPA has classified chloroform as a Group B2, probable human carcinogen."[166] If you're showering daily in city or county tap water, you most likely are inhaling and absorbing these chemicals.

Most public facilities measure the amount of THMs that are present at the facility. It must be below certain levels, or "action" needs to be taken, but there is no mandatory testing for chloroform gas in the air due to showering in unfiltered water in private homes, so the safe bet is to assume that if you're showering in water from a public supply system and you're without a filter, you might be at risk.

There are also companies that specialize in installing whole-home carbon filters inside water treatment or water softening systems. These remedies may seem expensive on the surface, but at what expense is your health, long-term health worth? Well or preventative care can be a lot less than the costs associated with sick care.

Want some amazing filtered water drinks called elixirs? You got it! Head on over to the Elixir section of the recipe book and play around with some warming ideas! You've reached the culminating section to round out your new diet, uh hem, excuse me, lifestyle!

perfectly plated

[recipes

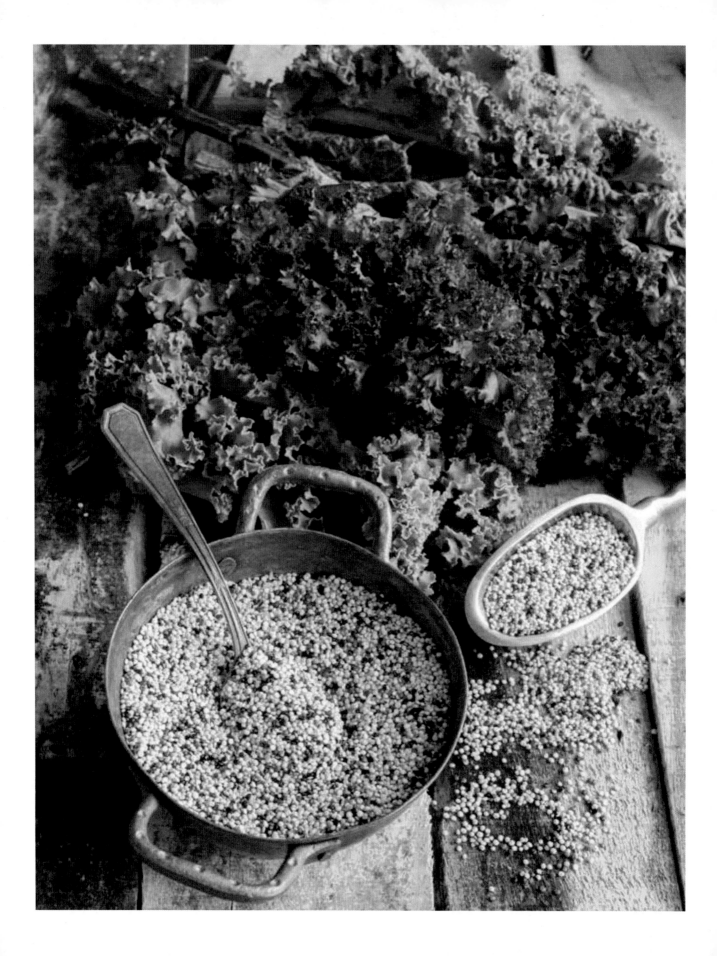

introducing kale & quinoa

Why start with kale and quinoa? Well, for starters, kale and quinoa boast numerous health benefits, too many to list them all! But it's not just about the nutrients; it's about other equally important nutrition information like, drum roll please, quinoa is a complete protein *and* a seed (not a grain), making it a nutritiously dense, gluten-free alternative food.

Quinoa is a good source of calcium, B vitamins, manganese, vitamin E, fiber, and even omega-3 fatty acids. Kale, on the other hand, packs a punch in surprising areas rivaling oranges with its vitamin C and beta carotene. Kale is part of the cruciferous family and contains sulforaphane, which helps lower the risk for certain types of cancer. Kale is also known as a powerful antioxidant.

But that still begs the question, why here and why together? In addition to a remarkable resume, they're easy to find and easy to prepare. They're a great duo as a supporting dish and even better as a main dish due to its dense nutrient profile.

Both kale and quinoa are quite adaptable in recipes, taking on flavors of herbs, spices, and dressings. They're fairly mild in flavor and favorable in texture. Kale can sometimes have tough leaves, but with some gentle massaging of oils, a squeeze of lemon, or a dash of raw apple cider vinegar, the cellulose breaks down,

morphing the once bitter and chewy leaves into a sweeter and more pliable leaf. Chomp on that for a minute!

For the best outcome, always remove the spine prior to preparing. You can either discard the kale spines or use them in a veggie broth. Cooking kale alters its natural flavors producing a pungent flavor due to the sulforaphane while lowering its touted health benefits, but overall cooked kale is a better alternative than no kale!

Both kale and quinoa are colorful, vibrant, easy to prepare, and hold up well when stored. They're relatively inexpensive considering their dietary significance! The Internet is full of recipes calling for kale and quinoa, making them an easy duo to canvass, experiment with, and refine. They are a reliable combination when embarking on a lifestyle and dietary change.

Quinoa seeds are processed to remove a natural phytochemical property and anti-nutrient called saponin, which is the plant's natural defense system to protect itself from infections by parasites. All commercial quinoa sold has had saponins removed by mechanical means or mixed-washing. Some suggest a vigorous rinse in the sink as an added measure. For those who currently suffer from gut issues, sprouted quinoa is a great choice! Sprouted quinoa has gone through a germination process, assuring you of all the good stuff and none of the bad.

Since quinoa seeds are invariably tiny, they can slip through the holes of most colanders. A handy tip would be to purchase a sieve for rinsing, which can easily be found in many grocery stores.

Have no fear or apprehension in purchasing quinoa. The process of cooking quinoa is very similar to that of cooking rice. Looking for a mild flavor to start? Try the white variety as it's the mildest. Rule of thumb, the darker the variety, the nuttier the flavor.

Kale varieties do matter when it comes to preparation. The most common kale varieties are green curly kale, lacinato (dinosaur, Tuscan), red Russian (ragged Jack), redbor, and lesser-known Siberian kale.

Curly kale is the most preferred and widely available kind. You can put it in salads (using the softening tips above), sauté, toss it in a bowl of hearty bean soup, or blend it in a fruit smoothie. For a colorful dish, add the redbor or red Russian kale together with the green for a colorful and vibrant salad.

Lacinato kale looks more like savoy cabbage with its rounded leaves and reptilian in texture. This is incredibly dense kale with a deeper flavor than curly or red kale. It is best suited in soups or down the chute of a juicer! It offers no bulk in a salad, and it is quite difficult to mask its flavor.

All kale and quinoa, regardless of color or texture, are a great addition to any healthy diet. Their growing popularity makes kale and quinoa a socially acceptable and mainstream dish to serve that's sure to impress!

quinoa & arugula salad dressed in cumin-lime vinaigrette

INGREDIENTS:

1 cup dry no-rinse quinoa

1 tbsp. coconut oil

1 ³/₄ c. water

1 can black beans, drained and rinsed

1 avocado, peeled, sliced into bite-size pieces

1 handful cherry or grape tomatoes, quartered

¹/₂ red onion diced

2 garlic cloves, minced or crushed

1 red bell pepper, diced

1 small handful cilantro, coarsely chopped

juice of 1 lime

¹/₂ tsp. ground cumin

¹/₂ tbsp. olive oil

salt, to taste

1 box baby arugula

This hearty and healthy quinoa dish is bursting with incredible southwestern flavors. It's substantial enough to stand on its own. Set over a bed of arugula, this dish one of my all-time favorites.

DIRECTIONS:

1. Warm the coconut oil in a medium saucepan over medium heat. Once it's hot, add the dry quinoa and toast for about 2-3 minutes until it takes on a nut-like fragrance. Add water, stir, cover, and simmer using the suggested cooking instructions found on the box or bag.

2. While the quinoa is cooking, prepare all other ingredients.

3. For the dressing, combine the olive oil, lime juice, cumin, and salt. Whisk briskly. Adjust seasoning to taste.

4. When the quinoa has finished cooking, remove it from heat and fluff with a fork. Add black beans and toss.

5. Let the quinoa cool for about five minutes and then add all the remaining ingredients, including the dressing. Mix through.

6. Serve over a bed of arugula and enjoy!

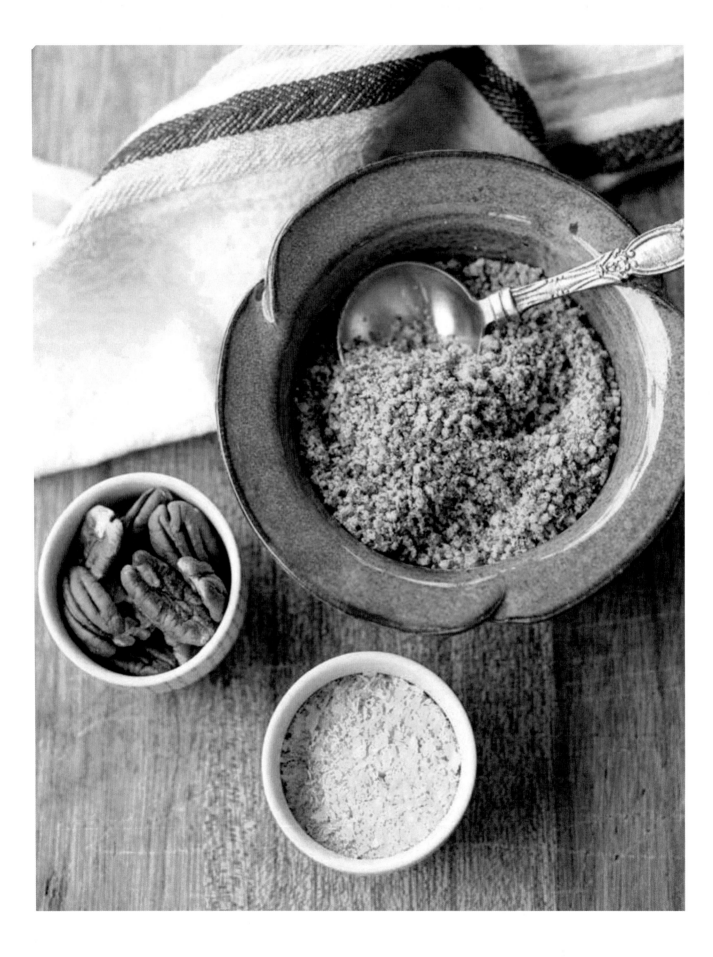

kale caesar with faux parmesan crumbles

This dish surely will not disappoint! The parmesan crumbles paired with the garlicky lemon and fibrous kale will have you feeling full without all of the bloat. It's simple and easy to make and stores well in the refrigerator. Keep the parmesan crumbles and the garlicky lemon dressing separate. Massage the kale with olive oil, place in a sealed container giving you a few ready-made salads at your fingertips!

INGREDIENTS:

2 medium bunches or curly or red kale
4-6 garlic cloves
juice of 2-3 lemons (resulting in 3/4 cup lemon juice)
1/2 cup extra-virgin, first cold-pressed olive oil
1/2 tsp. sea or specialty salt (not iodized table salt)
freshly ground pepper
For the crumbles:
2 cups raw pecans
6 tbsp. nutritional yeast

DIRECTIONS:

1. Preheat oven to 250° F.
2. Line baking sheet with pecans. Roast in oven for approximately 20-25 minutes or until slightly fragrant.
3. While pecans are cooking, de-spine kale, and rinse.
4. Juice lemons and set aside.
5. Peel skins from garlic cloves. Crush or mince and add garlic to lemon juice to marinate.
6. Take pecans out of oven and let cool.
7. Process pecans in food processor, pulsing for 5-second intervals into fine crumbles to ensure the oils don't separate from the meat.
8. Add the nutritional yeast and process twice more.

Preparing the salad:

1. Chop the kale into bite-size pieces and place kale in a large bowl. Drizzle with olive oil and massage into kale leaves.
2. Mix in marinated garlic and lemon juice and toss.
3. Add to a small bowl and add parmesan crumbles.
4. Optional additions: Add dried cranberries or protein of choice. However, leaving it plant-based is best!

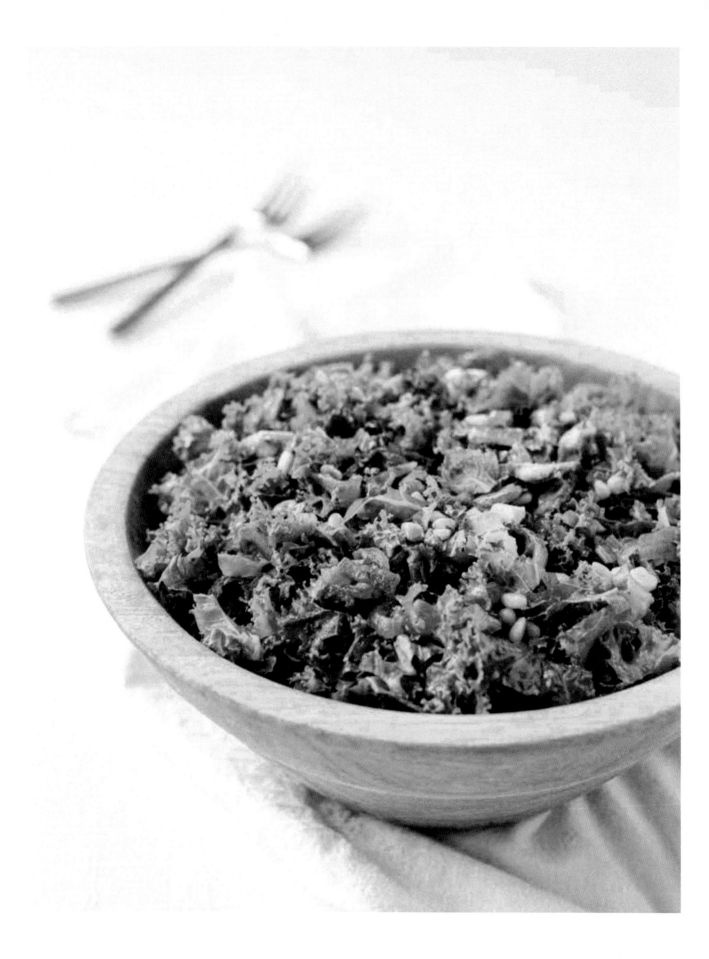

kale salad with toasted pine nuts and avocado

This is the very first salad I made for myself when I embarked on my health journey. Revamped a few times, this still is my original favorite. Not only did I love experimenting with raw kale, I never tired of it either. My plant-based repertoire of foods has certainly grown, but eating this salad never grows old! Using the freshest sun-dried tomatoes without the use of preservatives is best. They generally come in clear bags and are a deep maroon red. The vibrant red pre-sliced sundried tomatoes in air sealed packages usually contain chemicals to maintain their color! It's okay to skip on color in order to keep with healthy!

INGREDIENTS:

2 bunches kale, spines removed

1 red onion

6-8 sun-dried tomatoes (not packed in oil)

$\frac{1}{2}$ c. pine nuts toasted

1 avocado

$\frac{1}{2}$ lemon

$\frac{1}{2}$ c. olive oil plus 2 tbsp.

DIRECTIONS:

1. Remove spines from kale and coarsely chop. Rinse, drain, and pat dry with a paper towel. Set aside.

2. Chop red onion into small evenly cut pieces and sauté in 2 tbsp. of olive oil until browned (but not burnt). As the onions start to turn brown, they will develop a sweet flavor and aroma. Turn off heat, let sit.

3. Soak sun-dried tomatoes in clean water. Soak for 1 hour. Cut into thin strips. If already moistened in a flavor-stay pouch, do not soak.

4. Put pine nuts into a pan on low, periodically tossing nuts until light brown and aromatic making sure not to burn. Remove from heat.

5. Massage oil into kale leaves. Pour in juice from 1/2 lemon. Add in pine nuts, tomatoes, onions, and avocado. Sprinkle with salt and freshly ground pepper.

6. Optional additions: apple cider vinegar for a stronger bite or your favorite protein; however, leaving it plant-based is best!

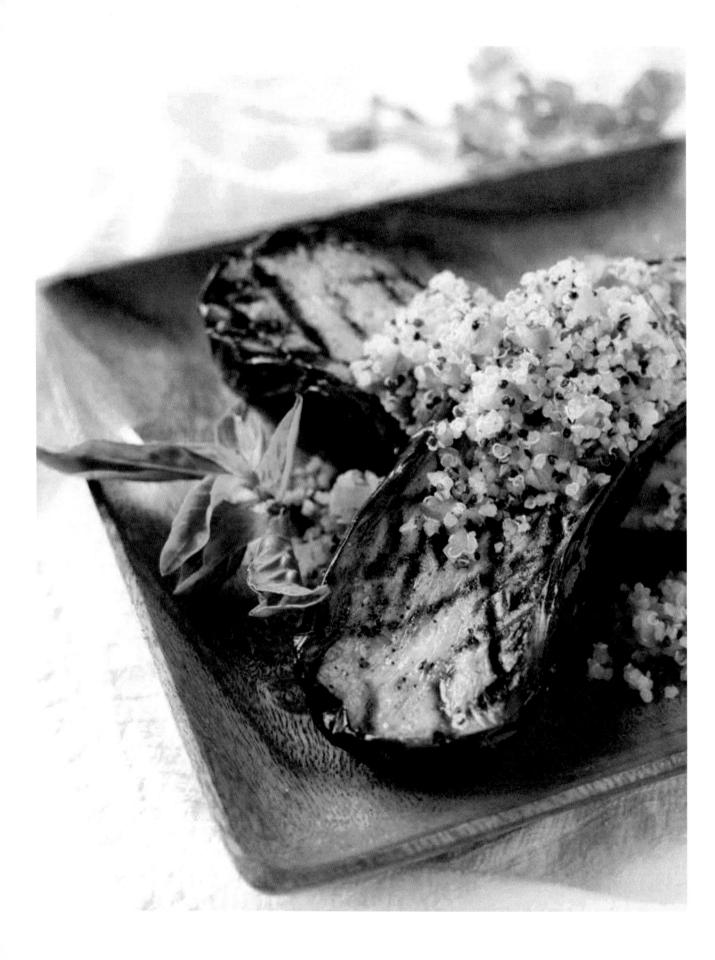

grilled eggplant with quinoa & red pepper salsa

With its deceptive meat-like consistency, this dish can be a great stand-alone lunch *or* dinner meal. Its hearty flavors pair well with freshly cut basil and cilantro. Crank up the summer barbie and bring on those summer vibes!

INGREDIENTS:

2 large or 4-6 small eggplants

1 yellow, 1 red pepper

handful of basil and cilantro leaves only

1 cup white quinoa cooked per direction on bag or box

1 lemon juiced

$\frac{1}{2}$ tbs. coconut oil (for high heat cooking)

1 tbsp. first-cold pressed olive oil (for salads)

2 garlic cloves, crushed or minced

DIRECTIONS:

1. Cook 1 cup white quinoa by following directions on box.

2. Wash eggplants, dry off and cut across the bias making round circles. Remove both ends. Rub coconut oil on both sides of eggplant patties.

3. Grill on medium heat until glistening and no longer firm. Turn over and cook until eggplants are soft and yellowing. Remove and set aside.

4. To make the salsa: removed stem and seeds from peppers and cut into bite-sized pieces. Coarsely chop cilantro leaves and slice basil diagonally into thin ribbons. Crush or mince garlic.

5. Add tbsp. olive oil and lemon juice to quinoa. Toss until mixed in. Add in the salsa.

6. Take each eggplant round and top with quinoa and salsa mix.

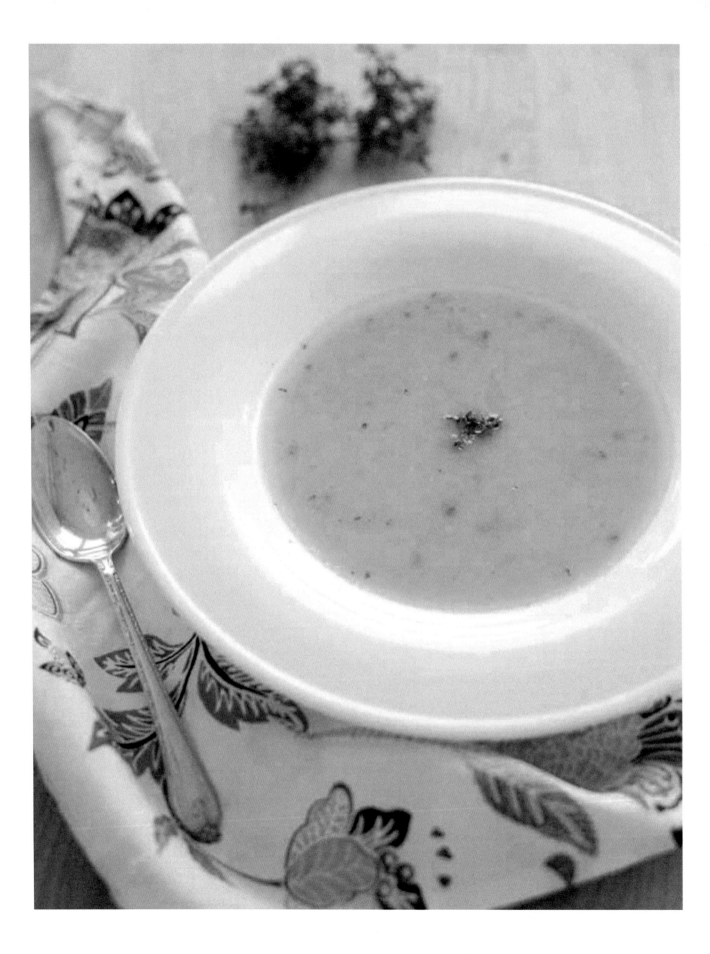

tuscan white bean soup with kale threads & fresh thyme

A fresh take on a traditional soup, this rendition can sure hold its own. As with most soups, the longer it sits, the better the flavors meld (blend) together. Want more heat, take the red pepper flakes up a notch and add a dash a cayenne. Want it mild, stick to the existing ingredient list. In any case, this soup is bursting with flavor, hands down!

INGREDIENTS:

32 oz. container vegetarian no-chicken broth or 32 oz. vegetable broth

1 can cannellini beans, drained & rinsed

1 large shallot coarsely chopped

4 garlic cloves, finely diced

4 cups kale, angled and chopped into thin threads

2 tbsps. fresh thyme pulled from stems

2 tbsp. olive oil

$1/2$ tsp. lemon zest

1 tbsp. fresh lemon juice

$1/2$ tsp. red pepper flakes

DIRECTIONS:

1. Sauté shallot in 2 tbsp. olive oil (for those seeking oil-free, sauté onions in 1/2 cup broth).

2. Add garlic and thyme and sauté until fragrant.

3. Once aromatic, add cannellini beans, red pepper flakes, and broth. Bring to a slight boil, cover, and let simmer on low for 10 minutes.

4. Using an immersion blender, blend beans to thicken into a soup-like consistency. Let cool.

5. Add kale threads, lemon juice, lemon zest, and let rest uncovered until completely cool.

Optional additions: Add faux parmesan cheese or top with your favorite protein.

For the best flavor, enjoy the next day!

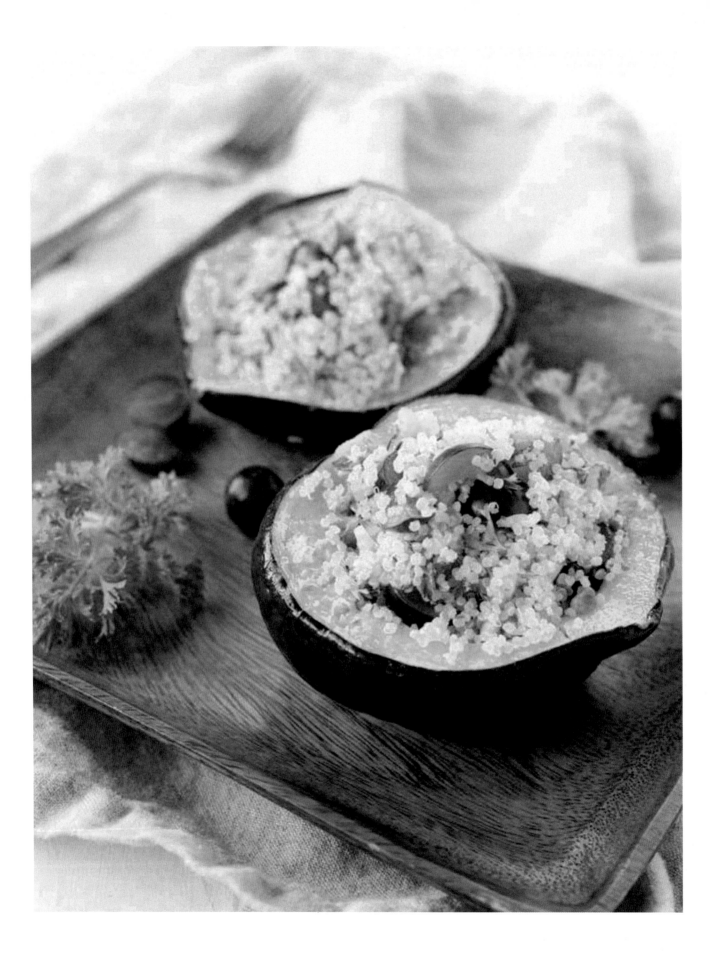

roasted acorn squash with pine nuts, grapes, and quinoa

Tired of the traditional acorn squash with butter and cinnamon? Turn this winter squash into a lighter Mediterranean feel with the rich flavors of olive oil, garlic, shallots, parsley, and thyme. Looking for a robust flavor, use flat-leaf parsley, which contains more of the essential oils than the curly variety.

INGREDIENTS:

2 small to medium-sized acorn squash

1 cup red grapes (or dried cranberries)

1 shallot

2 garlic cloves, peeled, left whole

$\frac{1}{2}$ cup quinoa (any variety)

$\frac{1}{4}$ cup walnuts, crushed

handful of fresh parsley, coarsely chopped

2 tbsp. thyme leaves pulled from stems

1 tbsp. sherry vinegar

DIRECTIONS:

1. Prep and cook the squash. Heat the oven to 400° F. Cut the acorn squash in half from stem to bottom point; scoop out seeds and discard.

2. Lightly oil the rim of the cut side of the acorn squash and place face down over each garlic clove.

3. Place in oven for approximately 30 to 35 minutes until soft to touch.

4. Cook quinoa per directions on bag or box. While the quinoa cooks, make the dressing using 2 tbsp. oil, vinegar, and stir until blended. Season with salt and pepper. Set aside.

5. Wash and dry parsley. Cut stiff stems off, roll parsley into a bundle and coarsely chop. Strip thyme leaves from stems, coarsely chop those as well.

6. Remove garlic from sheet pan and press garlic and shallots into the dressing. Mix walnuts, grapes (or dried cranberries), and herbs with the quinoa.

7. Transfer the stuffed squash to individual plates or a large bowl. Set quinoa salad in center of acorn squash.

Serve as a main dish or as a side. Not quite ready for strictly plant-based yet, top with feta or goat cheese, but remember plant-based is best!

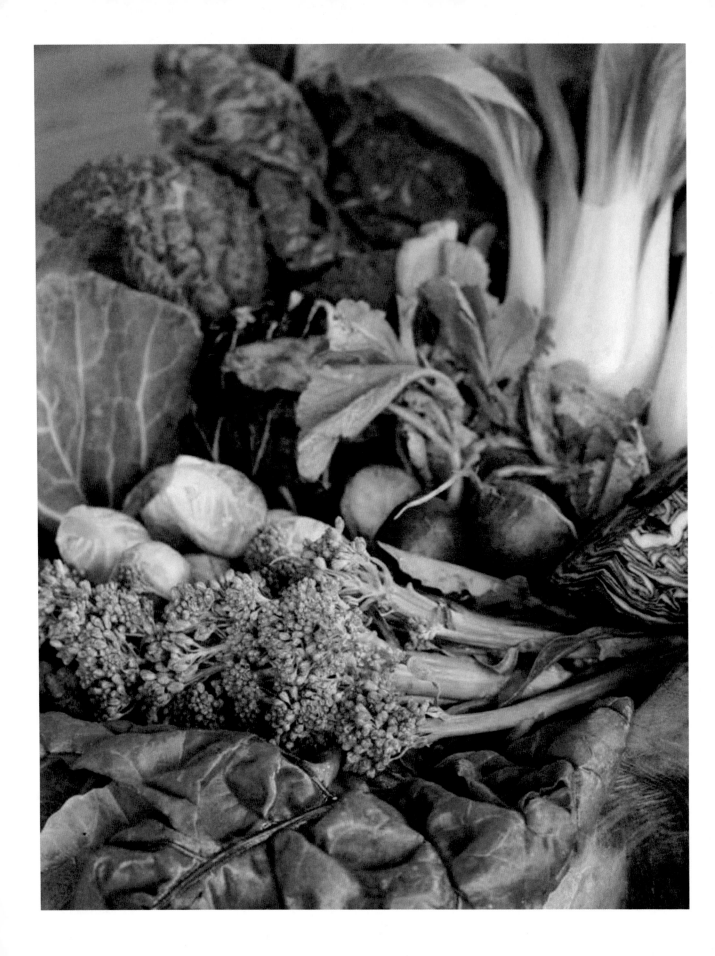

cruciferous vegetables

Cruciferous vegetables are a mainstay of a healthy diet! They are a must-have on any health regimen due to their numerous health benefits. Cruciferous vegetables are exceptionally alkaline, nutrient-dense, contain chlorophyll, and promotes the re-growth of oxygenated cells. They are widely known and touted as a cancer preventative food.

Cruciferous (or Brassica) vegetables add a considerable amount of value to any healthy meal. These vegetables contain substances that can lower the risk of developing cancer. The gassy and pungent smell you find when cooking cruciferous comes from a phytochemical called sulforaphane, which happens to be a well-documented cancer preventer. Studies have found that cruciferous vegetables may detoxify the body of recently ingested pollutants and carcinogens before they damage cells.

Eating raw cruciferous has been shown to promote healthy gut flora in the digestive tract. Researchers have found that the phytochemicals in cruciferous vegetables help protect the integrity of the stomach lining by preventing bacterial overgrowth of *Helicobacter pylori*, but just the concentrated fiber alone makes this food group a natural for digestive system support. If that wasn't enough to impress, Brassicas are replete with vitamins and minerals such as calcium (Got kale?) and even fats like omega-3s! The high vitamin K content helps the body to avoid chronic, excessive negative responses by the inflammatory system.

Add these hearty gems to your soups, sandwiches, salads, as a side dish, or even to all of your meals! Consuming cruciferous vegetables as an anti-cancer diet and potent detoxifier is a surefire way to maximize your health potential.

So if the pungent smell or bitter taste of cruciferous has been a turn off for you, the recipes in this section should get you to shed your former opinion about these dense yet delectable foods! The bold flavors of the cruciferous vegetables pair well with salt or the preferred choice, fleur de sel. When it comes to cruciferous, whether it be raw or cooked, adding fat, spice, and salt can balance or contrast its unappealing bitterness. Properly preparing and cooking brassicas will enlighten you with flavors you didn't know exist: complex umami flavors, undertones of sugary sweetness, and a hint of contrasting bitterness. Your palette awaits!

HOW TO COOK BRASSICAS

Steam, never boil, but try not to overdo it. Lightly steam and drop into an ice bath to abruptly end the cooking cycle. Not only will you avoid the proverbial nursing-home-green, but you'll also dodge the extreme bitterness that comes with overcooking these beauts as well. In a rush? Drizzle a good quality virgin olive oil accompanied by minced garlic. For salads, toss a handful of peppery, crisp Arugula, adorned with mustard vinaigrette and sliced avocado. Makes for a quick and easy side dish.

Brassicas step into their own when they're roasted in the oven (425°F). The natural sugars within them caramelize, negating any overt bitterness. Roasted cruciferous pair well with sugary root vegetables like beets, carrots, sweet potatoes, and squash. For a hint of added dimension and flavor, roast with quartered, bold-flavored onions.

LIST THEM FOR ME!

There are over 375 families and over 2,000 species of cruciferous vegetables. The most commonly consumed in the US are Arugula, broccoli, Brussels sprouts, cabbage, cauliflower, collard greens, kale, kohlrabi, mustard, rutabaga, turnips, bok choy, Chinese

cabbage, Mizuna, and tatsoi. Other brassica relatives are radish, horseradish, watercress, and swiss chard. This particular section contains an assortment of colorful and flavorful dishes dispelling the myth that cruciferous vegetables stink!

If you suffer from hypothyroidism or any other thyroid disorder and are concerned about adding cruciferous vegetables to your diet, you shouldn't be. According to Dr. Mercola, he points out that eating cruciferous vegetables like radishes, cabbage, broccoli, and kale can actually *improve* your thyroid function because they boost glutathione levels in the liver.

So, with ugliness and bitterness aside, these veggies can assist with detoxification and maximize your anti-cancer potential. In order to reap the digestive benefit and bypass any unintended consequences of digestive distress, be sure to reduce these veggies to a paste when chewing or opt for a good quality digestive enzyme to help breakdown the cellulose fibers in the digestive tract.

raw broccoli salad

INGREDIENTS:

3 cups broccoli florets, chopped into bite-sized pieces

1 red bell pepper, diced, stems, and seeds removed

$1/2$ cup raw sunflower seeds

$1/4$ cup chopped red onion

$1/3$ cup tahini

1 garlic clove crushed

$1/4$ cup lemon juice

$1/4$ cup olive oil

2 tbsp. wheat-free, low sodium Tamari or Nama Shoyu

When I first learned that a raw food-based diet was best for health, this was the first all raw dish I experimented with. I was completely sold on the idea of raw food, and even more so intrigued that I welcomed and embraced these deep, robust flavors. They felt healthy and fresh, like what I was eating was going to do its job! If you're new to eating raw vegetables, sometimes the gut takes time to catch up (if it's been sluggish and slow and churning imposter foods for a while). If that's the case, don't pass this salad up! Unsure at first glance? Lightly steam the broccoli and sub out the raw sesame tahini with your favorite Italian dressing. Remember, there's no right or wrong way to eat. As you begin to change your diet, transitioning may take some time adjusting.

DIRECTIONS:

1. Prepare vegetables and set aside in a bowl.
2. Whisk tahini, olive oil, lemon juice, and tamari.
3. Pour dressing over broccoli salad mix. Combine and serve.
4. Add sunflower seeds before serving.

Serve as a side dish.

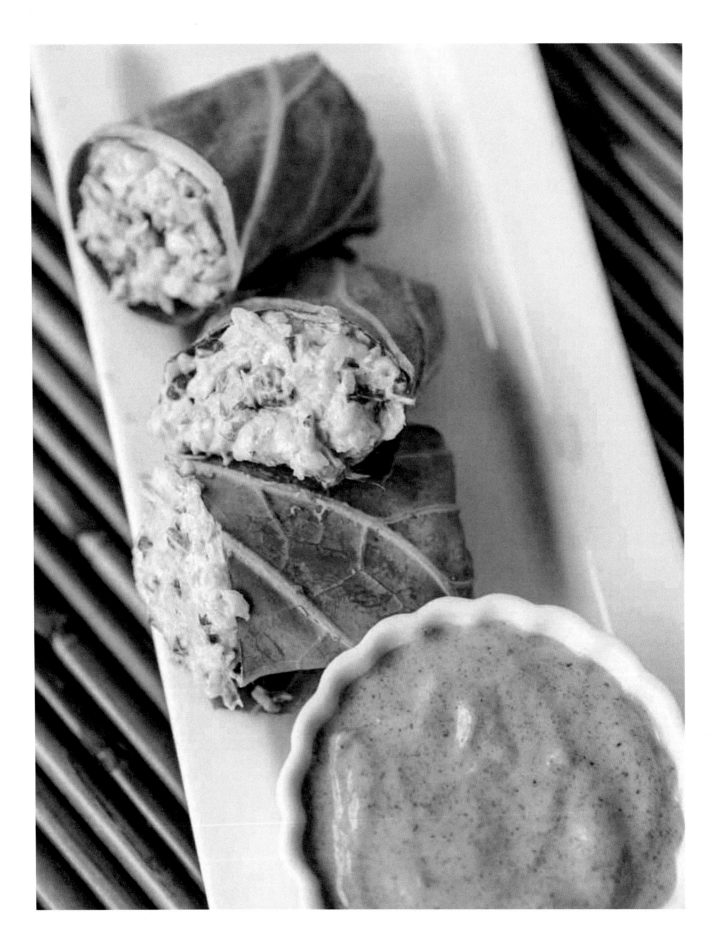

thai collard wraps with peanut sauce

INGREDIENTS:

1/4 cup raw pecans

1 tbsp. toasted sesame oil

1/2 tsp. sea salt

1/2 head Savoy cabbage, thinly sliced

Collard leaves cut in two and stems discarded.

1 cup matchstick carrots

1/2 jicama peeled cut into thin strips

1 ripe mango, peeled and cut into small cubes

3/4 cup chopped cilantro

3/4 cup basil, sliced into ribbons

1/2 cup chopped mint

For the Spicy Thai Sauce:

1/4 cup yacon syrup

1/2 cup lemon juice

1/4 cup water to thin the sauce

2 tbsp. grated ginger

1 tsp. dried Thai bird chile

1 1/2 tbsp. Nama Shoyu

3/4 cup peanut butter

By far, one of the best-kept secrets in the world of plant-based foods is the versatility of collards. Their flavor easily masked, and tough fibers effortlessly softened by acids contained within the wrap. The acid in this recipe? Luscious lemon!

DIRECTIONS:

1. In a small bowl, crush pecans with hands and mix together the chopped pecans with sesame oil and sea salt. Set aside.

2. In a blender, combine all ingredients for the Spicy Thai Sauce and mix well until smooth. Set aside. Thin sauce with water as needed.

3. In a large bowl, combine mango, carrot, jicama, cilantro basil, and mint.

4. In a separate bowl, combine 1/2 cup of Spicy Thai Sauce to shredded Savoy Cabbage and mix together, blending well. Reserve the rest for dipping sauce.

5. Clean and dry collard wraps and removing the spine with a knife leaving only the pliable leaves.

Place one half of the collard wrap on the cutting board. Place a small amount of pecan mixture on top of the collard green, then next layer the Savoy cabbage and the mixed mango, carrot, jicama, cilantro, basil, and mint. Roll like a wrap. Continue with remaining wraps and pieces.

Serve with a side of peanut dipping sauce.

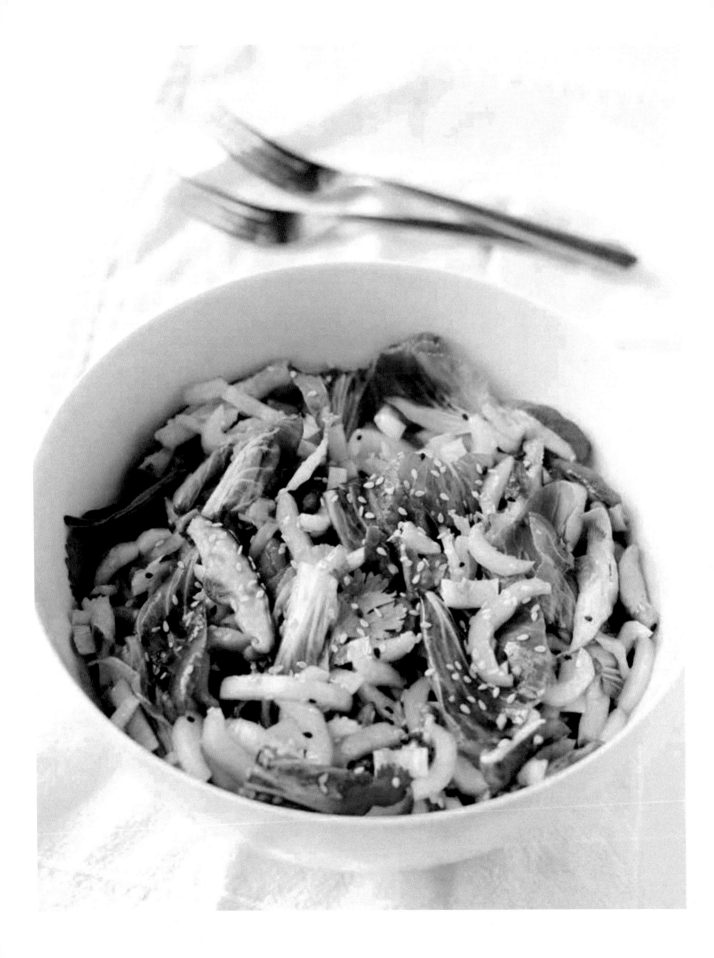

baby bok choy with shitake mushroom

INGREDIENTS:

4 cups baby bok choy or adult bok choy, greens sliced and stems chopped

1 bunch cilantro, chopped

1 cup shiitake mushrooms, stems removed and tops sliced into thin strips

$1/4$ cup sesame oil (raw, not toasted)

$1/2$ lime, juiced

2 tbsp. wheat-free, low sodium Tamari, Bragg's Liquid Aminos or Nama Shoyu

1 garlic clove, minced

1 tbsp. ginger, grated

1 tbsp. white & black sesame seeds

The beauty of this salad is its versatility! It can be prepared raw, which overall is best, or it can also be sautéed with your favorite protein and eaten as a main dish for dinner! Baby bok choy is the tender version of its mature counterpart. The leaves and stems are light green and trend on the sweeter side. All parts of the bok choy are used, including the leaves and stems.

DIRECTIONS:

1. Combine and whisk sesame oil, lime, tamari, garlic, and ginger in a small bowl. Set aside.

2. In a medium-sized bowl, add chopped greens. Pour dressing over greens and mix well.

3. Add in mushrooms and cilantro to toss. Top with white & black sesame seeds.

Serve as a side dish or as an addition to your favorite meal. While not necessary, you can add a desired protein to the side; however, plant-based is best!

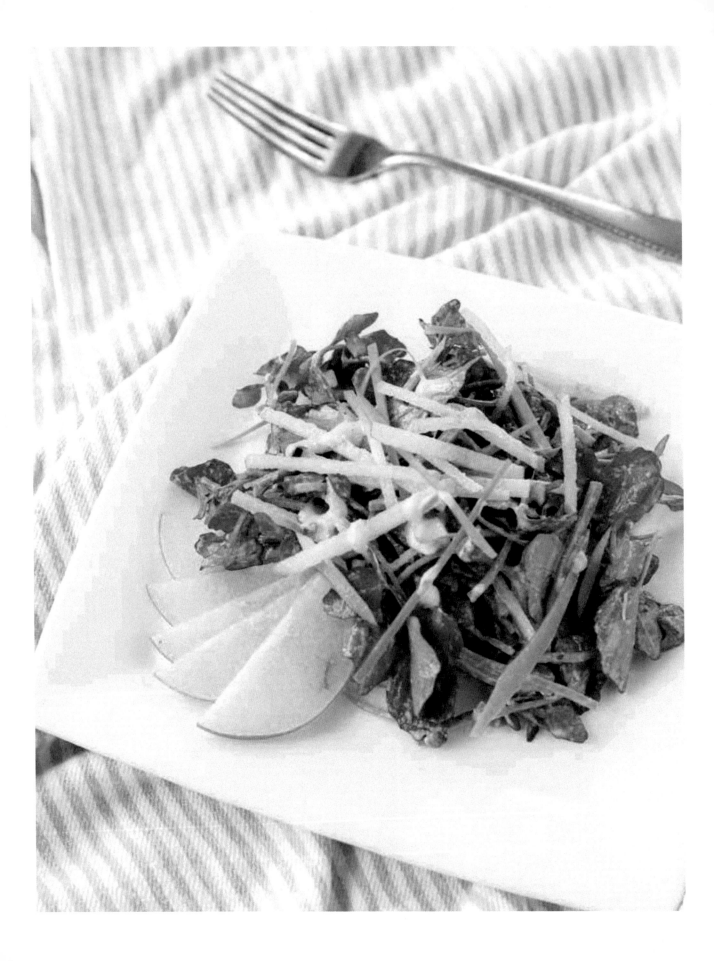

watercress salad with asian pear and tahini dressing

Watercress' peppery flavor lends itself to the likeness of arugula. Neither is part of the lettuce family. Instead, they are part of the cruciferous family and brimming with nutrients like beta-carotene, vitamin C. Watercress is a valuable source of vitamin K, thiamin, vitamin B6, potassium, and iodine. If you're new to eating watercress, I suggest finding leaves with delicate stems, which will produce a delicate aromatic flavor.

INGREDIENTS:

For the dressing:

1 knuckle (1-inch) ginger, skins removed and grated

¼ cup raw sesame tahini

3 tbsp. raw sesame oil

¼ cup unseasoned rice vinegar

1½ tbsp. sweetener of choice

2 tbsp. water to thin the dressing

1 tsp. Asian chile paste with garlic

½ tsp. Himalayan or Celtic sea salt

For the salad:

1 Asian pear, cored and cubed

4 cups trimmed watercress

1 carrot, shredded

DIRECTIONS:

1. Blend all of the ingredients for the dressing in a blender until smooth.

2. Cut the sides of the pear, discard the center core, and chop into bite-sized cubes

3. Using a cheese grater, shred carrot.

4. Trim watercress leaves from stems (for a more nutrient-dense salad, keep leaves attached to stems and coarsely chop)

5. Add watercress to bowl. Add carrots, pears, and toss.

Serve as a side salad or top with a favorite protein; however, leaving it plant-based is best!

detoxifying slaw

Prior to my health journey, there wasn't a cruciferous vegetable I liked. It's not that I didn't like vegetables, just not the notoriously bitter cruciferous ones. Fast forward to today. You'll find me ingesting some form of cruciferous, whether it be in the form of a juice, salad, or roasted veggie daily! Knowing their numerous health benefits, it's much easier to appreciate their boldness. I find they pair well with many foods, which complement their pungent flavors. There are cabbages that trend sweeter, and I find purple cabbage to be one of them, especially when thinly sliced. This has to be one of my absolute favorite raw cabbage slaw salads. It's not only detoxifying from the cabbage, scallion, and cilantro but contains heart-healthy omega-3s in the way of hemp seeds coupled with some satisfying fats from the avocado. It can be a stand-alone dish or paired with your favorite protein.

INGREDIENTS:

4 tbsp. olive oil

4 cups shredded purple cabbage

2 carrots, shredded

1 red bell pepper, seeded and diced

5 scallions, white part only sliced across the bias

Juice of 2 limes

1 ripe avocado, peeled and cubed

1 lg. handful cilantro, coarsely chopped

1/4 cup hemp seeds

DIRECTIONS:

1. Cut limes and squeeze lime juice into a small bowl.
2. Finely slice cabbage and set aside in a large mixing bowl.
3. Cut avocado lengthwise, around the pit. Discard the pit. Peel avocado skins off. Slice into cubes and set in bowl with lime juice to keep avocado from browning.
4. Rinse and remove dark green ends. Slice white and light green across the bias into thinly sliced circles.
5. Cut the end off of the pepper, discards seeds, and dice. Set aside.
6. Using a cheese grater, shred carrots.
7. Place carrots in a large bowl with cabbage. Add in hemp seeds.
8. Toss cabbage with oil. Add in red pepper, scallions, and mix until completely coated.
9. Gently mix in lime juice, avocado, and sprinkle with cilantro.

Serve as either a side or main dish. Top with your favorite protein, but remember, plant-based is best!

chicory-leek soup with black caviar lentils

INGREDIENTS:

4 tbsp. virgin coconut oil

2 large leeks, white and light green parts only

$1/2$ tsp. celery seed, whole

$1/2$ tsp. caraway seed, whole

1 bunch chicory (or endive, escarole, frisee), outer leaves removed, white end discarded

2 quarts no-chicken broth

2 tbsp. apple cider vinegar

2 tbsp. sweetener of choice

$1/4$ cup dry black caviar lentils rinsed thoroughly

$1/4$ tsp. Himalayan salt and freshly ground pepper

DIRECTIONS:

1. Cut dark stems off of leeks. With a knife, slice a line down the white and light green part of the leek and rinse folds under cold water until clean. Slice leeks into half-moons and set aside.

2. Discard outer leaves of chicory and cut white ends off, leaving only leaves.

3. Prepare an ice bath in a large bowl with ice cubes and water. Set aside.

4. In a small saucepan, bring lentils in 1/2 cup water to a quick boil and lower heat, simmering on low for 15 minutes. Once cooked, drain and rinse. Black lentils may also be found canned.

5. In a large pot of boiling water, blanch the chicory for 1 minute, then transfer chicory to an ice bath. Take chicory and squeeze to eliminate the water and coarsely chop. Set aside.

6. Melt coconut oil in a large saucepan on medium heat. Add the leeks, celery seed, and caraway seed until leeks are fragrant and slightly translucent. Be careful not to burn.

7. Add in the no-chicken broth and bring to a slight boil and lower heat to a simmer for 5 minutes. Do not cover.

8. Add the chicory and turn the heat off. Add in sweetener and vinegar.

9. Using an immersion blender, puree soup, or instead, take half the broth and puree in a blender. Return to a large bowl.

10. Add in cooked, rinsed lentils.

11. Sprinkle with Himalayan salt and freshly ground pepper.

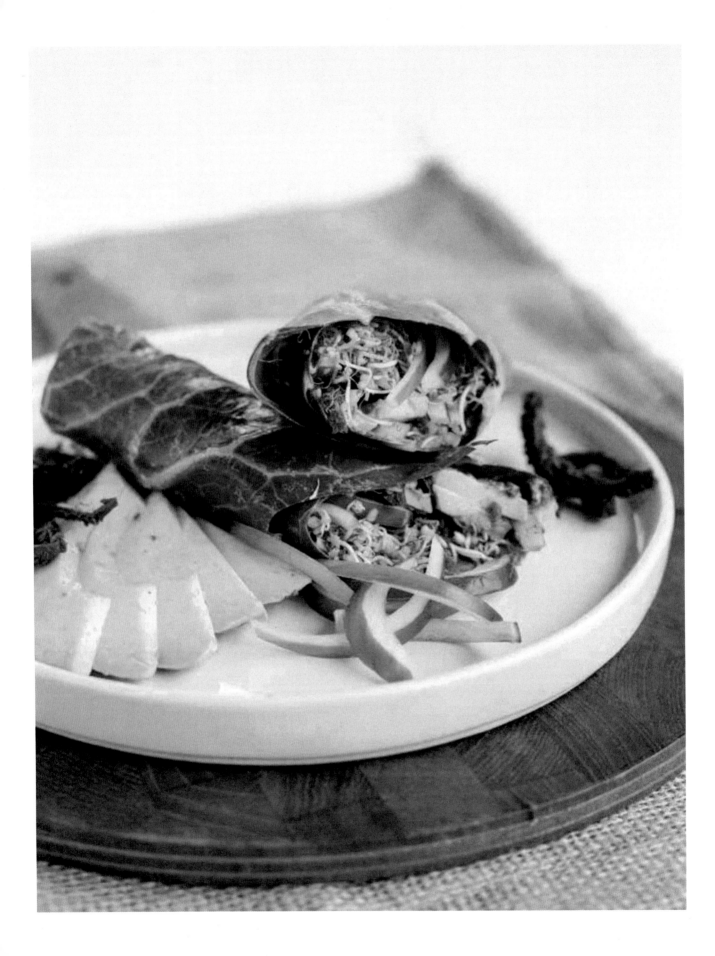

collard wraps with pesto and broccoli sprouts

Prior to my intense training at Hippocrates Health Institute, I feverishly tried to find a way to eat healthy without sacrificing the intensely rich flavors found with using fats and oils. Oddly enough, these wraps were it! One wouldn't suspect that these wraps could hold their own in "that" way, but they do. And they surely won't disappoint. The key to this dish? Freshly prepared pesto, heavy on the garlic, and some extra lemon to break down the toughness of the raw collards. You won't view collards the same way again!

INGREDIENTS:

Organic sundried tomatoes (not in oil)

1 Spanish/red onion

1 package Broccoli sprouts

1 bunch organic collard greens

1 ripe avocado

For the Pesto:

2 cups fresh Basil leaves

3 tbsp. lemon juice from fresh lemon

3 garlic cloves crushed

$1/2$ cup pine nuts

2 tbsp. olive oil

DIRECTIONS:

1. Soak sundried tomatoes in clean, cold water for 1 hour. Slice into thin strips. Do not soak if already softened in a flavor-seal pouch.

2. Slice red onion into thin slices.

3. Cut avocado in half. Discard pit. Remove skins and cube.

4. Prepare basil pesto. Add pesto ingredients in a small or mini food processor. Set aside.

5. Clean and de-spine collard leaves. Set collards on a clean tray or cutting board.

6. Layer each collard leaf with pesto, raw onion, avocado, sundried tomatoes, and sprouts. Roll tightly. Prick with a toothpick to keep rolled.

Additional option: Add your favorite protein inside the collards before rolling into wraps, but keep in mind plant-based is best!

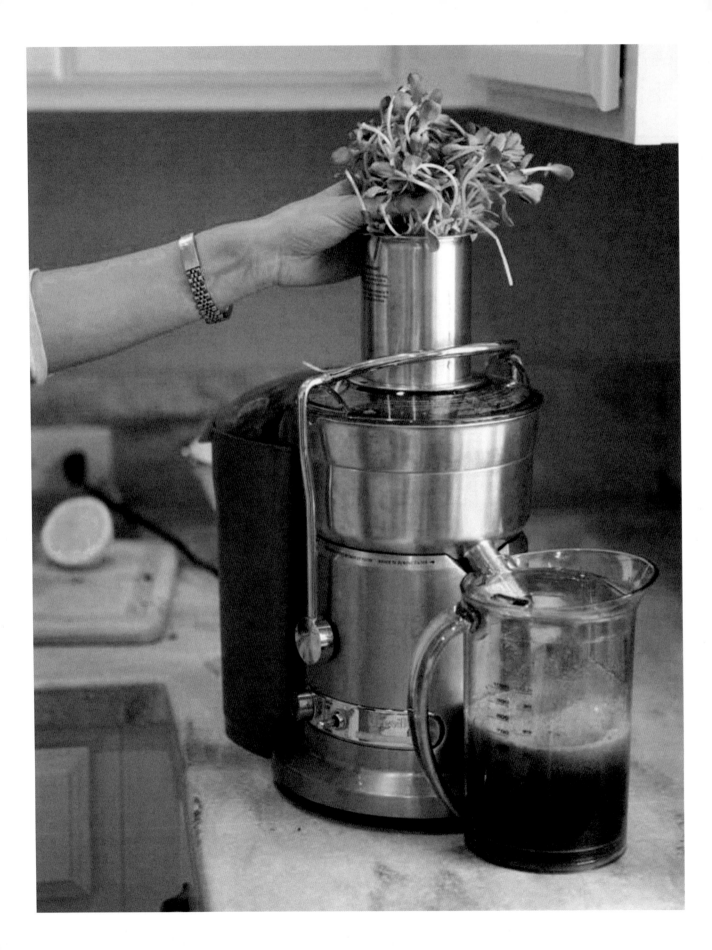

vegetable juicing

The Ultimate Fast Food

If you trend away from eating vegetables or have a lifestyle that limits the consumption of vegetables, juicing is a quick and easy way to get chlorophyll packed foods into your diet. Highly regarded as a superfood, chlorophyll's distinction comes from its blood building, heavy metal chelating, and antioxidant properties. Remembering from earlier in the chapter here, chlorophyll is the green pigment in plants responsible for photosynthesis – the growth that comes from the absorption of light and energy. Both land and sea vegetables contain chlorophyll, and those with the deepest green colors contain the highest concentrations of it. Chlorophyll is a dietary "must-have" when it comes to optimal health.

By adding vegetable juices to a diet already inclusive of cruciferous veggies and kale/quinoa blends, you are beginning to build an arsenal of nutrient-dense meals. You'll begin to notice your diet is more about quality rather than quantity, discovering quite possibly that you were overfed yet undernourished. In this case, less is more!

Juicing is not a replacement to eating greens but satisfies a 'better than nothing' approach to getting nutrition from organically grown plant-based foods. The dark leafy greens benefit the body in both whole food and supplement form (but don't go supplementing just yet). Juicing is fiercely rewarding when it is *in addition* to your 6-8 daily servings of vegetables. So, when the goal is to maintain a balanced diet, eat your veggies too!

Juicing affords us the opportunity to consume a wide variety of raw vegetables one would not typically eat nor ordinarily eat in one sitting. As your juicing prowess progresses, you may find yourself concocting juices containing beet greens, fennel, dandelion, and even broccoli stems. Maybe not all together, but with a well-intentioned juicing practice underway, you may begin to find these foods customary.

Another significant benefit to juicing is that it gives your digestive system a break. Being without fiber, the nutrients get absorbed within minutes. Without any fiber to break down and digest, the green liquid loaded with nutrients, minerals, phytochemicals, and chlorophyll is easily absorbed without any stress to the bodily system. Hence the term, "the ultimate fast food."

If consumed on an empty stomach, the body absorbs the nutrients almost immediately (approximately 15 minutes). There is no digestive wait time because the stomach is empty. This is important because many of us have an impaired digestive system from years of less-than-optimal food choices. An impaired digestive system means it is unable to absorb all of the nutrients from the vegetables. Leaving the fiber out solves this problem because the juice is being used for preventative, reparative, and detoxifying purposes. It's the quickest way to get the nutrients into the cells while receiving the maximum benefits. It's a short cut to health!

How and when to juice

Juicing is best consumed first thing in the morning, between meals, and before bed. It should be drunk approximately 15-30 minutes before meals depending on how quickly or not so quickly your body digests liquids. Conversely, do not juice until several hours after eating a meal. You want your juice to be immediately absorbed by your system rather than waiting in line for your previous meal to digest.

How many ounces to drink and how many juices.

How many ounces and the number of juices depends on your preferences, budget, and schedule. Two, 8-12 ounce juices daily do the trick. If embarking on a juice cleanse, 16 ounces is a favored size.

What to add to juices.

An array of juice recipes can be found online, but juicing is an art form. The best juice to consume is absent of fruit, with the exception of lemons and limes. Adding fruit to juices has deleterious effects. While sucrose from fruits isn't bad when the fiber remains intact, sugar from fruits in juices can increase your insulin levels. Insulin is a critical hormone that encourages our cells to consume glucose that flows through our bloodstream after eating. However, too much insulin becomes a drain on the pancreas. The sole purpose of having a vegetable juice is to gravitate away from bodily stressors.

If the taste of 100% vegetable juice is unappealing at the start, then add some low sugar fruits like apples or citrus or some root vegetables such as carrot and beets. Over time as your taste buds adapt, you'll be able to enjoy the taste of 100% green juice. It is sometimes easier to take the green plunge rather than weaning yourself off of those sweeter fruits and veggies mixes, but do whatever it takes to start juicing! The recipes contained here within have some low sugar fruit options. A hint of sweetness is harmless and a better choice than the alternative. Just be mindful of the purpose of your juice. Add fruits to smoothies and try to keep the fruits to a minimal in juices.

One day fasts

Whether your decision is based on health, weight loss, or spiritual reasons, a one-day juice (nourishing) fast is a purposeful part of an optimal diet. Fasting requires determination, discipline, and commitment. Cleanses are not anything new and have been around for centuries. Giving your overworked digestive system a break will make you feel lighter, happier, and more focused.

Fresh juices are an elemental tool in restoring health to a fatigued, sick body as well as an immune-boosting and balancing practice for a healthy individual. Putting into practice a weekly one-day cleanse is a fantastic jump-start to healing and a prescription for longevity.

What should I do prior to a cleanse?

Tip #1

Add freshly-squeezed lemon juice to daily water

Eat less or no dairy products, red meat, alcohol, coffee, black tea, tobacco, candies, soft drinks, junk foods, or gluten

If you eat meat, use pasture-raised eggs, wild-caught fish, limit poultry and minimize red meat

Eat 6 to 8 servings of vegetables and fruits per day—eat at least 50% raw.

Do not overcook! Only lightly cook your foods such as sautéed, steamed. Never boil.

Chew your foods a long time to stimulate enzymic breakdown at the mouth.

Eat organic foods as much as possible. The diagram shown provides the list of foods to avoid, if not organic, dubbed "the dirty dozen." Immediately to the right is "the Clean 15," a list of foods regarded as having low-pesticide residue and considered acceptable to buy if not organic.

How should I expect to feel?

Tip #2

Symptoms vary greatly from person to person. You may also experience more negative symptoms if you haven't geared up for your one-day juice cleanse, so do yourself a favor and utilize Tip #1 about five to seven days prior to a juice cleanse, which will help minimize possible adverse symptoms.

Here are some typical symptoms one may experience during a nourishing fast:

Headaches	Body Aches
Fever	Nausea
Dizziness	Irritability
Nervousness	Intestinal Gas
Skin Breakouts	Rashes
Intense Food Cravings	Loss Of Appetite
Runny Nose	Increase Phlegm
Constipation/ Diarrhea	Feeling Overwhelmed

If your energy does get low by the end of the day, then make sure to take it easy!

Don't worry. You won't feel all of these symptoms at once or possibly not at all. Generally, the longer the fast, the more "cleaning up" your system is doing, and the more likely you'll experience the symptoms listed above. A one-day juice fast is less likely to produce any flare-ups. For optimal health, longevity, and a digestive sweep—embark on a ritualistic once a week, one-day liquid fast.

So, I just drink these juices, and I'm done? Well, almost! Follow the advice below!

Tip #3

1   Have six, 16-ounce. drinks available or make them throughout the day.

2   Start your morning out with warm lemon water and a dash of cayenne. The goal is to alkalize your body, and this is the best way to start the day!

3   Drink your morning green juice. Do not chug. Take the time to drink slowly and possibly "chew" your drink to stimulate enzymic activity in your mouth. Don't forget, enzymes help aid in digestion.

4   Drink your second and third green juice between the hours of 10:00 a.m. and 2:00 p.m.

5   The afternoon may become a little difficult. This may be the best time to incorporate different electrolyte drinks like coconut or cactus (prickly pear) water or a root vegetable juice like beets and carrots or have your fourth green juice that contains just a little bit of low-sugar fruits.

6   For dinner, drink your fifth green juice.

7   Before bed, but with enough time to digest, you try either nut milk, a smoothie, a blended soup, or your sixth green drink will do.

Please remember while doing your fast that you will need to drink purified water throughout the day. Try to avoid filtered refrigerator or tap water. Use one of these options: distilled water, reverse osmosis with minerals added, alkaline water, or Artesian Well water such as Fiji brand. You'll want to consume half of your body weight of water in ounces. Water is an essential key to flushing the body of toxins.

You will need to make sure your bowels are moving. If you naturally move your bowels on a daily basis, then great. If not, you may want to try psyllium husk or magnesium supplements to keep your bowels moving because you are NOT ingesting any fiber necessary to keep the colon moving.

So, what to eat the next day?

Tip #4

Your digestive system has been on a much-needed vacation. Give it time to adjust. The best approach to take is to follow the recommended diet in Tip #1.

What type of juice fast (cleanse) should I be doing?

You should only do a vegetable/fruit juice cleanse. If you want to "beef" up your juice cleanse or extend it, try consuming wheatgrass juice, liquid blue-green algae, and/or a 2-ounce. shot of whole leaf aloe vera juice before bed. As with all dietary adjustments, it's recommended that you consult your physician prior to embarking on any juice cleanse.

But this begs the question—what juicer do I use?

Here are some helpful suggestions when thinking about purchasing one of the very important and much-needed kitchen basics for juicing.

CENTRIFUGAL JUICER

A centrifugal juicer spins at high speeds rotating around a central axis point. The vegetables are basically ground to a pulp. The spinning motion forces the juice away from the pulp, ejecting it into a waste receptacle out the back while simultaneously forcing juice through a spout out the front into a pitcher.

Centrifugal juicers are very affordable and can be found in many discount department stores. As a side note, a centrifugal juicer cannot juice wheatgrass, a very beneficial addition to a wholly-healthy diet. While this juicer offers a great flavored juice similar to that found in juice bars, it may not make sense to purchase if you intend to incorporate wheatgrass as part of your health regimen. If wheatgrass is for a later date, then the centrifugal is a fantastic option. There are a few high-quality, inexpensive juicers like the Breville Juice Fountain Plus for under $150. Use a 20% coupon at Bed, Bath and Beyond, and it's worth every penny. There are different Breville models to choose from, but the Fountain Plus will give you what you exactly what you need.

MASTICATING JUICERS

A masticating juicer squeezes the juice out through the slow grinding, chewing motion of a gear. Mastication means "to chew" and works the same as our mouth when we chew food. The gear or gears knead the vegetables into a pulp rather than through centrifugal force and sharp edges. A masticating juicer requires a little bit more of a financial investment and a little bit more time to juice as the vegetable chute is generally quite narrow in diameter.

A few important things to consider would be: cost, cleaning the juicer, and amount of pulp ejected after juicing. First, discern between a single and double auger (gears) juicer.

SINGLE AUGER MASTICATING JUICER

Many of the single auger juicers are moderately priced, making them appealing due to their affordability. While they take less time to clean than a double auger juicer, one drawback is the pulp that is ejected can be wet, creating more waste. To maximize results, the pulp can be sent through a second time for further extraction. This technique works quite well.

DOUBLE AUGER MASTICATION JUICERS

Double auger juicers are more efficient considering the ratio of juice to pulp. Double auger juicers expel a dry pulp, putting more of the juice into your cup. The one drawback to a double auger juicer is that it can take considerably more time to juice and more effort in cleaning than a single auger juicer. On average, it takes 3-5 minutes longer to clean a double auger juicer than a single auger juicer. On average, that's about 10 minutes more than a centrifugal juicer. Additionally, double auger juicers are considerably more expensive than single auger juicers.

COLD PRESSED JUICERS

Cold-pressed juicers have exploded over the past decade, offering convenient, freshly prepared juices in a variety of flavors and combinations. Most cold-pressed juices (not to be confused with high-pressure processing juices) can be refrigerated safely for up to 3 days offering the same distinct flavor you'd find in a freshly prepared juice minus the wait! Cold-pressed juicers are different from your typical juicer giving the resultant juice a longer shelf-life. With cold-pressed juicers, the process uses a dual-stage compression technology, which translates into a high power/low-speed method—this type of technology results in a juice that preserves valuable enzymes and vitamins longer than traditional juicers.

WHAT DO JUICERS COST?

A durable double auger juicer like the Green Power juicer comes in a variety of colors and is priced anywhere from $499-$600. Green Star belongs to the Green Power family and is priced a little bit more favorably. The Green Power produces excellent quality juice and expels very dry pulp leaving more juice in your cup. Your savings equate to having to purchase less produce, of course, depending on what is purchased, and can be quite a cost savings. Generally speaking, double auger gears use less plastic and more metal in their gears, making it more durable in the parts department.

Omega juicer models 8000 and above generally cost between $249 and $299, respectively. Omega juicers are single-auger juicers, produce a great juice, are easy to clean, and moderately priced. Oddly enough, the newly released H3000D Omega Cold Press 365 carries retail price at the writing of $149, a significant bargain over traditional juicers while yielding a juice with the potential of a 3-day shelf life. However, that does not come with a health and safety guarantee. Some of the drawbacks with Omega juicers are the fragile plastic attachments (I have had to replace a few parts at no cost due to the juicer still being under warranty). Omega's customer service is outstanding.

If the plan is to juice fruits/vegetables without wheatgrass in the near future, then a centrifugal made by Breville would be my recommendation.

If you're new to juicing, I'm excited for you! It's a great permanent addition to a healthy diet!

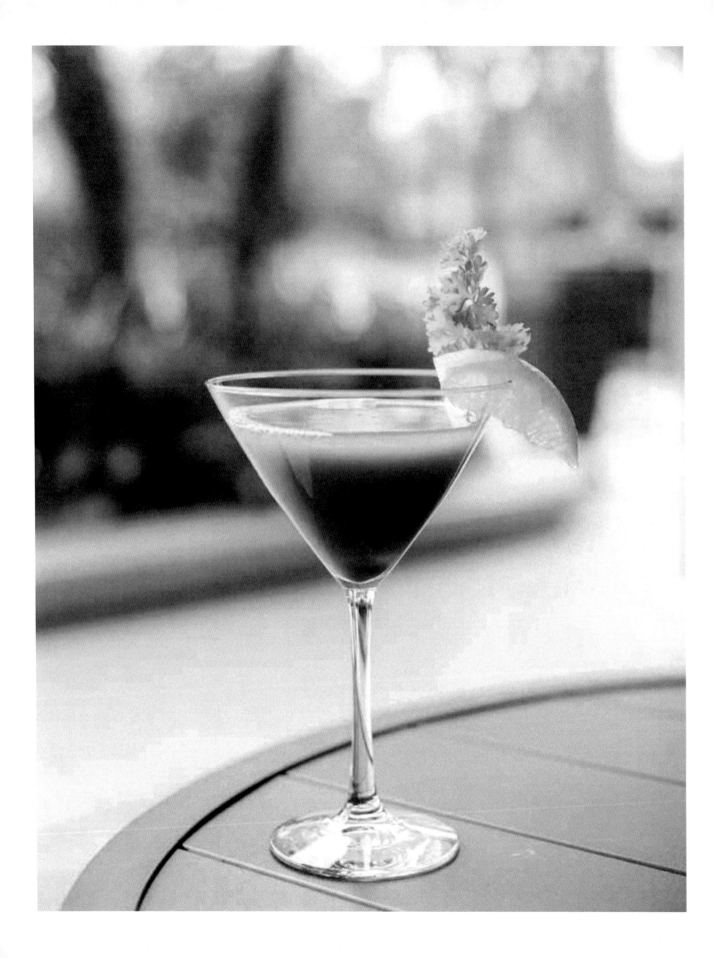

the southwestern

INGREDIENTS:

1 1/2 cucumbers

2 celery ribs

1 red pepper, seeds and
stems removed

Handful of cilantro leaves

1-2 cloves raw garlic

Optional:

Handful of kale or spinach

Raw garlic in juice? First drink of the day, you say? No way! This juice has to be the #1 favorite with just about every client! The nutrients in this drink will astound you, and the flavor surprise you! Cilantro is a known heavy metal detoxifier, garlic a blood cleanser, and the vitamin C in the red peppers is equal to 160% of RDA and the beta carotene content, which is sure to excite your skin's cells! Don't think you can muster up the desire to make it a daily first? Try then for a 4 pm afternoon pick-me-up!

DIRECTIONS:

1. Wash and prep all ingredients.

2. Send all vegetables through juicer chute.

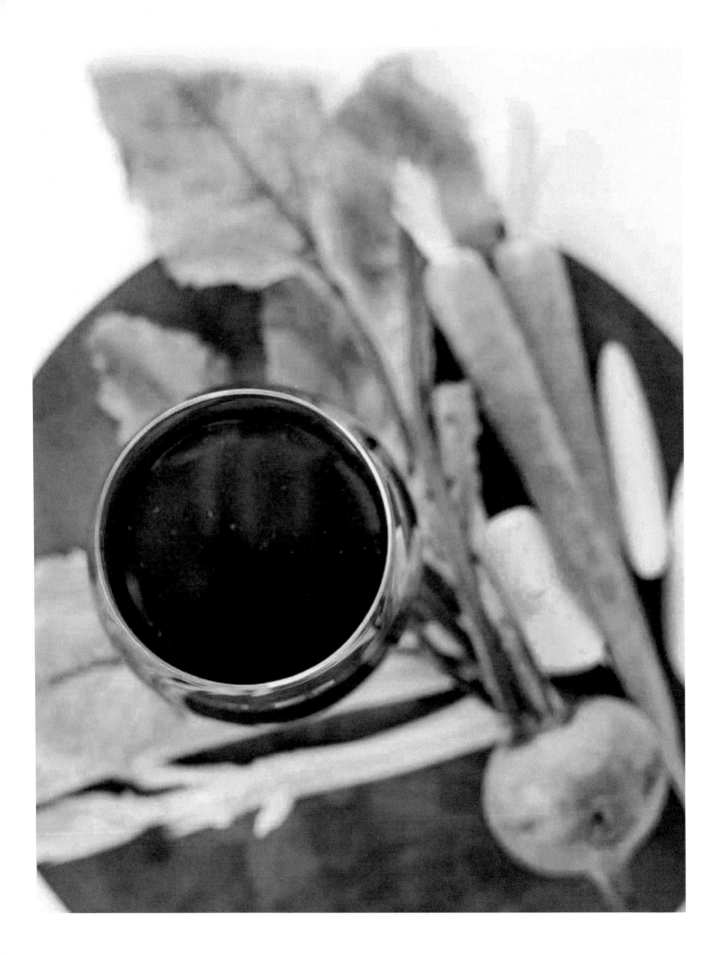

roots and shoots

For those beet lovers, this one's for you! With an impressive amount of folate (B9), manganese, potassium, iron, and vitamin C, beets have been associated with improved blood flow, lowers blood pressure, and offers increased exercise performance by way of nitrates. As a cautionary measure, don't drink beetroot juice regularly if you have low blood pressure & be sure to monitor your blood pressure carefully. Beets are high in oxalates, so if you're prone to kidney stones, make this your occasional drink

INGREDIENTS:

4 small beets, scrubbed, tops removed

2 carrots

1 red apple, cored

1 celery rib

Lemon wedge

DIRECTIONS:

1. Rinse carrots and beets thoroughly and scrub. Beets and carrots can also be peeled. Cut in half.
2. Rinse apple and core to remove seeds
3. Cut a small lemon wedge from the whole lemon
4. Rinse inside of celery rib. Keep celery tops intact.
5. Send through the juicer, one item at a time.

the daily green

INGREDIENTS:

1 cucumber

2 celery ribs

1 bunch parsley

1 lemon wedge

3 leaves lacinato kale or

1 handful spinach

This is the perfect "go-to" daily drink! Change it up a bit! Interchange spinach with Lacinato kale or use them both! For a bigger bite, try a small piece of ginger!

DIRECTIONS:

1. Wash and prep all vegetables
2. Send vegetables through juicer chute.

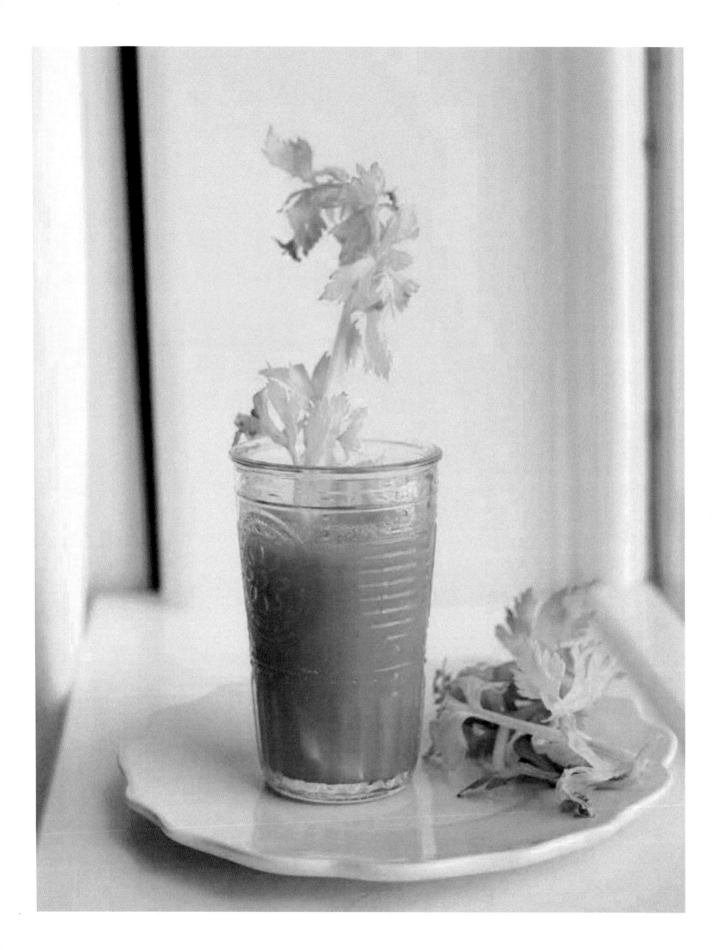

tums away!

You got that right! Send those Tums away! This drink is sure to settle the stomach among a plethora of other health benefits! Surprisingly, celery leaves, while not orange nor red, contain a high amount of beta carotene! The stems contain vitamins B1, B2, B6, and C and also include a significant amount of potassium, folate, calcium, magnesium, iron, phosphorus, and sodium. Celery also includes a multitude of essential amino acids. Nutrients in the fiber are expelled during the juicing process, which will aid in urination and bowel movements. Due to its natural diuretic properties, starting at 2 ounces is a great place to start. The sodium in celery is unlike table salt, which is harmful to those with high blood pressure.

Four to six ounces is a perfect amount to drink. Start slowly consuming 2 ounces at first and moving up to 6 ounces.

INGREDIENTS:

All Organic Ingredients:

1 celery stalk including leaves (approximately 10 ribs)

DIRECTIONS:

1. Wash and prep all ingredients.
2. Clean each celery rib and send it through the juicer chute.

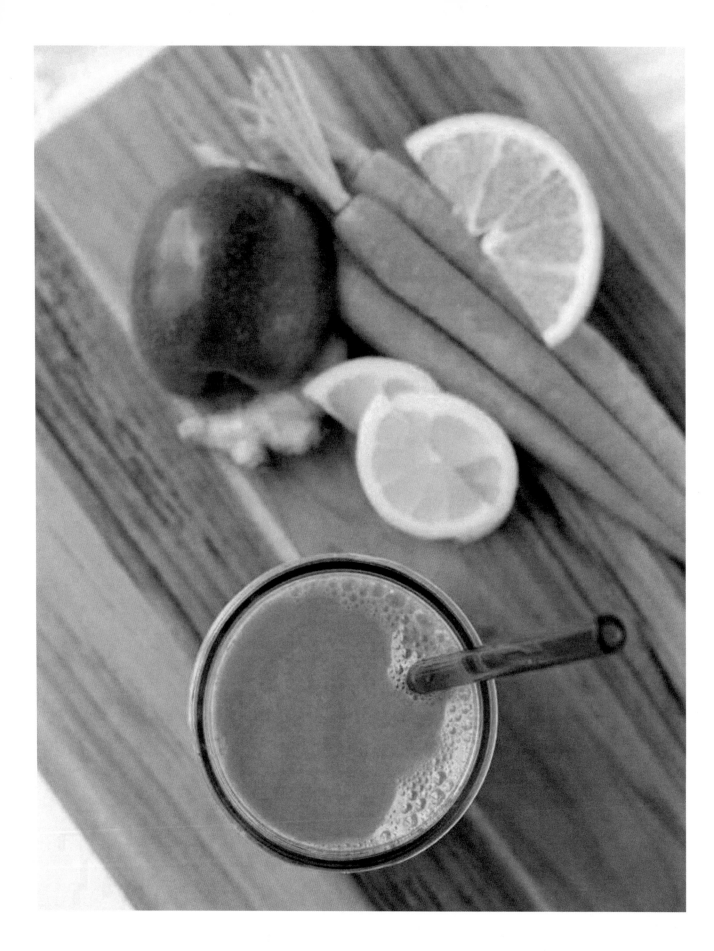

glow

INGREDIENTS:

8 carrot sticks

1 red apple (cored)

$\frac{1}{2}$ lemon

knuckle of ginger

$\frac{1}{2}$ orange

Enjoy the skin-boosting benefits of beta-carotene, the precursor to vitamin A, in this delicious carrot drink!

DIRECTIONS:

1. Wash carrots but do not peel as many of the nutrients are found in the skins.

2. Core the apple. Seeds should not go through the juicer due to the possible arsenic content in apple seeds. They are not lethal and pose no harm, but, as do-gooders-do, leave them out of your health drink.

3. No need to peel skins off ginger but cut off ends that may have developed any mold.

4. Make sure all produce is organic to avoid ingesting any unwanted pesticides.

5. Enjoy on an empty stomach and wait 15 or so minutes before consuming food.

sour apple

ALL ORGANIC INGREDIENTS:

1 $\frac{1}{2}$ organic cucumbers, skins on

$\frac{1}{2}$ lemon

2 in. piece fresh ginger, skins on

1 green apple, cored

If you like the taste of Green Jolly Ranchers candies, then this is the drink for you! For a bit more sour, add in 1/2 green apple and a whole lemon. It's best served with a 1-ounce drizzle of wheatgrass!

DIRECTIONS:

1. Wash and prep all vegetables

2. Put vegetables through the juicer.

Optional:

Drizzle with 1 oz. wheatgrass for a delicious flavor and pour over ice.

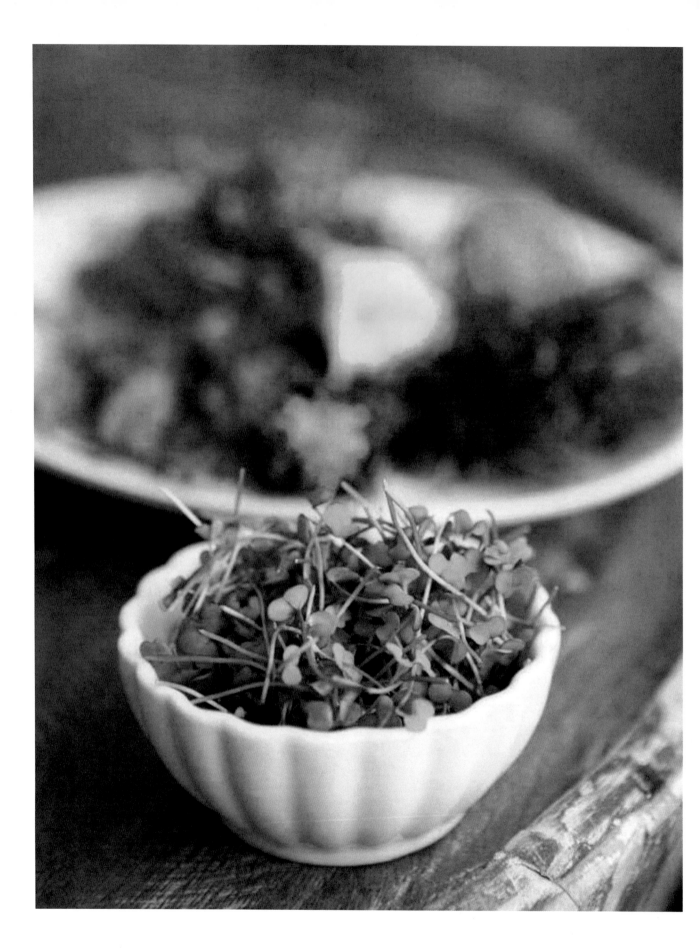

colors of the rainbow

The Many Benefits of Phytochemicals

Ever wonder where the term "eat the colors of the rainbow" comes from? It has little to do with the culinary attractiveness of foods (although the colors are certainly attractive) but everything to do with phytochemicals, the disease protective compounds responsible for the color, flavor, and odor of plants. Phytochemicals are non-essential nutrients that may play a key role in reducing the risk of chronic disease. Studies have shown that we may reap the benefit of vital plant chemicals when we consume those very same foods that contain them. Plants are the only natural source of phytochemicals[167] and can be found in such foods as herbs, spices, teas, fruits, nuts, seeds, legumes, and grains.

There are over 25,000 known phytochemicals, all with distinct chemistry and varying disease-fighting potential. Listed below are the top ten most widely known benefits.

- reduces inflammation
- acts as an anti-microbial, antiviral, and antiparasitic infection
- protects against heart disease
- protects against cancer
- improves vision
- offers neuroprotective effect
- lowers LDL cholesterol
- stimulates the immune system
- improves the cognitive function of the brain
- helps to lessen the severity of the menopause phase

Not mentioned yet is the contrarian view of phytochemicals. What I mean by that is the same phytochemical properties that provide us with the beneficial phytonutrients found in plants also contain powerful anti-nutritional effects. These are often referred to as anti-nutrients.

The natural world provides phytochemicals in order to protect plants against insects, viruses, mold/fungus, and to protect them while lying dormant waiting to be germinated. If consuming some of these foods on a regular basis, we need to remove phytates and other anti-nutrients to make them more digestible. There's an easy way to do it!

When it comes to lowering the content of "bad" anti-nutrients that are more harmful than beneficial, preparation methods such as soaking, sprouting, and fermentation are an effective means of minimizing phytate count. Within the sprouting process, there is a lessening of starch while at the same time, a marked increase in protein, fat, amino acid composition, and B vitamin content. Through the enzymatic action that occurs with sprouting, the anti-nutrients are significantly decreased, making the seeds more easily digestible.

How to do this at home:

• Soak dry beans, legumes and nuts, and seeds in filtered water between the temperatures of 72ºF – 92ºF using a facilitator such as apple cider vinegar or lemon juice. Kombu seaweed can also assist with phytic acid removal in water as well!

• After 24 hours, rinse liberally then prepare to cook (beans and legumes only – cooking does not apply to nuts and seeds). A little time consuming, but it's pretty easy actually!

• If wanting to germinate nuts and seeds, rinse in a colander, cover with a cheesecloth or keep in a sprouting jar rinsing liberally 4x daily for three days. Some nuts and most seeds will begin to sprout, some with tails, while others do not produce a sprouted tail. You can eat them raw, germinated, or continue with your process to cook them, but don't forget, you lose the valuable digestive enzymes you just spent time trying to create!

• If choosing to ferment, a culture starter is needed, such as yeast, rye, a probiotic, or even lemon. Generally, the fermentation requires room temperature of 72ºF or up to 118ºF to culture and ferment. This process can take anywhere from 24 hours to 3 days and is also known as souring when fermenting grains.

• Soaking, sprouting, and fermenting beans, legumes, seeds, and nuts become easier to digest, and your body can access their full nutrient profile. I hate to provide short cuts, but in a pinch or when traveling, it's safe to consume digestive enzymes to assist with digestion. Individuals who have good intestinal flora will have an easier time digesting food containing phytic acid.

When it comes to soy, organic, non-GMO fermented soy products like miso, Nama Shoyu, and tempeh are best. It is not advised to use soy as the preferred choice for protein replacement in a holistic diet. There are countless other ways to include protein into the diet! If you're a tofu lover, we have included a few recipes for you. The age-old advice has always been to eat in moderation, and that goes for soy as well!

Enjoy the easy to make and flavorful recipes in the next recipe section. They contain a varietal number of herbs, spices, beans, legumes, and root vegetables.

kitchen gadgets and small appliances

THE ESSENTIALS OF HOME COOKING

Removing phytic acid from nuts, seeds, grains, beans, and legumes require a soaking process since phytates interfere with mineral absorption in the gut. If you prefer to DIY, you will most likely need sprouting containers and/ or a dehydrator.

There are kitchen gadgets that can make the process a little easier and a bit more organized when using counter space. When it comes to nuts, seeds, beans, and legumes, a large glass bowl with a colander is sufficient. If you plan to sprout in your home, glass mason jars with holed screw-on tops are best, or Sproutman containers work great too. They are super convenient, but they are made of plastic, which is a turn off for some super focused on health.

Nowadays, it's very easy to find packaged nuts and seeds that read "sprouted" on the front of the packaging. While these products may be pricier than raw or roasted/salted, the phytates have already been removed, so please take advantage! Since sprouted beans, legumes, and seeds are considered raw (haven't been cooked over 118°F), you can eat them right out of the package, reconstitute in water or cook them. Cooking is fine as the anti-nutrients have been removed for you, but you will lose the beneficial enzymes in doing so. Either way, you're on to a more nutrient-dense diet. Kudos to you!

THE HOLISTIC HOME CHEF

DEHYDRATORS

A dehydrator acts like a countertop toaster oven with the exception of heating at temperatures lower than 170°F *and* removes moisture. The object of a traditional oven is to heat at high temperatures while sealing in moisture. The purpose of a dehydrator is to "cook" at temperatures below 118°F, keeping the enzymes alive in our food. Remember from Chapter 1, the importance of preserving enzymes is for aiding digestion. Many of us have compromised digestive systems, oftentimes leading to inflammation, immune, and allergy issues. The key to optimal health is through optimal digestion; therefore, the process of soaking, sprouting, and dehydrating is an ideal way to preserve living enzymes as well as remove the harmful anti-nutrients found naturally in nuts, seeds, and grains. Fermentation, a step beyond germinating, is another way to improve the digestibility of plant foods.

With the advent of modern-day appliances and electricity, a dehydrator is your most convenient option, although not the most svelte appliance in your kitchen ensemble. Functionality is at the core of this beast. The Excalibur brand is the preferred choice of dehydrators, but a refurbished Waring brand is available at a fraction of the cost of an Excalibur. If you don't plan to live 100% on dehydrated food items, the Waring is a fine option.

MILK BAGS FOR NUT "MYLKS"

In order to make homemade nut "mylk," you'll need a specific type of bag to separate the nut pulp (also called meal) from the liquid, which ultimately becomes your mylk. The most commonly used bag is made from fine-mesh nylon, which is stretch resistant, meaning that your bag will remain in good condition for quite some time. Nylon bags do not easily pick up odors and are also resistant to stains. These bags are machine washable, making post-straining cleanup a breeze!

There are organic cotton bags on the market for those who want to keep synthetic chemicals out of the diet altogether. Even the sewing threads and drawstring on most organic cotton bags are made from organic material. To further ensure your food avoids chemicals altogether, you'll also want to make sure it's glue-free.

FOOD PROCESSORS

If you plan to make more food at home and spend less time eating out or grabbing packaged food from the pantry, a food processor is an incredibly handy, multi-purpose small appliance that will assist you for years. Food processors are excellent for tasks that call for chopping, slicing, grinding, and puréeing. If you purchase a higher-end model food processor, you can also use it to make salsas, mix the batter for crackers and knead the dough. If you don't already own one, you may want to invest in a food processor. It's a fun tool for those who love food prep.

Pull up a website for food processors, and the choices can be overwhelming. There are dozens of sizes, speeds, and prices. It can be difficult to find the model that's right for you.

The best choice depends entirely on how large your family is or how many people you usually cook for. In general, it's best to choose a bowl that holds at least nine cups. In that same vein, if you're only cooking for one or using the processor to make small amounts of food, a bowl that holds three cups (mini) is fine, but I reserve a mini-food processor for smaller projects like pesto or aromatic bases for soups and stews. My favorite is the Cuisinart 11-cup, which has lasted me for over 20 years. Occasionally, a plastic part will break, but it is easy, convenient, and inexpensive to order replacement parts.

HIGH-SPEED BLENDERS

The next item essential to holistic cooking is a high quality, high-speed blender. A blender is one of the most versatile appliances on your kitchen counter. With a good countertop blender, you can whip up smoothies, creamy soups, gravies, salad dressings, dips, and salsas. And with the right model, you can even make puddings or hot soup.

Shopping for a blender, though, can be frustrating. Like food processors, there are so many options on the market it's hard to know which features are worth the extra investment and which features you can live without.

My preference is a refurbished standard series product by VitaMix (with the exception of their personal blender, which is an expensive version without the power). BlendTec is my second choice. Honestly, the difference is like choosing a Toyota or a Honda. It's more about preference.

A certified refurbished VitaMix is tested and certified by the manufacturer or by a third-party to look and work like new, with limited to no signs of wear. The refurbishing process includes functionality testing, inspection, reconditioning, and repackaging. The product ships with relevant accessories and a minimum 90-day supplier warranty. Accessories may be generic, though, and not directly from the manufacturer, but overall, it is still worth the discounted price.

A great place to find a refurbished product is at Amazon. If a refurbished price tag still gives sticker shock, then a personal-sized Nutribullet, another brand name blender, is a fine option. The only drawback to a Nutribullet (if using it for more than just smoothies) is that the blade and gear are screwed together on the top of the pitcher,

requiring you to turn the container upside down to blend. With an enclosed container, it doesn't allow access to eliminate air pockets. Not having the ability to release air means the gears end up spinning air and not your ingredients. If that occurs, you have to take it out, unscrew the top, give it a shake, and then repeat the process. Despite a little inconvenience at times, it's a great blender with an even better price tag.

Steer clear of deeply discounted inexpensive blenders, as they will not do what you are expecting and will end up disappointing in the end.

WHAT WILL ALL OF THIS COST?

Given the numerous kitchen items needed for purchase, the order in which you would most likely want to purchase would be:

- Blender as it will be a much-used item (Vitamix, BlendTec, Nutribullet)

- Food processor (Cuisinart 8- or 9-cup, and add a mini to your wish list)

- Dehydrator (Excalibur or Waring)

- Milk Bags

- Sprouting Containers

All in all, being a savvy shopper, researching online, using coupons, or buying refurbished, all of the above items fall under $375 total (not including tax and shipping). Not bad considering all that they can assist with. The appliances will last for decades and is an investment well spent. It's essentially investing in your daily healthcare! It's an investment in YOU!

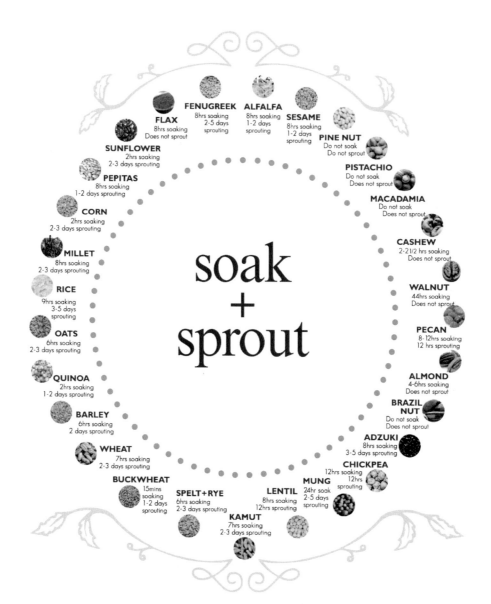

soak
+
sprout

FLAX
8hrs soaking
Does not sprout

FENUGREEK
8hrs soaking
2-5 days
sprouting

ALFALFA
8hrs soaking
1-2 days
sprouting

SESAME
8hrs soaking
1-2 days
sprouting

PINE NUT
Do not soak
Do not sprout

PISTACHIO
Do not soak
Does not sprout

MACADAMIA
Do not soak
Does not sprout

CASHEW
2-2 1/2 hrs soaking
Does not sprout

WALNUT
44hrs soaking
Does not sprout

PECAN
8-12hrs soaking
12 hrs sprouting

ALMOND
4-6hrs soaking
Does not sprout

BRAZIL NUT
Do not soak
Does not sprout

ADZUKI
8hrs soaking
3-5 days sprouting

CHICKPEA
12hrs soaking
12hrs
sprouting

MUNG
24hr soak
2-5 days
sprouting

LENTIL
8hrs soaking
12hrs sprouting

KAMUT
7hrs soaking
2-3 days sprouting

SPELT+RYE
6hrs soaking
2-3 days sprouting

BUCKWHEAT
15mins
soaking
1-2 days
sprouting

WHEAT
7hrs soaking
2-3 days sprouting

BARLEY
6hrs soaking
2 days sprouting

QUINOA
2hrs soaking
1-2 days sprouting

OATS
6hrs soaking
2-3 days sprouting

RICE
9hrs soaking
3-5 days
sprouting

MILLET
8hrs soaking
2-3 days sprouting

CORN
2hrs soaking
2-3 days sprouting

PEPITAS
8hrs soaking
1-2 days sprouting

SUNFLOWER
2hrs soaking
2-3 days sprouting

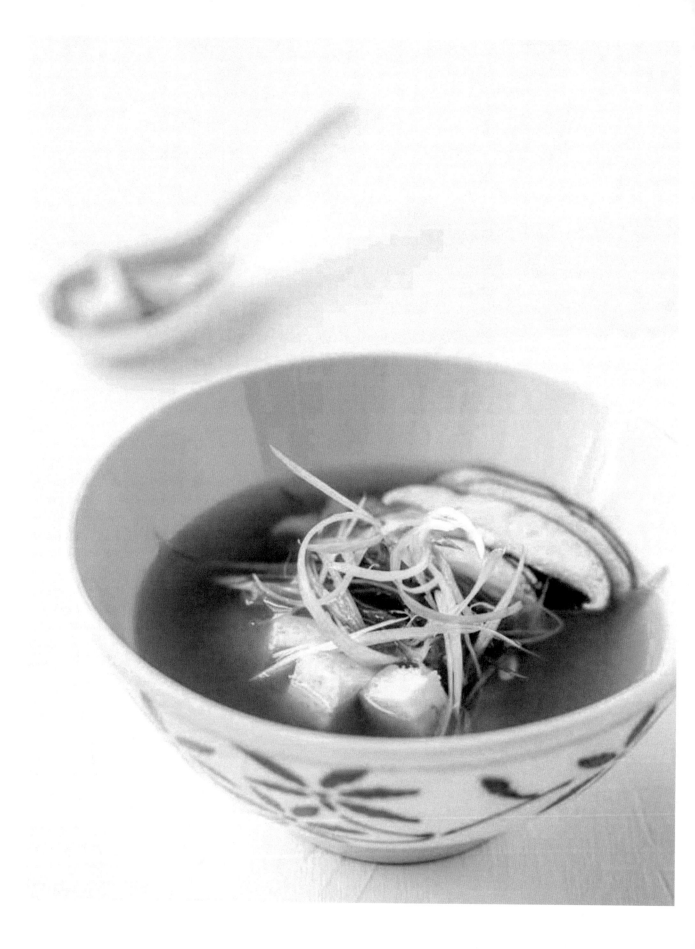

miso soup

INGREDIENTS:

1 tbsp. dried wakame seaweed

1/2 oz. dried kombu about one piece rinsed in cold water

32 oz. cold water

4 oz. firm tofu, drained and cubed

1 tbsp. mellow white miso

2 scallions, white and light green parts only, sliced on the bias or shaved with a vegetable peeler

For the Vegan Fish Sauce:

3 cups cold, filtered water

3 dried shiitake mushrooms, left whole

2 tbsp. salt

2 tbsp. Nama Shoyu

Probably, the best vegan miso ever made. Wait? Definitely the best. Creating a vegan fish sauce is the most important part of getting the umami flavors just right. Instead of twirling traditional soft tofu, we just cubed extra firm tofu and set it in bowls when ready to serve. The broth was clear, and let's say full of umami!

DIRECTIONS:

1. To make the fish sauce: combine the water, shiitake mushrooms, salt, and soy sauce. Simmer until reduced by half. (May be saved for 4 weeks in refrigerator). Set aside when done.

2. Meanwhile, put wakame in a small bowl with enough cold water to cover and let stand until about 10 minutes to soften and release salt.

3. In a medium saucepan, combine kombu with 3 · cups cold water and cook over medium heat until water just begins to boil. Remove kombu with tongs and discard. Add vegan fish sauce and bring to a boil over high heat. Reduce and simmer dashi for 10 minutes.

4. Drain wakame, rinse, and coarsely chop. Add to dashi along with cubed tofu. Set over medium heat until warmed through. Do not stir.

5. In a small bowl, whisk miso paste with a small amount of warm dashi to dissolve into a thin paste.

6. Remove dashi from heat and very gently stir in miso paste.

Ladle soups into a bowl, garnish with scallions and serve immediately.

root vegetable salad with organic sweet sauce

INGREDIENTS:

For the Dressing:

¼ cup freshly squeezed lemon juice

¼ cup raw, organic sesame oil

¼ cup organic olive oil

¾ tsp. fresh ginger, grated

¼ tsp. Himalayan salt

1 tsp. cinnamon

¾ tsp. pumpkin pie spice

½ tsp. agave

1 tbsp. Madagascar vanilla extract

For the Base:

1 small butternut squash (already cubed or whole)

1 sweet potato, peeled

1 juicing carrot (carrot without top)

2 tbsp. raisins

½ cup roasted, chopped pecans

1 crisp red apple, cored and chopped

It's funny how some recipes get noses snubbed when mentioned. This is, without a doubt, one of them! It certainly won't disappoint, guaranteed, especially for those sweet lovers. An idea? Make it a breakfast dish, a dessert, or a Thanksgiving side. Enjoy its skin-boosting benefits!

DIRECTIONS:

1. Prepare the dressing first by combining all ingredients. In a bowl, whisk dressing to smooth consistency. Set aside.

2. In a food processor with a shredding blade, send squash, sweet potato, and carrot through the chute.

3. Toss in pecans, apples, and raisins.

indian spiced root vegetable curry with creamy coconut

INGREDIENTS:

4 cups peeled and diced root vegetables of your choosing (turnip, parsnip, rutabaga, carrots)

4 tbsp. olive or coconut oil

3 large garlic cloves

1 red Thai bird chili, roughly chopped, seeds discarded

1 small can of diced tomatoes

1 bunch freshly chopped cilantro

2 cinnamon sticks

3 tsp. Madras curry powder

1 tsp. fennel seeds, crushed with mortar and pestle

1 in. fresh ginger, grated

Juice of 1 lime

1 can of coconut milk

Salt and pepper to taste

DIRECTIONS:

1. Preheat oven to 375º F. Place roasting tray in oven to preheat as well.

2. Clean root vegetables and dice into squares and put into a bowl. Coat with 2 tbsp. olive oil and season with salt and pepper. Put the vegetables onto the tray when hot and shake to distribute evenly. Roast for approximately 15 minutes while prepping sauce.

3. Mix curry and crushed fennel seeds.

4. Put the chopped chili, ginger, crushed garlic, and onion in a blender or mini-food processor and puree.

5. Add 2 tbsps. of olive oil in a pan on medium heat. Stir in the puréed mix, curry, and fennel.

6. Stir in the coconut milk a nd tomatoes. Add the cinnamon sticks, simmer stirring often.

7. Pour the mixture over the roasted vegetables in a baking dish. Bake for another 20 minutes until vegetables are tender and sauce has thickened.

8. Garnish with cilantro and fresh lime juice. Serve immediately.

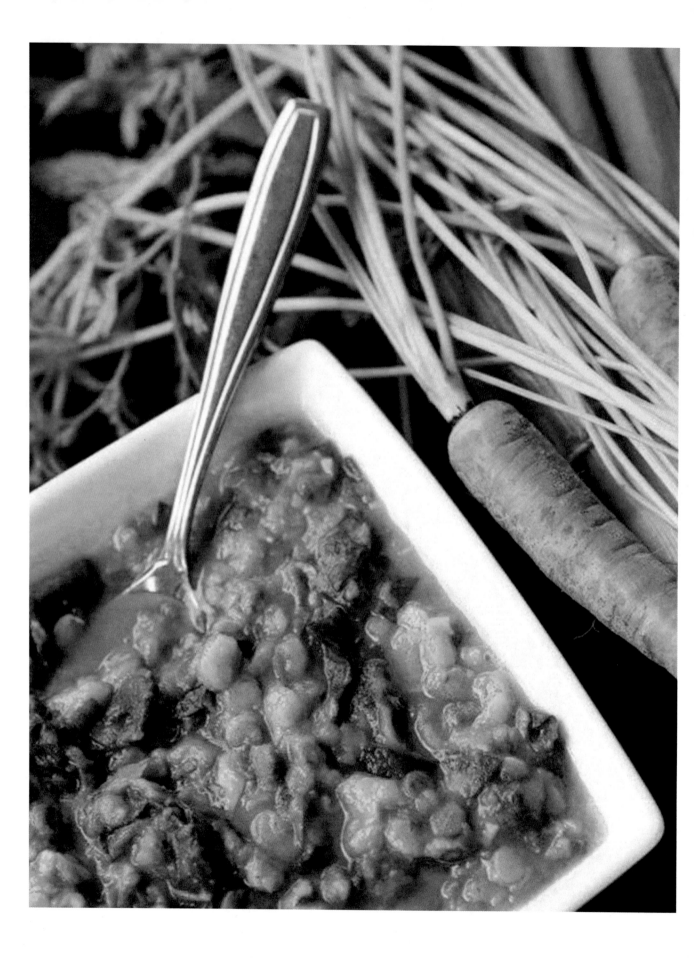

curried lentils and sweet potatoes

INGREDIENTS:

3 tablespoons extra virgin olive oil

1 large onion, diced

4 garlic cloves, minced

1-inch piece fresh ginger root, peeled and grated

2 teaspoons garam masala

2 teaspoons curry powder

1 jalapeño pepper, seeded if desired, then minced

6 cups vegetable broth as needed

2 pounds orange-fleshed sweet potatoes, peeled and cut into $1/2$-inch cubes

1 cups dried lentils

1 bay leaf

1 pound Swiss chard, center ribs removed, leaves coarsely chopped

1 teaspoon salt, more to taste

$1/2$ teaspoon ground black pepper

$1/3$ cup chopped fresh cilantro

Finely grated zest of 1 lime

Juice of $1/2$ lime

What is garam masala? Garam masala is an all-purpose spice mix used in small quantities in a variety of dishes used in Pakistani and North Indian cooking as well as other nearby countries. Garam masala refers to a mix of spices, whereas the spices give heat to the body, according to Ayurvedic principles. Garam means hot. The "garam" spices typically contain black pepper, cumin, cloves, bay leaves, nutmeg, mace, cardamom, and cinnamon. The heat blending properties of the combination of spices are what make it 'garam.' It makes for a wonderful fall and winter dish.

DIRECTIONS:

1. In a large saucepan, heat oil over medium heat. Add onion and sauté until translucent, approximately 5 to 7 minutes. Add garlic, ginger, garam masala, curry powder, and jalapeño. Cook only until fragrant. Be careful not to burn.

2. Stir in 4 cups broth, sweet potatoes, lentils, and bay leaf. Increase heat to high and bring to a quick boil, then reduce heat to medium.

3. Partially cover and simmer for 20 minutes, periodically adding 1/2 cup broth every 5 minutes.

4. Add chard, salt, and pepper, and continue cooking until lentils are tender and chard is cooked about 30 minutes total. Do not cover.

5. Just before serving, stir in cilantro, lime zest, and juice. Spoon into a large shallow serving dish.

6. Garnish with scallions.

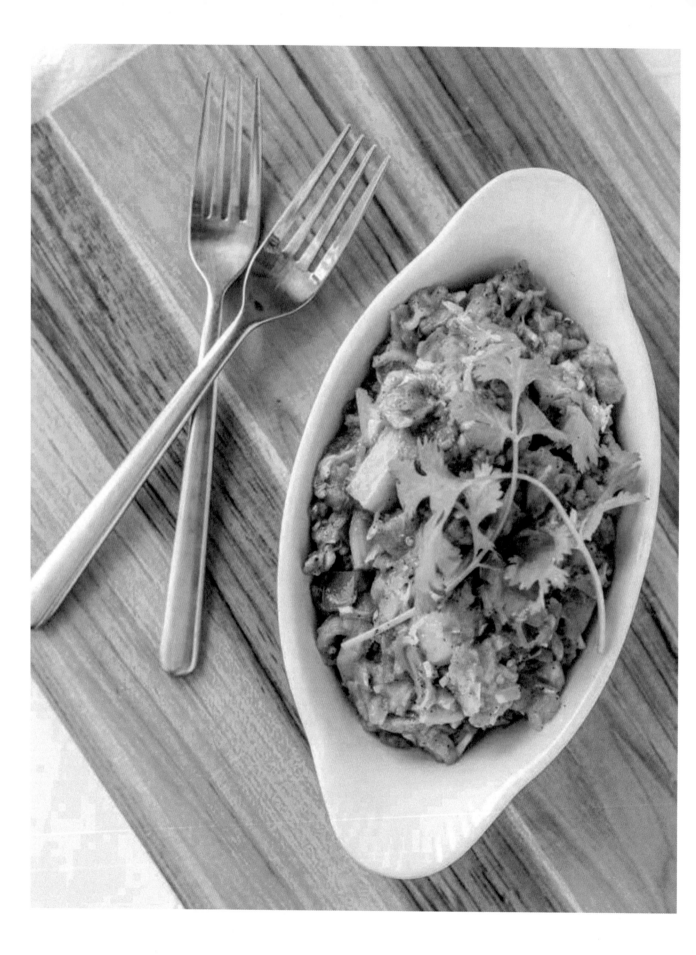

baingan ka bharta

Traditionally prepared, but without the use of dairy. Its vegan preparation is bursting with incredible flavors and mild heat. It can be eaten alone, with rice, naan, or try with a side of sautéed spinach and let the eggplant be your starch.

INGREDIENTS:

2 tbsp. mustard oil

2 medium-sized eggplant

1 can organic diced tomatoes

1 medium red onion finely chopped

2 cloves garlic

1-inch piece of ginger, grated

1 green chili pepper, seeded

1 tsp. whole cumin seed

$1/2$ tsp. ground turmeric

$1/2$ tsp. red chili powder

2 tsp. coriander powder

To prepare the eggplant:

1 tsp. salt for flesh

1 tbsp. olive oil

DIRECTIONS:

1. Preheat oven to 350°F.

2. Prepare the eggplant by slicing lengthwise in half. Thoroughly salt the eggplant flesh and set aside for 10 minutes or until it sweats. Remove the sweat with a towel and then rub with olive oil. Put the eggplant face down on baking sheet. Roast for approximately 20-30 minutes. For larger eggplants, add more time.

3. To make the bharta, start by heating the mustard oil in the pot. When the oil is hot enough, add the cumin seeds. They should crackle right away.

4. Add the onions and cook until translucent. Then add the ginger, garlic, and green chili pepper.

5. Add the tomato and gently mix into the bharta. Cover the pot for 2-3 minutes so the tomatoes can cook.

6. Meanwhile, using an oven mitt, remove the eggplant and scrape the insides with a fork or spoon. Place the insides of the eggplant into the pot. Add the remaining spices.

7. Add salt according to your taste and thoroughly combine everything in the pot.

8. Cover and allow the bharta to simmer on low heat for 5-7 minutes.

9. Garnish with cilantro and serve with rice or Naan.

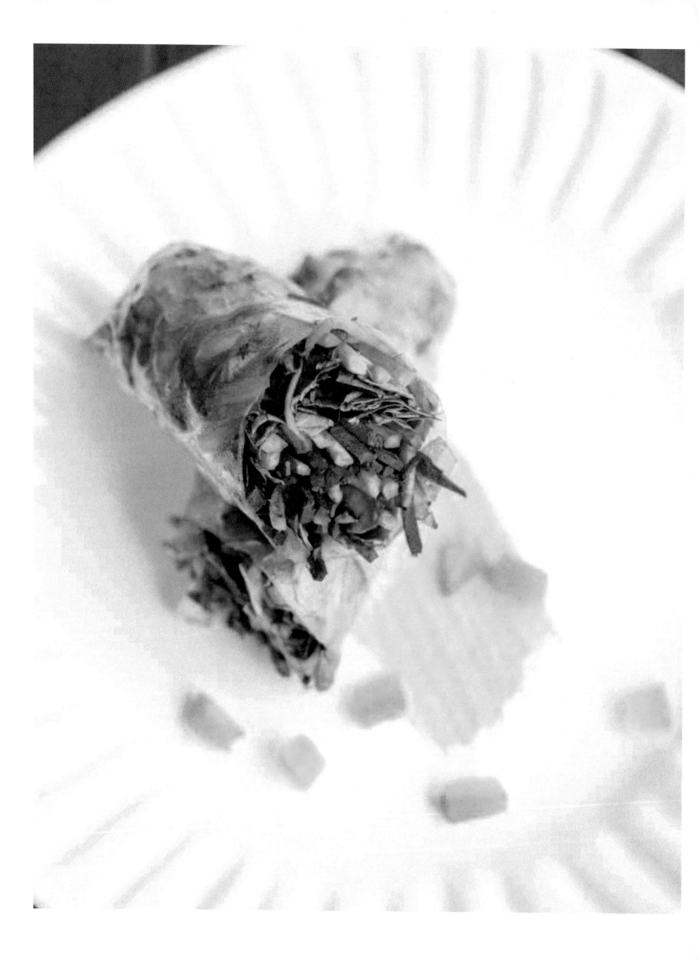

rainbow salad in rice paper with sesame tahini dipping sauce

INGREDIENTS:

Asian rice paper wraps

1 bunch rainbow chard; rinsed, de-spined, and finely chopped

1 bag matchstick carrots

1 beet, sliced on a mandolin or shredded

handful of basil, shredded

small bunch mint leaves

finely chopped chives

To make the sauce:

1/2 cup sesame tahini

2 tbsp. yacon syrup

3 tsp. Nama Shoyu

2-inch wedge of ginger, skins removed

1/2 jalapeño, seeded and chopped

juice from one lime

water to thin as needed

Not only filling, but these wraps contain vital nutrients, antioxidants, and phytochemicals. The name is in the title—eat the colors of the rainbow! These delicious and tasty wraps not only feed your cells but your heart and soul too!

DIRECTIONS:

1. Put all ingredients for sauce in a blender and blend until creamy smooth. If too thick, add water to thin as necessary.

2. Rinse and finely chop all ingredients for wrap. Toss lightly in a bowl.

3. Take rice wraps and rinse under warm water to soften. You've got a time limit with these finicky little things. Wrap too early, and they won't stick. Wait too long, and they wither away and stick to your fingers like tape. After a few good tries, I'm confident you can master these wraps!

4. Line your glass container with parchment paper, so the rice paper doesn't stick to the container. Add your rolled rice wraps one by one. After one row is complete, line the next with parchment paper and repeat.

5. Store the dressing in the refrigerator for up to one week. Best to consume fresh wraps within 2-3 days.

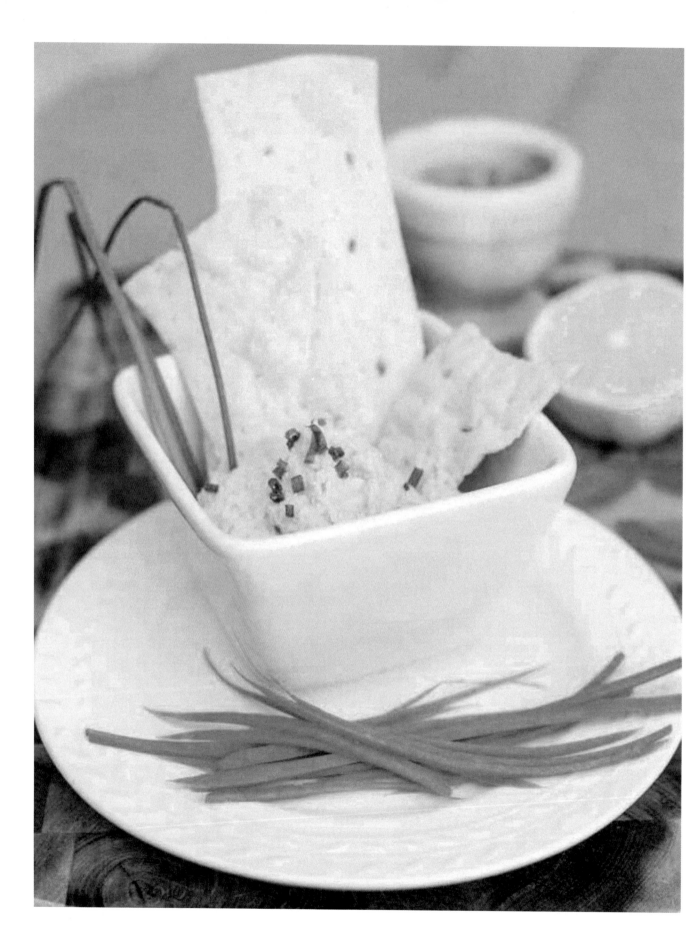

detoxifying sides

Side dishes are an easy-to-make addition to your daily meal. Love how these dishes taste? Turn them into a main dish or throw them on top of salads.

These dishes are densely packed with phytochemicals, a plethora of nutrients, and, if kept raw, enzymes that assist in digestion all the while keeping you satisfied throughout the day. These detoxing sides are designed to hook you on health at first bite. They're made from whole foods and clean ingredients. Best of all, they're simple to make.

Delve into a fantastic and easy array of both raw and cooked side dishes while immersing your palette in nature's delightful pleasures.

traditional hummus recipe

INGREDIENTS:

2 (15.5-ounce) cans no-salt-added chickpeas (garbanzo beans), rinsed and drained

2 garlic cloves, crushed

1/2 cup water

1/4 cup tahini

3 tbsp. fresh lemon juice

2 tbsp. extra-virgin olive oil

3/4 teaspoon salt

1/4 teaspoon black pepper

1 tsp. ground cumin (optional)

DIRECTIONS:

1. Place beans and garlic in a food processor; pulse 5 times or until chopped. Add 1/2 cup water and remaining ingredients; pulse until smooth, scraping down sides as needed.

Serve with your favorite snacks. Being that hummus is considered a starchy dish, try scooping with carrot, red pepper, and cucumber sticks for an alkaline and super healthy snack!

simple sautéed mustard greens

INGREDIENTS:

2 tablespoons olive oil or grapeseed oil

2-3 cloves garlic, minced

4 large bunches mustard greens, stemmed and chopped

Kosher, sea or Himalayan salt and freshly ground black pepper

$\frac{1}{4}$ cup organic low-sodium vegetable broth

1 tsp. red pepper flakes

1 tbsp. stone-ground mustard

Sauteéd mustard greens are a great addition to an evening meal. Not the norm for some, I'm sure, but incorporating cruciferous vegetables is a great way to give your body the right types of food that can work for you! Mustard seeds contain high amounts of selenium, which is a big boon for thyroid health!

DIRECTIONS:

1. In a large pan, turn on medium heat add the oil. When the oil is warm, add the garlic to the oil. Sauté until just softened and has infused the oil, about 1 minute. Do not let the garlic brown as it will taste bitter.

2. Add the red pepper flakes. Season the greens with salt and pepper, and sauté while tossing to wilt. Once wilted, add the vegetable stock and stir. Raise heat to a simmer, then lower and cook for about 5 minutes more.

3. Add the stone ground mustard.

4. Remove from heat and let stand to cool.

cauliflower-spinach purée

INGREDIENTS:

1 head cauliflower, rinsed and quartered

6 cups baby spinach

2-4 garlic cloves

1 teaspoon onion powder

$1/4$ teaspoon nutmeg

$1/4$ cup cashew butter

Move over mashed potatoes; cauliflower has replaced you! The cashew butter makes this mashed madness a true dinnertime champion!

DIRECTIONS:

1. Steam cauliflower and garlic for about 8-10 minutes or until tender. Drain and press out as much water as possible in a strainer. Set aside.
2. Add spinach to steamer and wilt slightly.
3. Place cauliflower, garlic, and cashew butter into a blender or food processor and blend until desired consistency.
4. Add seasoning and adjust to suit your taste.
5. Mix puréed cauliflower with wilted spinach. Serve hot or warm.

fresh okra with tomatoes and ginger

INGREDIENTS:

1 lb. fresh okra

2 garlic cloves, crushed

2-inch piece ginger, peeled and minced

2 tablespoons olive oil

$1/4$ tsp. cayenne pepper

3 large tomatoes, cored and quartered

$3/4$ teaspoon Himalayan salt

$1/4$ teaspoon pepper

Think okra is just known as a southern dish? Think again. The lycopene from the tomatoes gives it a monster-sized cancer preventative touch. And okra? Yes, the lectin in okra![168]

DIRECTIONS:

1. Pulse tomatoes with salt and pepper in a food processor until coarsely chopped and set aside.
2. Add olive oil to a large skillet and add garlic, ginger, and 1/2 of the cayenne to taste and cook over moderate heat, stirring, until slightly fragrant about 30 seconds.
3. Stir tomatoes into skillet cooking uncovered over moderate heat, stirring occasionally, 10 minutes.
4. While the tomatoes are cooking, trim ends off of okra and discard. Slice okra into 1/2 inch rounds and set on a platter.
5. Top fresh okra with tomato mixture and serve.

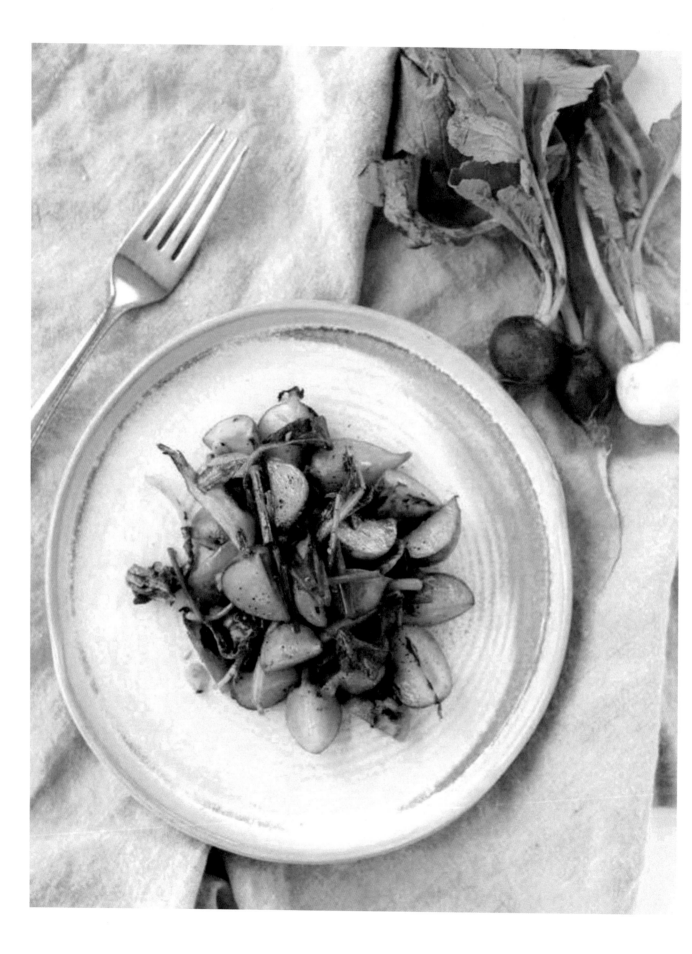

sautéed radishes with radish greens & chives

INGREDIENTS:

3 small bunches radishes with greens attached (2 lbs.)

2 ¹/₂ tablespoons coconut oil

1 teaspoon Himalayan salt

2 garlic cloves minced

3 tablespoons chopped fresh chives (garnish)

One of the best foods for skin! And we don't stop there! We kept the greens in with the dish. Amazingly, the greens contain more nutrients than the radish root itself! The greens are an excellent source of vitamin A, C, B6, magnesium, potassium, folic acid, phosphorus, iron, and calcium. They also contain antioxidants such as sulforaphane indoles, including the chives! Try eating the radishes raw, with a touch of salt, or whip up this delectable and amazingly healthy side dish!

DIRECTIONS:

1. Cut greens from radishes and coarsely chop. Rinse through a colander.

2. Trim radishes and cut into quarters

3. Heat 1 1/2 tablespoons coconut oil in a 12-inch heavy skillet over moderately high heat but not smoking.

4. Sauté radishes with salt, stirring until crisp-tender about 10 minutes. Transfer to a plate and keep warm.

5. Sauté garlic in remaining tablespoon of coconut oil over moderately high heat, stirring until fragrant, about 30 seconds. Add greens and sauté, stirring until wilted about 1 minute.

6. Return radish slices to skillet and stir in chives.

7. Serve warm.

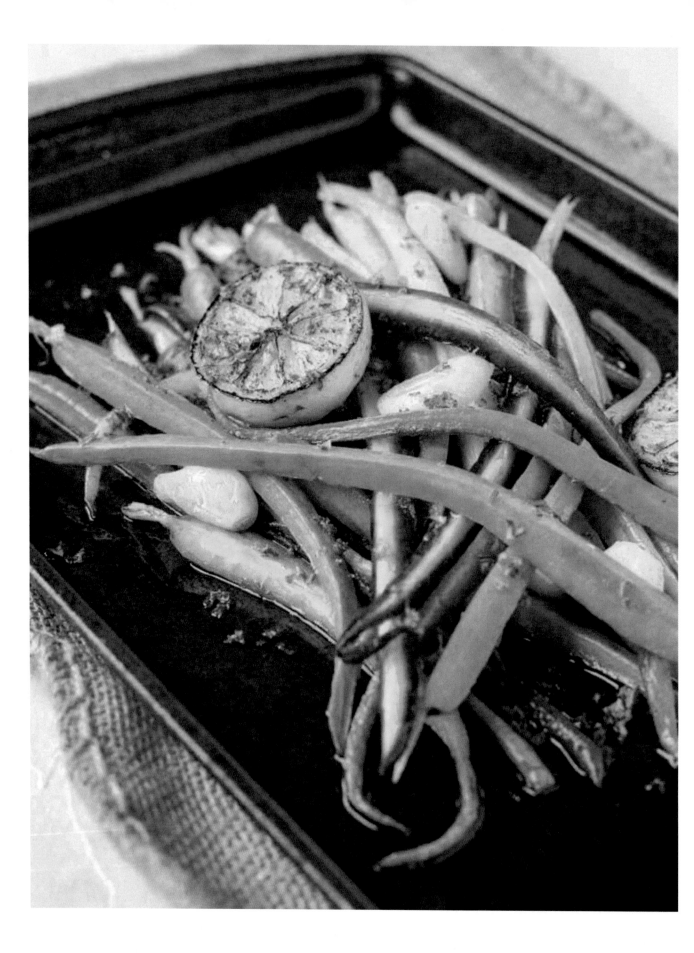

roasted rainbow carrots with roasted garlic and lemon

Carrots are highly nutritious and a good source of beta carotene, fiber, vitamin K1, potassium, and antioxidants. Their beta carotene antioxidants have been linked to a reduced risk of cancer. The compounds in garlic and lemon are also beneficial in reducing the risk of cancers, including certain types of brain and lung cancers. Garlic also has a positive impact on high blood pressure and high cholesterol.[169]

We used rainbow carrots with tops and quartered, charred the lemon, and roasted garlic. It's incredibly tasty and, best of all, healthy! You may find you never have any leftovers!

INGREDIENTS:

1 lb. small garden carrots, tops removed, sliced lengthwise into quarters

2 tbsp. extra-virgin olive oil

5 cloves roasted garlic

1 lemon, halved

Finely diced parsley

DIRECTIONS:

1. Preheat oven to 450°F.

2. To roast the garlic, take 5 cloves of garlic still inside their skins and set inside aluminum foil with olive oil until soft.

3. Scrub, rinse, and dry carrots. Cut lengthwise into quarters. Arrange in a single layer on a baking sheet. Cut lemon wedge in half. Add olive oil, salt, and pepper to carrots and lemon. Set lemon face down on baking sheet. Add carrots to oven with garlic and bake until tender and beginning to brown, approximately 20 minutes.

4. Remove carrots and roasted garlic from oven. When cool, remove garlic from skins and add to carrots.

5. Squeeze lemon over carrots. Garnish with parsley.

Serve immediately.

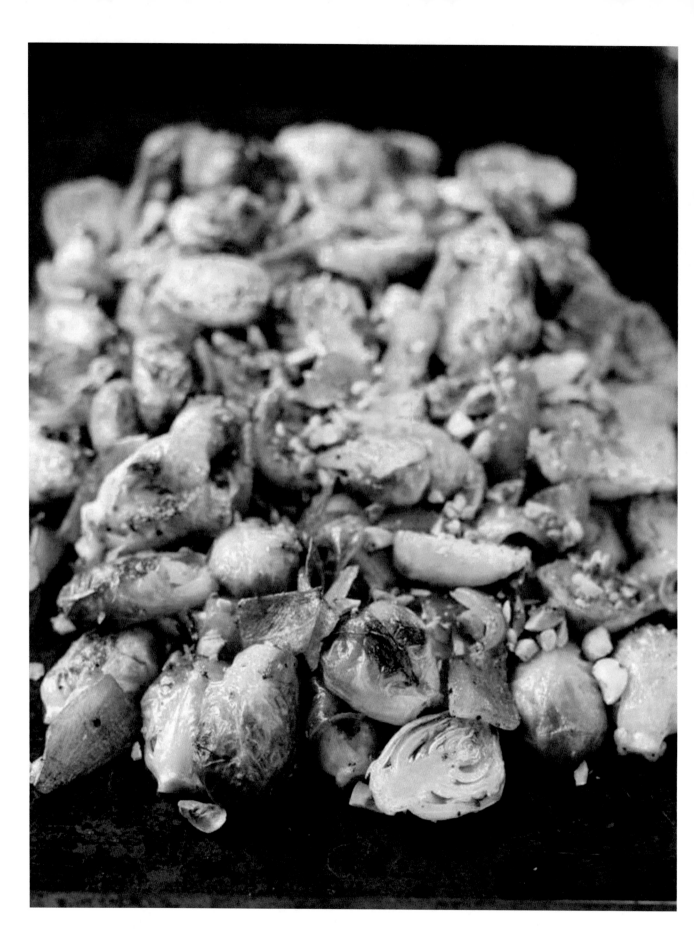

roasted brussels sprouts with hazelnuts

For anyone who has never tried brussels sprouts or insists they don't like them, think again! Brussels sprouts, part of the cruciferous family, are known for their distinct taste and smell from the sulforaphane, a powerful phytochemical in the plant, but when prepared correctly at high heat, brussels sprouts release their sugars, making them an incredibly tasty and satisfying dish. Add in a bite of apple cider vinegar and a touch more sweetness from the maple syrup, and this dish is sure to sway the non-believer! Boasting with 88g of protein in 1 cup, brussels sprouts also meet the recommended daily requirement of vitamin C and K! Consuming these mini cabbages may have the potential to decrease the risk of certain diseases like heart disease and some cancers.[170] And don't forget, we added another powerful cancer preventative, especially in regards to stomach and colorectal – the red onion – part of the allium family.[171]

INGREDIENTS:

1/2 cup whole hazelnuts

6 cups Brussels sprouts, trimmed and halved

1 small red onion, cut into 1-inch wedges

4 tbsp extra-virgin olive oil

1/2 tsp. salt

1/4 tsp. pepper

1/4 cup maple syrup (optional)

2 tsp. cider vinegar

DIRECTIONS:

1. In a small metal cake pan, toast hazelnuts in oven at 350°F until fragrant, 5 to 10 minutes. Transfer to tea towel; rub off as much of the skins as possible. Coarsely chop and set aside.

2. In roasting pan, toss together Brussels sprouts, onion, oil, salt, and pepper. Roast in 425°F oven, stirring occasionally until tender and edges are browned, about 20 minutes.

3. Add hazelnuts, maple syrup, and vinegar; toss to combine. Roast for 5 more minutes.

In a pinch? Don't have time? Can't find hazelnuts? Just halve brussels sprouts and quarter onions, toss with olive oil, salt, and pepper. Roast in oven for 25-30 minutes and serve immediately. You'll still get the amazing benefits from the fabulous cruciferous Brussels!

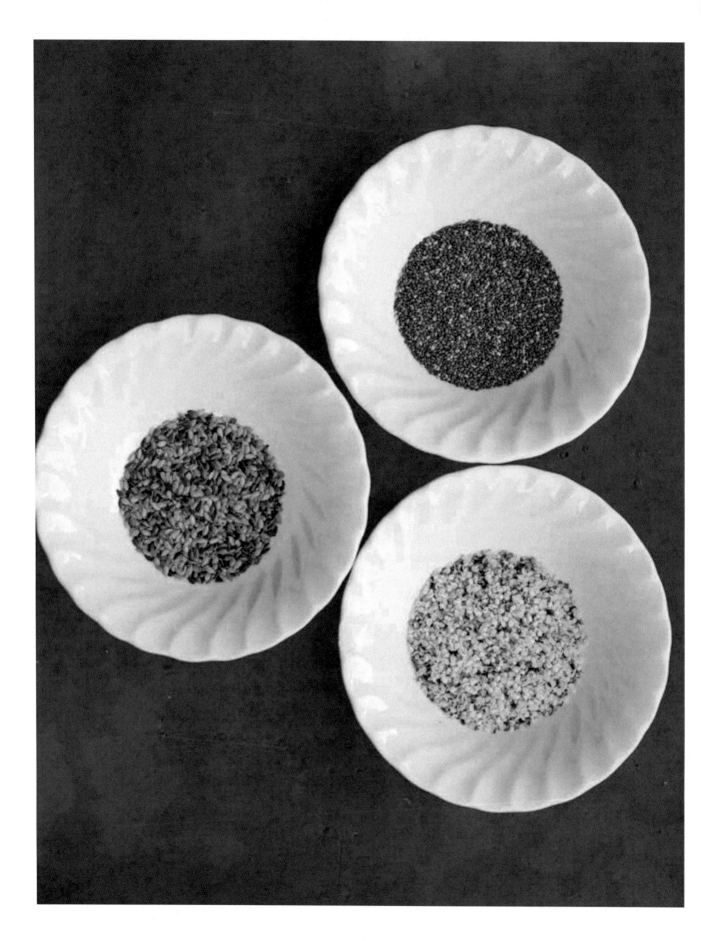

the health benefits of good fats

OMEGAS 3-6-9

Fats are an integral part of overall health, but we learned that not all fats are created equal. And that goes for preparation and storage as well. Knowing a little bit about the preparation, cooking, and storing of fats and oils can give you a clearer understanding of how to best preserve the unique qualities each one of them possesses. If the state of your heart, your brain, and your mood are important to you, then this is the recipe section for you.

There are four types of fat, but we will only be incorporating 3 out of 4 of them for the obvious reasons!

- Trans fats
- Saturated fats
- Monounsaturated fats
- Polyunsaturated fats

SATURATED FATS

The most celebrated of all the saturated fats is coconut oil! Some experts say the body handles the medium-chain fatty acids (MCT) found in coconut oil differently than the longer-chain fats found in liquid vegetable oils, dairy, and fatty meats. MCT is readily used by the body for energy rather than stored as fat. MCTs are also helpful for ridding the gut of harmful microorganisms like pathogenic bacteria, viruses, fungi, and parasites and contain antioxidant and anti-inflammatory properties. It is no wonder coconut oil tops the chart as a helper and healer. When buying high-quality coconut oil, stick to organic, virgin, and unrefined, not the unhealthy refined version (historically used as hydrogenated oils in industrial baked goods).

MONOUNSATURATED FATS

The highly-rated, heart-healthy omega-9 can be found in olive oil, avocados, and nuts (except macadamia and walnuts). The Mediterranean diet contains a significant amount of these oils. They are good for you and are a great part of a healthy diet.

POLYUNSATURATED FATS

The other omega's #6 and #3 are polyunsaturated and not produced by the body, which means it must be taken in through diet. Of the two, omega-6 oils are consumed to excess in our diet. Too much omega-6 causes inflammation, while omega-3s reduces inflammation. Currently, much attention is being paid to both omega-3s and omega-6s for that reason.

The omega-3 oil is believed to play a role in the prevention of cardiovascular disease and necessary for proper brain and nerve development.

Where do you find rich dietary sources of omega-3?

You will find an abundance of omega-3 in:

Flaxseeds   Walnuts

Hemp Seeds   Soybeans

Green Leafy   Green Algae

Vegetables   Chia Seeds

Chlorella   Primrose Oil

Seaweed   Pumpkin Seeds

In seeking a healthy balance, experts site anywhere from 4:1 or as low as 1:1 omega-6s to omega-3s ratios in food.

The culprits of high omega-6s include:

Corn Oil   Cottonseed Oil

Safflower Oil   Canola Oil

Sunflower Oil

Corn oil's omega 6-to-omega-3 ratio is 49:1. Talk about out of balance!

COOKING AND STORAGE

Polyunsaturated oils, including the omega-3 fats, are easily damaged by heat, light, and oxygen; therefore, omega-3 oils are kept in dark-colored bottles with tightly fitting lids stored in the refrigerator. Omega-3s are generally not used for cooking because heat alters the delicate chemical make-up. Omega-3s are better suited in salads or raw recipes.

Grapeseed oil, avocado oil, and coconut oil are chemically stable in contact with high heat and make for a healthier alternative when cooking.

Increasing your intake of omega-3s through plant-based foods and minimizing your intake of omega-6 oils and foods by eliminating processed foods and refined oils may significantly reduce the risk of inflammatory ailments. A relief for many! A good rule of thumb is to vary your oils in order to give the body a wide range of nutritional benefits and to minimize oxidation when cooked.

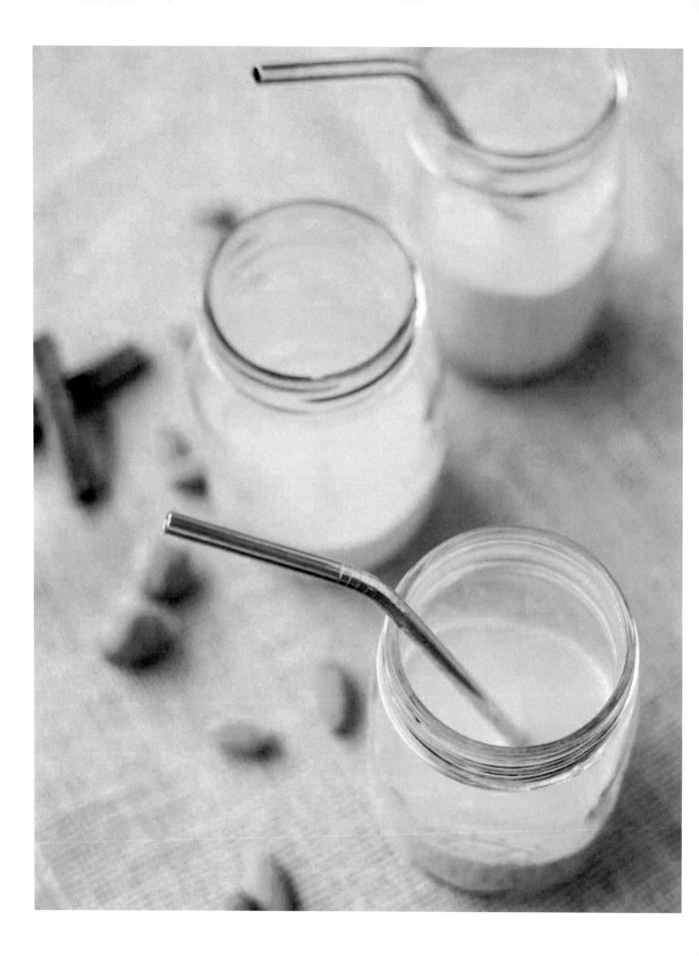

nut "mylk" shake

WHAT YOU'LL NEED:

High-speed Blender

Nut Mylk bag

Wide mouth glass bowl with pour spout.

INGREDIENTS:

1 cup raw almonds

1 cup brazil nuts

4 cups water

3 black mission figs

1 date – pitted

1 tsp. vanilla extract

1 tbsp. yacon syrup

1 tsp. cinnamon

We chose to mix up calcium loaded almonds and pair it with the healthy fats from brazil nuts (which is technically a seed and not a nut!). What do you also get with all that richness? Selenium! Selenium plays an important role in reproduction, metabolism, and immune health and may even help improve mood. Brazil nuts contain polyunsaturated and monounsaturated healthful fats, which can help improve cholesterol levels.[172] And best of all? It is incredibly creamy and delicious. By far, one of our favorite nut mylks!

DIRECTIONS:

1. Blend nuts and water in a blender.

2. Pour half nut mylk mixture into nut mylk bag and squeeze down on the mylk bag to draw down liquid into a wide mouth bowl with pour spout.

3. Either discard remaining nut meal or dehydrate in a dehydrator.

4. Pour the rest of the mixture into mylk bag and repeat process.

5. Return nut mylk to blender. Add black mission figs, date, vanilla extract, yacon syrup, and cinnamon. Blend on high for 1 minute.

6. Store in a glass carafe.

Serve immediately.

Store your nut mylk in the refrigerator for up to 3 days.

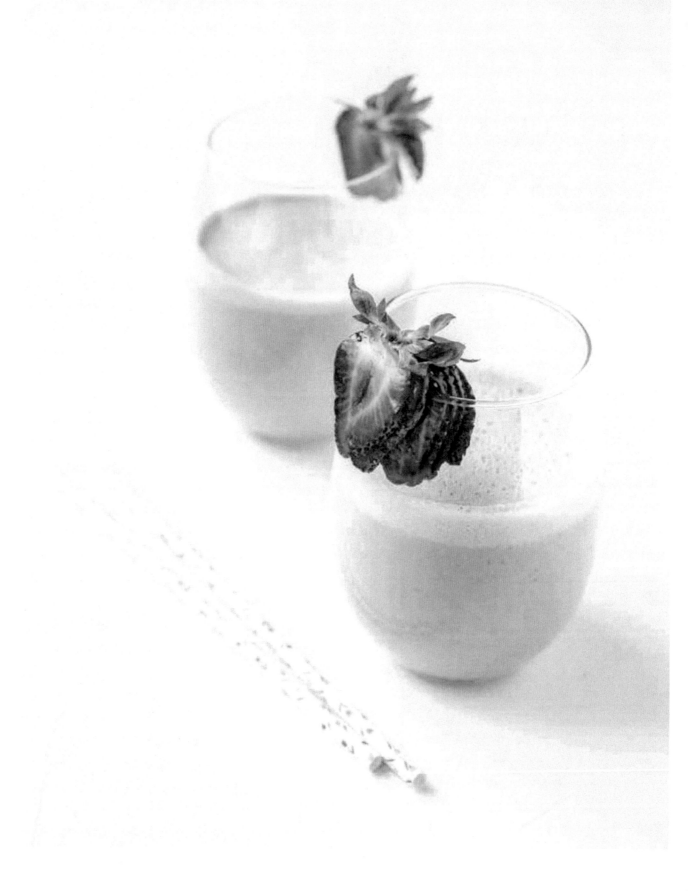

strawberry cashew milkshake

INGREDIENTS:

2 cups raw cashews soaked, at least 4 hours or overnight

4 dates, pitted

½ lb. fresh strawberries, rinsed, tops removed

1 tbsp. raw honey or sweetener of choice

2 cups filtered water

Another Brazilian nut, the cashew, is high in monounsaturated and polyunsaturated fats as well as a good source of protein. According to Medical News Today, consuming a high proportion of plant-based foods appears to reduce the risk of many lifestyle-related health conditions.[173] As if you needed convincing now!? Cashews are known to be a good source of magnesium, which plays an important role in over 300 enzymatic reactions within the body.

And since we focus heavily on digestive health, eating just less than one cup of strawberries per day could improve the symptoms of inflammatory bowel disease. The mixture and combination of this recipe could be a big boon to your health! Cheers!

DIRECTIONS:

1. In a high-speed blender, add rinsed, soaked cashews, strawberries, dates, water, and sweetener until smooth.

2. Serve immediately or store in the refrigerator for up to 3 days.

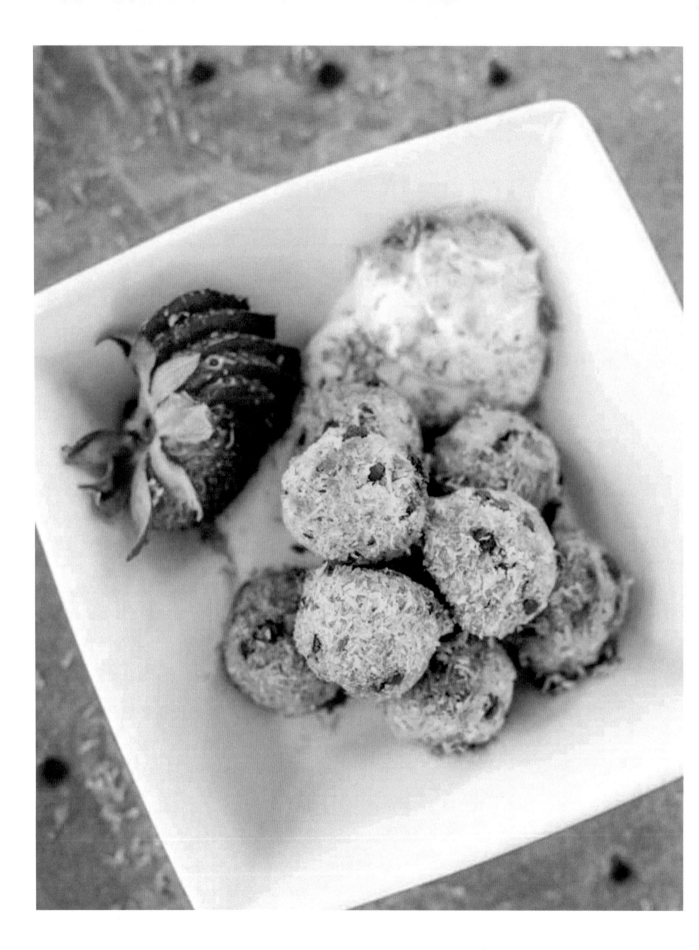

chocolate chip macaroons

INGREDIENTS:

1 1/4 cups unsweetened shredded coconut, fine

3/4 cup almond or gluten-free all-purpose flour

1/2 cup extra virgin coconut oil (unrefined)

1/4 cup coconut butter

2 tbsp. ground chia seeds

1/3 cup agave syrup (light, not amber)

2 tsp. Madagascar bourbon vanilla extract

1/2 teaspoon sea salt

1/2 cup vegan mini chocolate chips

1/2 cup toasted coconut flakes, fine

Coconut butter, unlike coconut oil, is made from whole coconut flesh. It's made using a special blending process that transforms raw coconut into a buttery texture. It is typically found in specialty grocery stores. Coconut butter can be found on an aisle shelf, usually near cooking oils or baking products, but beware, it has an unbelievably decadent flavor!

DIRECTIONS:

1. In a medium bowl, mix together 1 1/4 cups of the unsweetened coconut, almond flour, coconut oil, and coconut butter. Using bare hands, massage the coconut oil and butter into the coconut flakes. The warmth of your hands will help soften the coconut oil and butter to facilitate the process.

2. Add the remaining ingredients and stir together until well incorporated.

3. Shape into small bite-size balls.

4. Put 1/2 cup toasted shredded coconut in a small bowl.

5. Place 3-4 truffles in the bowl with the toasted shredded coconut and roll around until lightly covered with coconut.

6. Store in refrigerator.

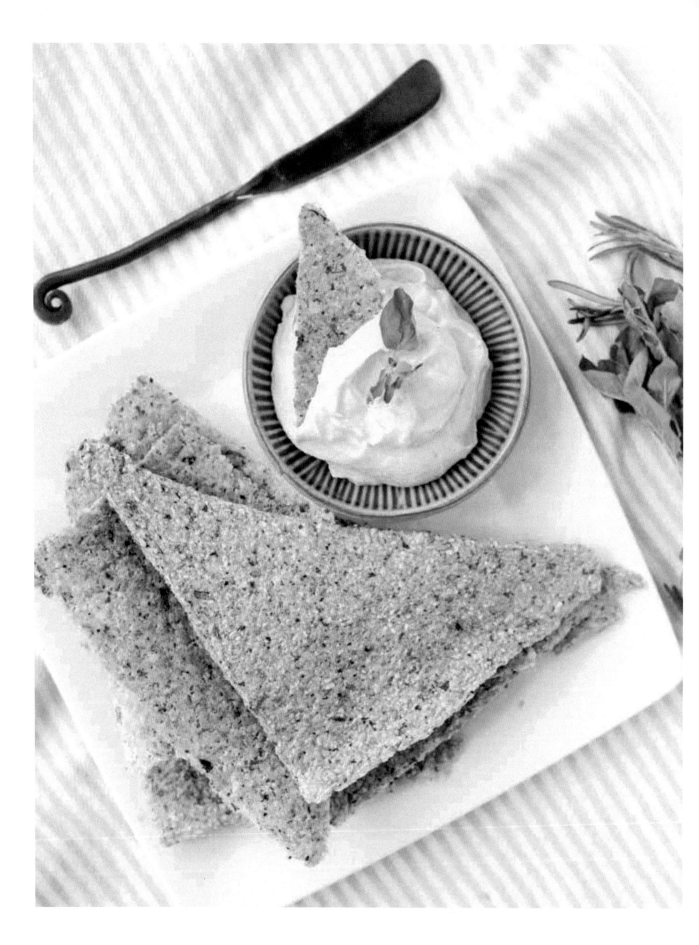

dehydrated herbed flax crackers with lavender buds

INGREDIENTS:

$1/2$ cup flax seeds, soaked overnight in 1 cup water

$1/2$ cup almonds, soaked overnight

$1/2$ cup sunflower seeds, soaked overnight

2 cups roughly chopped zucchini (approx. 1 lg. or 2 small zucchini)

4 small garlic cloves, minced

$1/2$ tbsp. onion powder

2 tsp. Lavender buds

2 tbsp. chopped fresh basil

1 tsp. fresh oregano

2 tsp. fresh rosemary, chopped

$1/4$ tsp. Himalayan salt plus $1/2$ tsp. for sprinkling

The nutrients in flaxseed include lignans, antioxidants, and, of course, beneficial omega-3s! The lignans in flaxseeds appear to have antioxidant properties, ridding your body of the bad stuff while bringing on the good! The omega-3s may help prevent different types of cancer cells from growing. And here I just thought they were delicious! Talk about a functional snack!

DIRECTIONS:

1. Place almonds and sunflower seeds in a food processor and pulse until granular.

2. Add zucchini and continue to pulse until blended.

3. Add coagulated flax seeds and rest of ingredients and blend until smooth.

4. Divide batter onto 2 (possibly 3) Teflex sheets and spread evenly and thinly.

5. Lightly salt crackers.

6. Score crackers into diagonals or squares using a plastic dough scraper.

7. Dehydrate at 115ºF for 4 hours.

8. Take tray out of dehydrator and cover crackers with another tray with plastic mesh liner only. Keeping trays held tightly together, flip trays over. Peel Teflex sheet off the underside of crackers and dehydrate for another 3-4 hours until crispy.

9. Store in plastic Ziploc bags or a sealed glass container in the refrigerator to keep its crunch for up to one week.

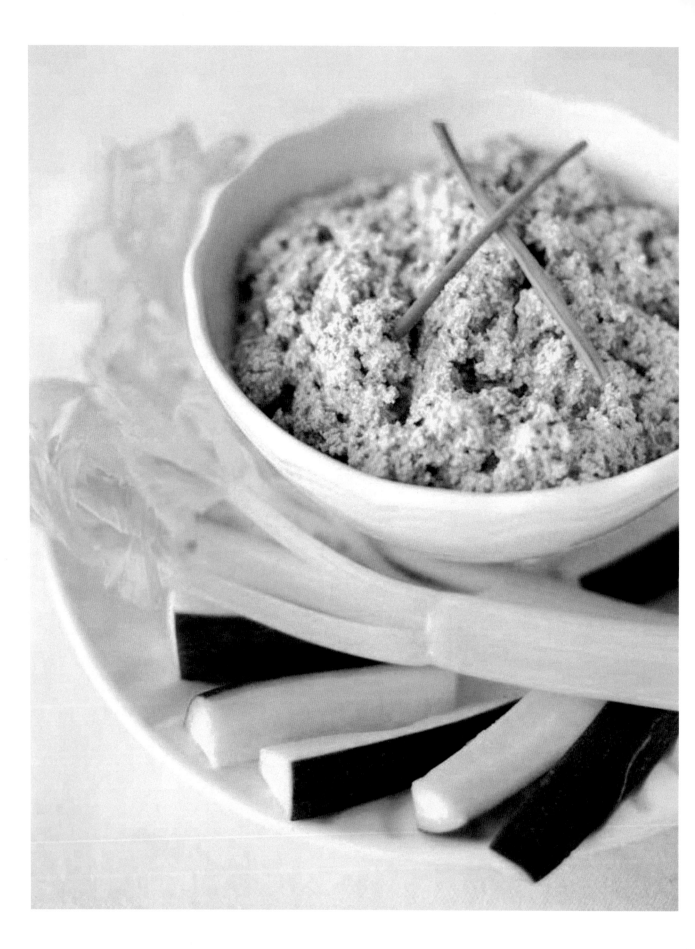

curried almond pate

INGREDIENTS:

1 cup raw almonds

1/2 cup raw sunflower seeds

1/4 cup raw sesame tahini

1/4 cup fresh squeezed lemon juice

1 celery rib chopped

2 tbsp. scallion bottoms (white and light green parts only), sliced on the bias

1/4 cup roughly chopped cilantro

1/4 cup water to thin the pâté as necessary

1 garlic clove minced

1 tbsp. Madras or good quality curry

1/4 tsp. Himalayan salt

Almonds contain numerous vitamins, minerals, including protein! Almonds are also high in the good unsaturated fats, therefore possibly improving one's blood cholesterol. Almonds and sunflower seeds can also increase vitamin E levels and lower the risk of Alzheimer's disease as well as lower the risk of breast cancer.[174] Pungent in taste and numerous in health benefits, curries have been around for centuries originating from ancient India and Thailand. This dish is both satisfying and brimming with health benefits.

DIRECTIONS:

1. Soak almonds and sunflower seeds in filtered water for 12 hours

2. Take all ingredients and add to food processor and process until a smooth, cream-like consistency.

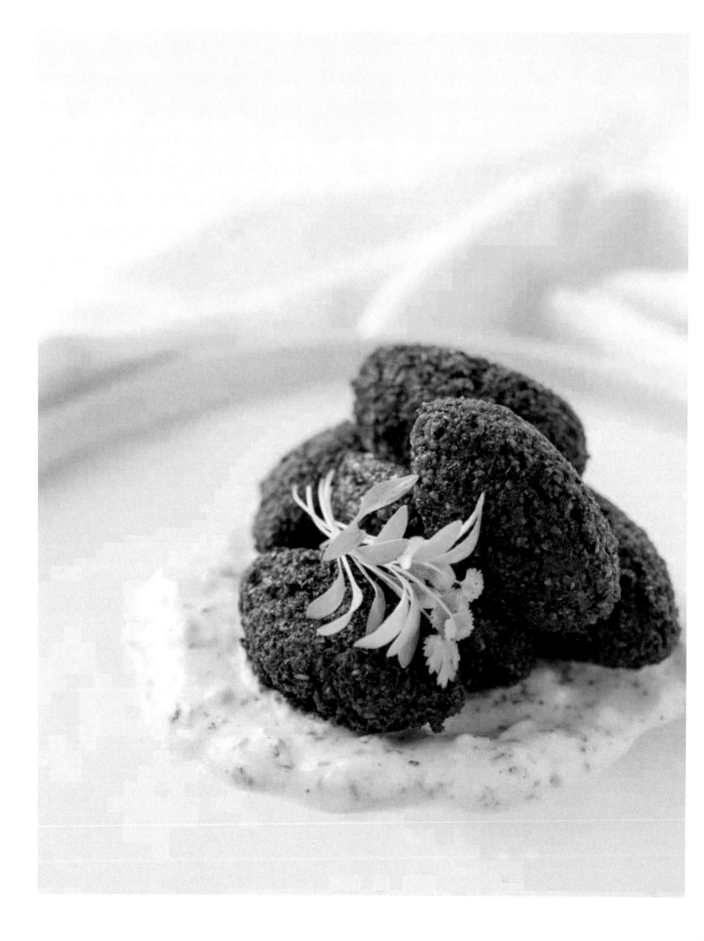

falafel with tzatziki sauce

INGREDIENTS:

For the falafel:

1 cup dried chickpeas, soaked overnight, rinsed 3 times

1 1/2 cup coarsely chopped parsley, stems removed

1 sweet onion diced

5 cloves of garlic, minced

1 tbsp. finely diced jalapeño

1/2 tsp. cumin powder

2 tsp. baking powder

Salt and pepper to taste

High heat oil for frying

1 seedless cucumber (optional)

1 red pepper (optional)

For the tzatziki sauce:

2 cups organic, plain almond or coconut milk yogurt

2 tbsp. chopped parsley

Juice from 1/2 lime

2 garlic cloves, minced

2 tbsp. small diced onion

Salt and pepper to taste

Traditional preparation minus the dairy in our rendition of this amazing Tzatziki sauce!

DIRECTIONS:

1. One day prior (18-24 hours), soak the chickpeas in enough water to completely submerge them to allow for expanding. Add 1 tsp. of baking soda.

2. Rinse the chickpeas and dry with a towel or cloth.

3. Place the chickpeas, onions, herbs, spices in the bowl of a food processor with the S-blade. Initially, pulse the mixture then run approximately 20 seconds at a time until well-combined.

4. Transfer mixture to a refrigerator and let sit for at least one hour. In the meantime, prepare the tzatziki sauce in a medium-sized bowl.

5. Add oil to a medium-sized saucepan about 3 inches up (less than halfway), making sure you have on a hand a metal slotted spoon (not plastic) to remove falafel balls from oil.

6. Heat oil on medium-high until bubbling just a bit. The temperature of the oil is vitally important to cooking thoroughly without burning.

7. Add 1 tsp. baking powder to mixture. Roll into balls just before frying.

8. Drop falafel balls into oil one at a time, frying until golden brown and crispy. Remove with slotted metal spoon into a colander or plate lined with paper towels to drain the excess oil.

9. Serve falafel with tzatziki sauce, cucumbers, and red pepper slices.

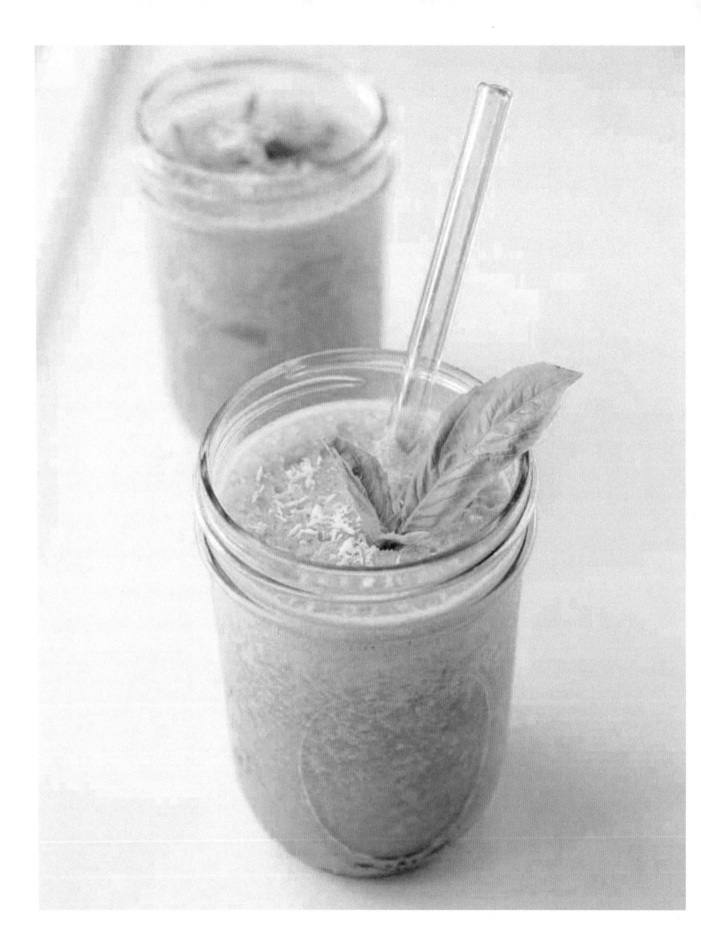

superfoods & smoothies

Superfoods have the characteristics to assist in the prevention and elimination of disease and premature aging. They are meant to help with efficient elimination and promote the presence of healthy intestinal flora. Superfoods are an excellent, permanent daily dietary choice. No food, however, no matter how "super," can stand alone or replace a complete and well-rounded diet.

The foods used in the following section are not new and have been around for centuries. They're also super delicious!

The Super-charged, Super-powered, Super-food Smoothie

What's in your Base?

The recommendation would be an unsweetened organic milk alternative without carrageenan as a thickening agent. Derived from red seaweed, carrageenan has been used for decades as an effective means to thicken a multitude of products. Before 2016, it was allowed in organic foods, but has since been demoted to a "food additive." Its unique chemical structure that makes it quite appealing as a choice of thickening agents also happens to be the same chemical structure that causes an immune response in some people (especially the gut). Dr. Andrew Weil states when in doubt, avoid it altogether.[175]

There are excellent national and regional brands of nut milk. If you find one with the least amount of ingredients, go for it! Products also come and go and even change formulas, which is why I choose not to recommend a specific brand. The key factor to remember is organic, minimal ingredients, minimal sugar, and zero carrageenans. Raw is best but only lasts 3 days and is quite expensive and time-consuming to make at home but certainly worth giving it a try.

Good milk alternatives:

Hemp	Brazil Nut
Rice	Pine Nut
Almond	Coconut
Hazelnut	Buckwheat
Cashew	Oat
Walnut	Flax

protein powders

There are several varieties and choices in brands. Here is what you should look for...not one that is a complete meal or All-In-One shake as fruits are combined with vegetables, a case for digestive upset or worse flatulence! Look for simple organic vegan protein powders using the vegan protein sources listed below. You don't need to find all of the ingredients in one powder as it most likely doesn't exist, but feel free to rotate protein powders and find ones that are appealing to your taste buds. If you're not used to vegan powders and are weaning yourself off whey, the taste and texture are quite different. Some vegan protein powders taste "chalky" and don't blend well. It all comes down to preference and your flavor palette. The key point: do not use whey. Oy vey!

Hemp

Sunflower

Rice

Pea

Quinoa

Artichoke

Goji

Amaranth

Chia

VEGETABLES

If you find it difficult to eat a multitude of greens, add them to your smoothies. Dropping them into your blender is a great way to disguise their taste! Greens such as kale, spinach, and dandelion greens are a great addition to protein smoothies!

FRUITS

Many people love to sweeten their smoothies with fruits. If it can be avoided, I would avoid fruits altogether in a protein smoothie. Fruits have a quicker digestive time, so its best to chew your fruits and leave them out of juices and smoothies too!

Nut Butters and Nut Powders

Nut butters and nut powders are a great option in this type of smoothie!

SUPERFOODS

This makes smoothies so incredibly nutritious—the ability to load them up with superfood supplement powders, and there are several! Not sure where to buy? Just look them up on Amazon to narrow down your choices. Prefer to shop local? Check out your local organic grocer or health food store. Here are some incredible options:

Maca Root

Lucuma

Chlorella

Blue-Green Algae

Açai

Camu Camu

Spirulina

Mesquite

Cacao

Goji

Wheatgrass

Turmeric

Aloe Vera

Green Tea Extract

Fennel Powder

Nona

Barley Grass

Alfalfa

Coconut Meat

Maqui Berry

You have a variety of options to supercharge your superfood smoothie. Using a blender is best, but if mixing in powders, a shaker cup would work just fine. Find the combination of flavors that you like and stick with it until your supplies run out, then try a different combination of superfoods!

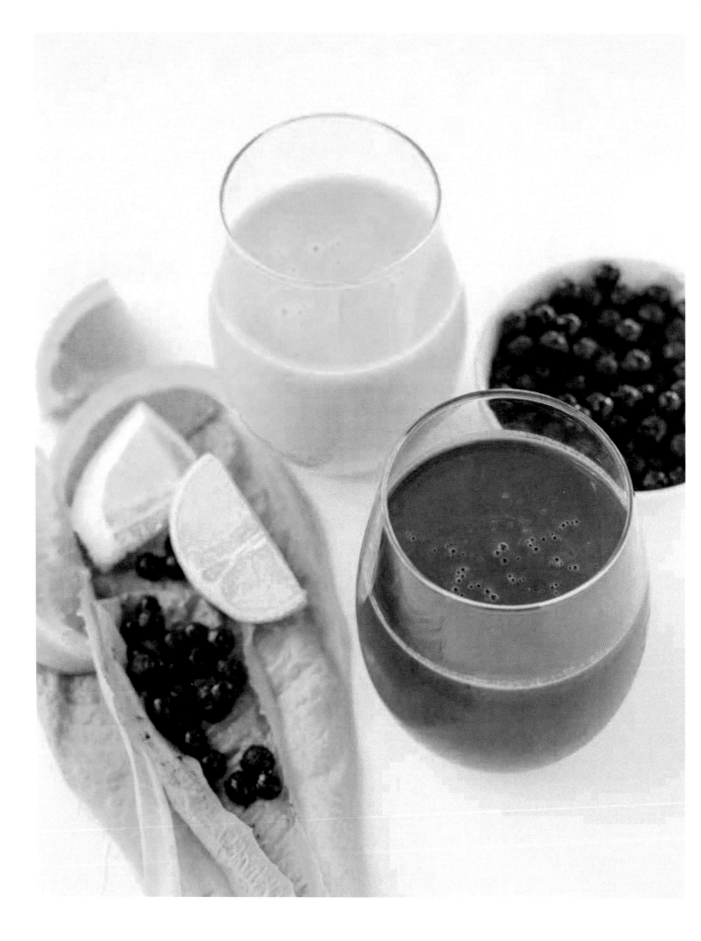

blueberry açai

INGREDIENTS:

$^3/_4$ cup blueberries

1 açai packet (Sambazon brand found frozen)

$^1/_2$ cup milk alternative (cashew, almond, walnut, coconut, rice, or hemp)

1 tsp. lemon juice

small handful sweet greens like romaine, buttercrunch, or leaf lettuce

DIRECTIONS:

Add all the ingredients to a blender and blend on high until smooth and creamy.

orange boost

INGREDIENTS:

1 nectarine

1 carrot

$^1/_2$ cup frozen pineapple

1 cup cactus water

$^1/_4$ cup coconut yogurt

1 small wedge of fresh turmeric root or

$^1/_4$ tsp. powdered turmeric

DIRECTIONS:

Add all the ingredients to a blender and blend on high until smooth and creamy.

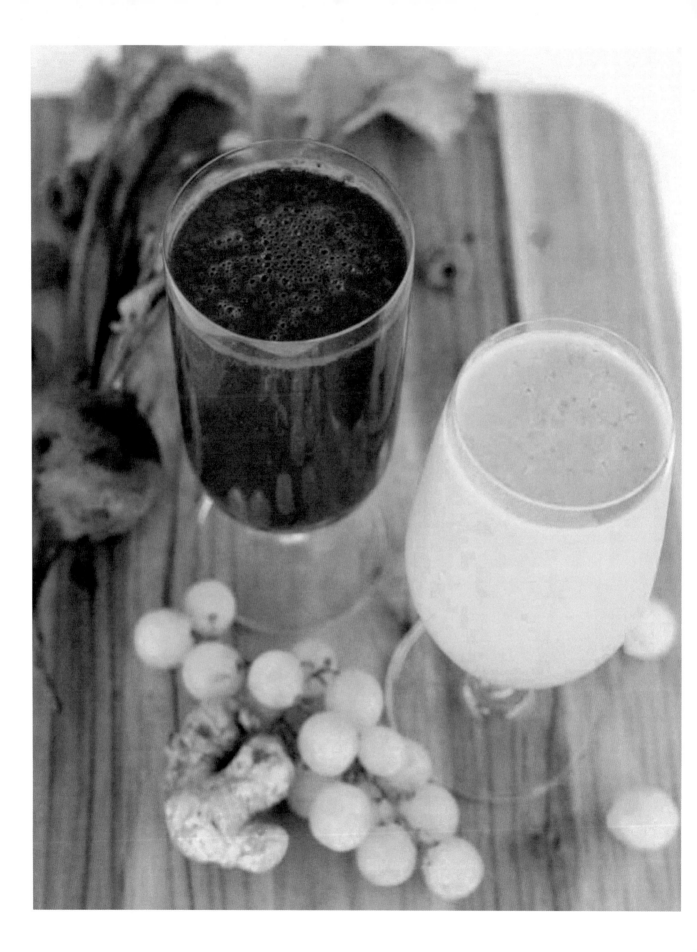

green goddess smoothie

INGREDIENTS:

1 scoop of Amazing Grass Greens or 1 handful of spinach

$1/2$ cup green grapes or $1/2$ cup pineapple chunks

$1/2$ cup unsweetened coconut milk beverage

$1/2$ avocado

juice from $1/2$ lime

$1/2$ tsp. peeled, grated ginger

$1/4$ tsp. sugar alternative like Monk Fruit sweetener

DIRECTIONS:

Add all the ingredients to a blender and blend on high until smooth and creamy.

beets and berries

INGREDIENTS:

1 small beet, stem removed, chopped

$1/2$ banana

$1/2$ cup frozen raspberries

$1/4$ cup cold water

$1/4$ cup plain coconut yogurt

DIRECTIONS:

Add all the ingredients to a blender and blend on high until smooth and creamy.

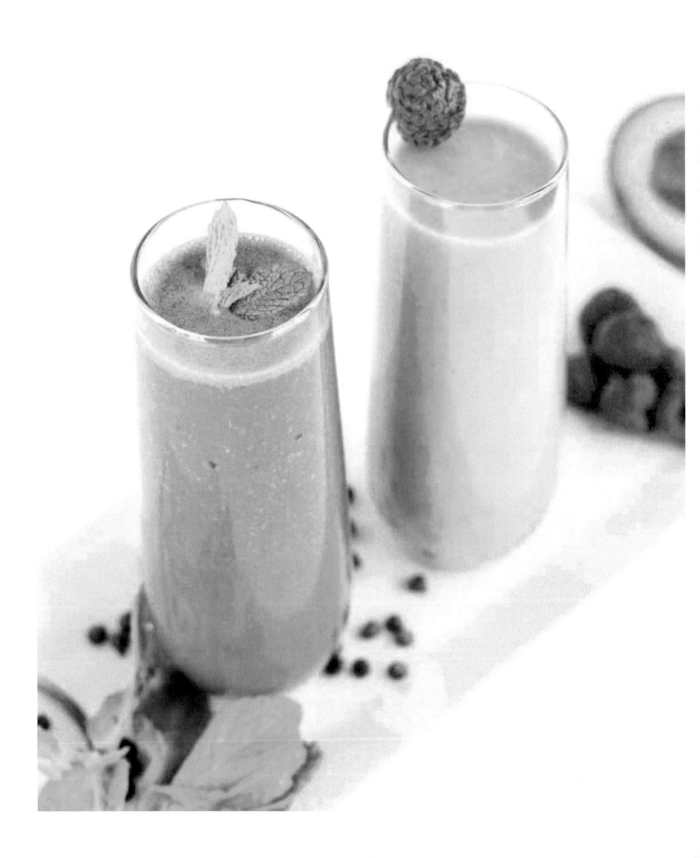

raspberry kisses

INGREDIENTS:

1 cup frozen raspberries

$1/4$ avocado

$1/2$ cup ice

1 tsp. Chia seeds

$3/4$ tsp. sweetener squeeze of lemon wedge

DIRECTIONS:

Add all the ingredients to a blender and blend on high until smooth and creamy.

mint madness

INGREDIENTS:

1 cup cashew milk

1 full dropper chlorophyll with mint

4 dark chocolate squares

1 banana

$1/2$ cup ice

DIRECTIONS:

Add all the ingredients to a blender and blend on high until smooth and creamy.

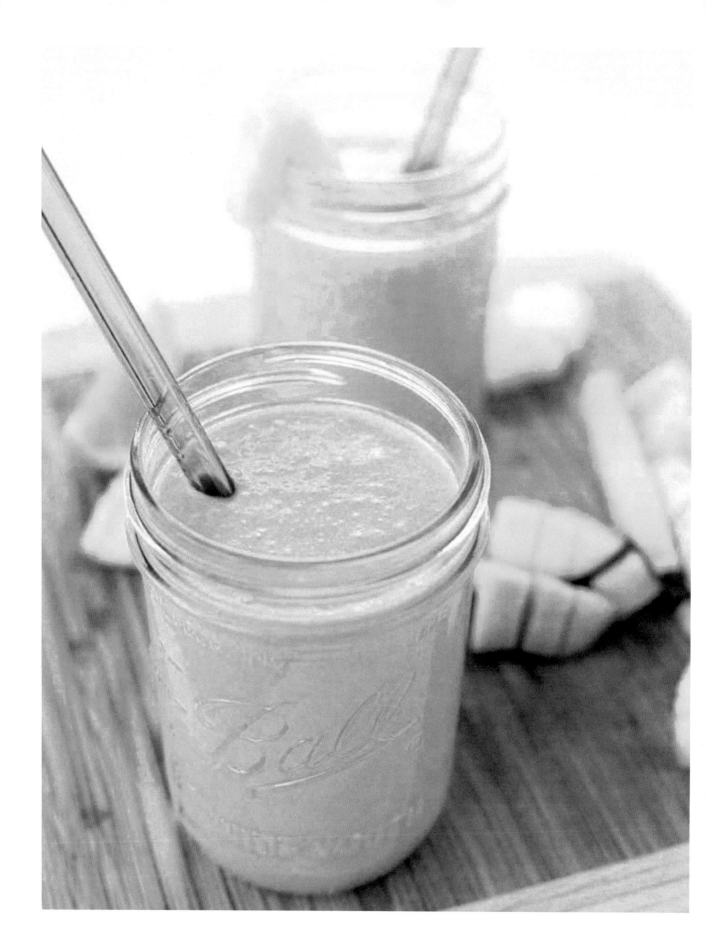

mango-coconut smoothie

INGREDIENTS:

2 cups fresh spinach leaves

1 cup frozen mango cubes

$^1/_2$ medium banana

$^3/_4$ cup light organic coconut milk
(canned)

juice of 1 orange

$^1/_2$ cup ice

DIRECTIONS:

Add all the ingredients to a blender and blend on high until smooth and creamy.

the palms

INGREDIENTS:

$^1/_2$ medium banana

1 cup frozen mango

$^1/_2$ cup frozen pineapple

1 tsp freshly grated ginger

$^3/_4$ cup light organic coconut milk

4 oz. coconut water

$^1/_2$ cup ice

DIRECTIONS:

Add all the ingredients to a blender and blend on high until smooth and creamy.

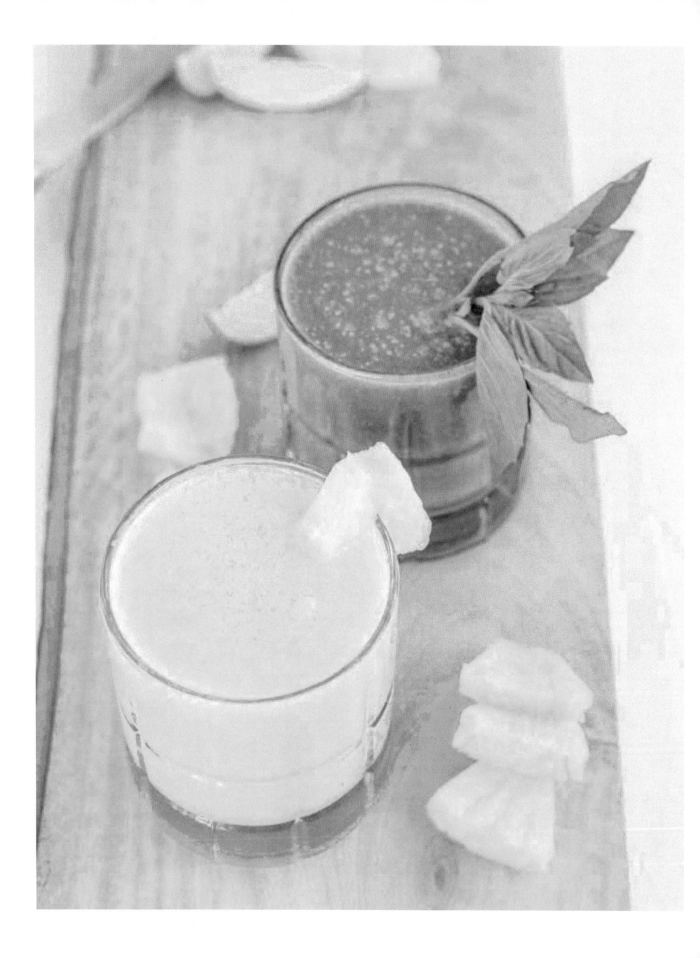

coconut coolada

INGREDIENTS:

1 cup coconut water
1 frozen packet Inner-Eco coconut
meat
5 pineapple chunks
juice of $\frac{1}{2}$ lime
1 tbsp. bee pollen

DIRECTIONS:

Add all the ingredients to a blender and blend on high until smooth and creamy.

hydrating smoothie

INGREDIENTS:

1 cup coconut water
juice of $\frac{1}{2}$ lime
2 handfuls spinach 4
basil leaves
5 pineapple chunks

DIRECTIONS:

Add all the ingredients to a blender and blend on high until smooth and creamy.

breakfast ideas

Breakfast is one of the hardest times of the day when trying to adapt to a new lifestyle. We have been trained to eat sweet foods and simple/complex carbohydrates for breakfast, such as whole-grain bars, cereals, waffles, pancakes, toaster pastries, bagels, muffins, granola, oatmeal, and a whole host of other on-the-go foods completely devoid of nutritional value.

One could look at the purpose of breakfast in a variety of ways, but, in spite of that, we are still going to have to shift our thinking away from the traditional "continental breakfast."

Breakfast is just that. It breaks the fast overnight. Intermittent fasting is a healthy and purposeful part of a daily and weekly diet. Fasting overnight is no different. It gives the bodily systems such as the liver, kidney, lymphatic system, and even the brain the ability to perform its natural metabolic processes and cleanse for the next day. The body does this without you having to do anything other than nourish it!

Upon waking, breakfast breaks that fast, but by using a variety of techniques, we can continue to assist the body with detoxification and carry that into the day.

The best morning cup is not a cup-of-joe but filled with lemon water and cayenne instead.

The capsaicin in cayenne is best known to boost metabolism, causing the body to produce extra heat and burn more calories for fuel.[176] Not only does it mirror coffee in that it starts the engine running, but it does so without any negative side effects.

Next on the list for the early morning routine would be AM juicing, either wheatgrass and green juice or some other form of tonic or elixir. We are still drinking liquids but not causing any stress on the digestive system or having blood sugar levels rise. We're at zero caffeine...and still keeping the body in balance.

About one-hour post juice, a fantastic digestive-supporting and nutrient-dense option would be to consume a smoothie. A smoothie can provide both the necessary vital fat for energy and focus and protein for muscle building and repair. The morning's juices, smoothies, and lemon water are an essential component to healthful living. The only foods consumed so far are the ones necessary for getting us through the busiest part of our day while providing us with energy and clarity.

For those who have a larger appetite or the desire to chew, a small salad or side of soup would be an optimal choice as this will hold the body over until post noon time where our HCL and digestive juices are high and ready to burn whatever we put into it.

As you can see, this morning line-up is far different than how we've been taught to eat, three square meals a day starting with simple carbs!

For a fresh start, a clear head, and a focused mind, the above schedule is worth trying out. There are different breakfast options to choose from in this section...some savory, some sweet, but none of them contain ingredients that will slow you down.

These foods will boost metabolism, fight aging, curb hunger, detoxify, nourish, hydrate, alkalize, and give the body energy.

They surely will do a body good!

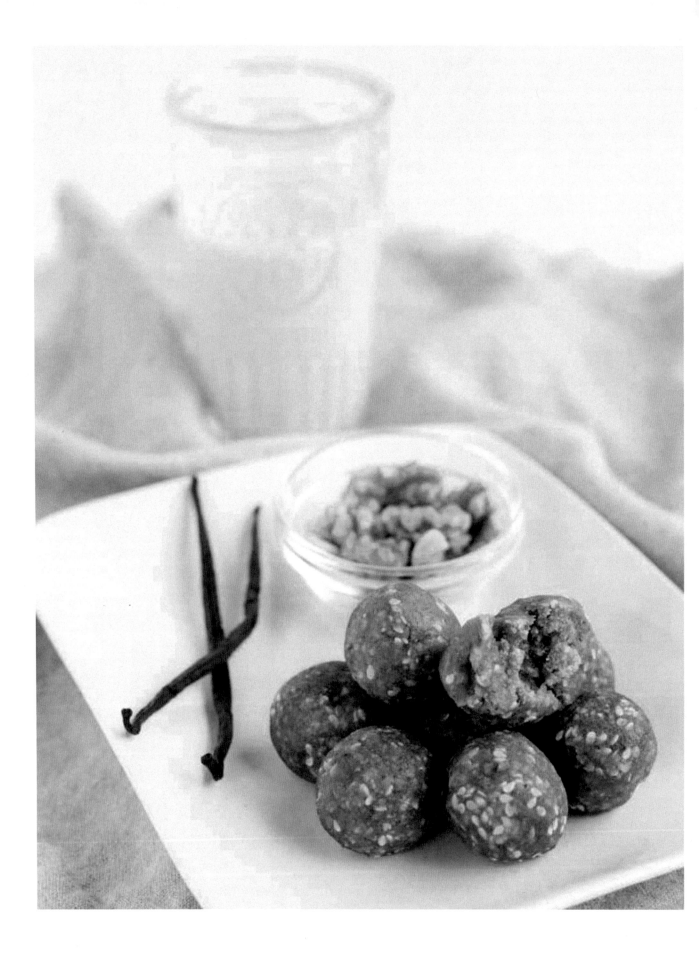

chocolate sesame energy bites

INGREDIENTS:

2 cups walnuts, soaked for 4 hours and rinsed

2 tbsp. raw cacao or cocoa powder

1 tbsp. vanilla

1/2 tsp. sweetener of choice

1/4 cup sesame seeds

1 tbsp. water to thin

High in protein and fats, walnuts and sesame seeds will give you the energy needed to start your day off right! Adjust any non-GMO sweetener to your liking. Not a fan of sugars, try soaking 2-3 pitted dates with your nuts and blend together, keeping the fiber intact with the plant. Or hey, why not make it paleo and omit the fruit/sugar altogether. Enjoy with your favorite nut mylk for breakfast....or even your favorite cup o' Joe! Being healthy doesn't mean 100% *all* the time!

DIRECTIONS:

1. Pulse walnuts in food processor until coarsely ground. Add water to thin as necessary.

2. Add raw cacao, sesame seeds, vanilla, and pulse until smooth.

3. Press mixture into a flat dish or roll into round balls.

4. Refrigerate or serve as is. Enjoy with your favorite nut milk for breakfast.

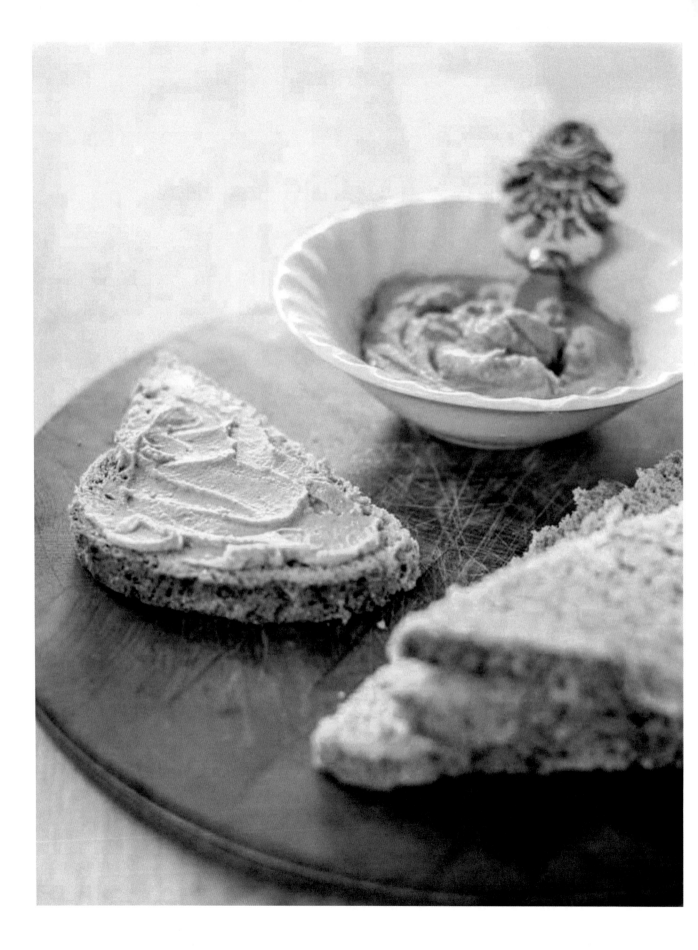

pumpkin pie spread

INGREDIENTS:

1 can organic pureed pumpkin (no sugar added)

⅓ cup coconut butter

2 tbsp. extra-virgin, unrefined coconut oil

1 tsp. pumpkin pie spice

2 tbsp. of your favorite sweetener

¼ tsp. Himalayan salt

Did you say the Paleo option again? You betcha! We're not a Paleo program, but we are definitely low to no grain! We offer in all of our recipes a sweetener of choice because sweetness is personal. If you want a sweet treat, there are numerous ways to make your treat sweet! Give organic stevia a try. Not a fan of stevia, then whole pitted dates work just as well or even monk fruit, a low-carb natural sugar. Another option to satisfy your taste is yacon syrup, one of the best sources of fructan and inulin (a fiber)!

DIRECTIONS:

1. Place all ingredients in a blender and puree until smooth.
2. Store pumpkin pie spice in a sealed container in the refrigerator.

For ease in spreading, take pumpkin pie spread out of the refrigerator 30 minutes prior to use.

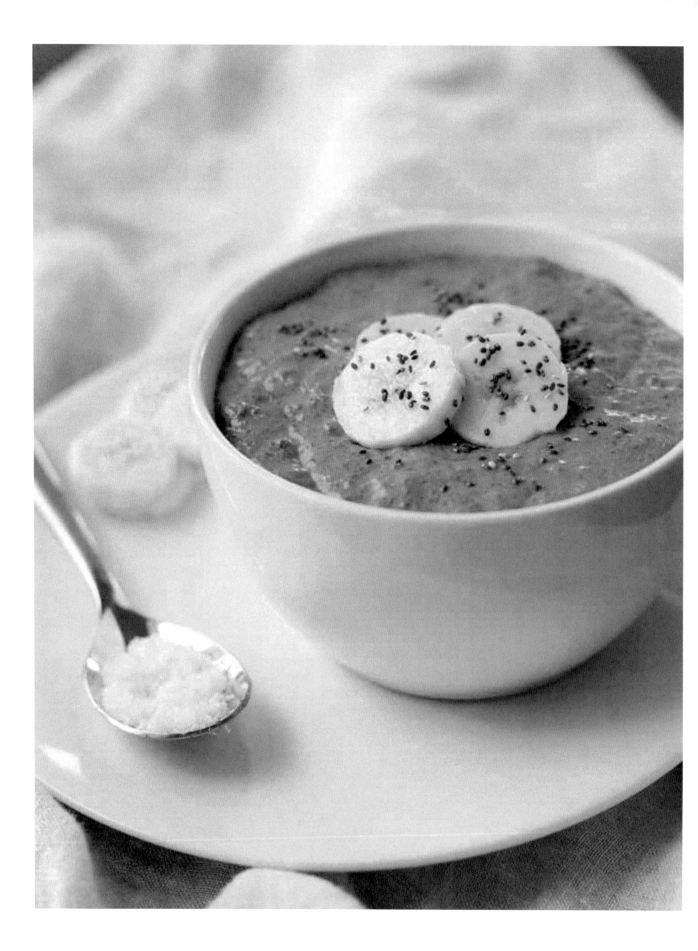

chocolate chia pudding

INGREDIENTS:

2-4 tablespoons ground chia seeds

1 can organic full fat coconut milk

2 tbsp. raw cacao

2 tbsp. sweetener of choice

Optional Additions:

pawpaw

lychees

soursop

star or jack fruit

bananas

Whether you like warm porridge or cold porridge, this is the healthiest porridge for you! You'll find the fat from the chia and coconut milk carry you throughout the morning while avoiding that caffeine or carbohydrate spike and crash. Best of all, it's healthy and delicious!

DIRECTIONS:

1. If using whole chia, grind the seeds in a blender with a grinder attachment like you would to grind coffee beans or grind in a coffee grinder.

2. Add the coconut milk to a medium saucepan and heat on low. You can omit this step if you want it to be a cold pudding.

3. Whisk the ground chia seeds into the liquid. Whisk again after a few minutes. Let cool.

4. Store in refrigerator for a few hours or overnight and serve with a drizzle of sweetener or your preferred fruit.

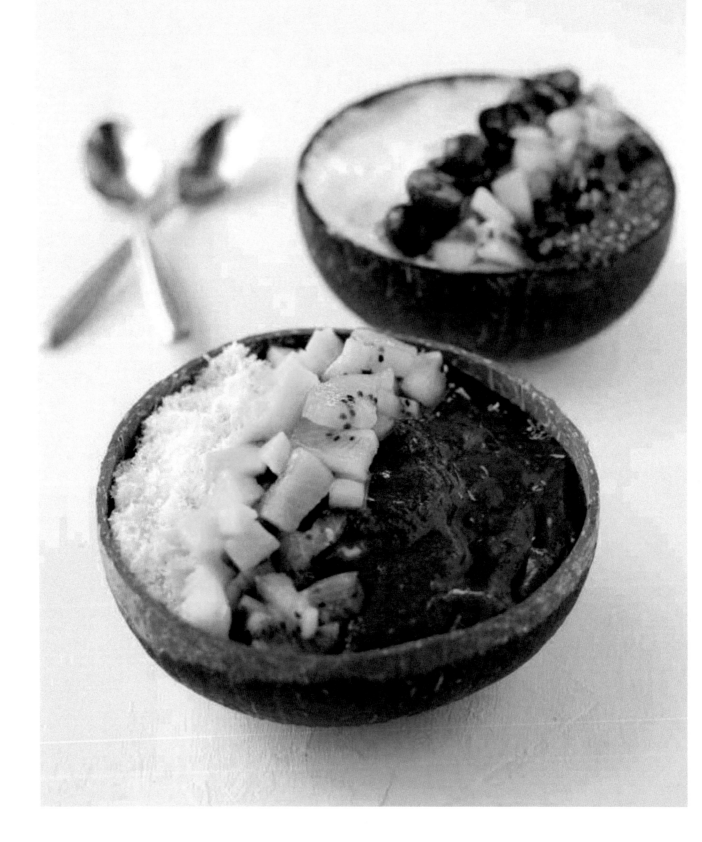

pitaya bowl

INGREDIENTS:

1 frozen pitaya packet or

1 cup frozen pitaya

½ cup unsweetened almond milk

1 tsp. ground yellow flax seeds

Top with:

Kiwi, mango and coconut flakes, fine

Beauty in a bowl. More for the sweet lover, these bowls are loaded with natural plant-based foods. All of the good stuff, none of the bad!

DIRECTIONS:

1. Add frozen pitaya, 1/2 cup almond milk, and blend in a high-speed blender until desired consistency making sure your base is thick enough to support toppings. Adjust mixture accordingly.

2. Top with toppings listed or using your favorite fruits

coconut bowl

INGREDIENTS:

2 frozen packs Inner-Eco young green coconut meat

4 oz. coconut water

2 drops sweet leaf stevia vanilla cream (optional)

Top with:

Chia seeds, kiwi, pomegranate seeds, and a frozen blend of cherries and blueberries

DIRECTIONS:

1. Add frozen coconut packets, coconut water, and vanilla drops into a high-speed blender. Blend until smooth and creamy or desired consistency making sure the base is thick enough to support toppings. Adjust accordingly.

2. Top with chia seeds, pomegranate, cherries, and blueberries.

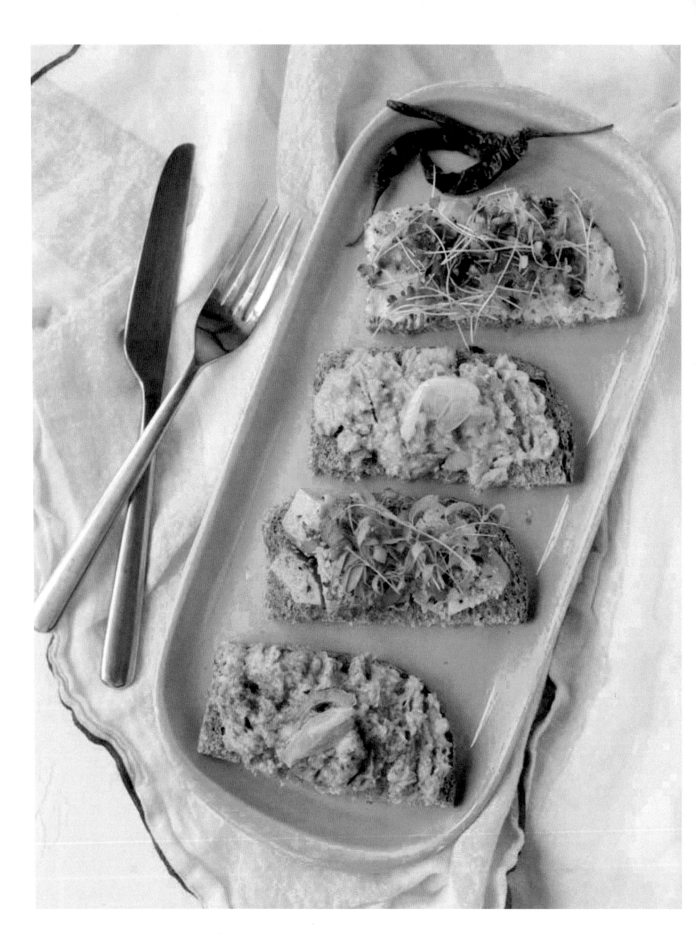

avo toast

INGREDIENTS:

1 medium-sized ripe avocado

1 tbsp. freshly squeezed lemon juice

Optional additions:

Hemp seeds

Olive, truffle, or flax oil

cilantro

pinch of cayenne pepper

red pepper flakes

broccoli microgreens

Vegenaise mayonnaise

Red onion

sea salt and pepper to taste

We do have a bread we like, but it doesn't contain processed grains. Instead, the grains used in Ezekiel bread have been sprouted, making it a flourless bread (remember we call it "the old fashioned way"), leaving the nutrients and fiber intact. Ezekiel bread is made without preservatives, so it's best kept stored in the freezer and taken out upon use. Enjoy the many varieties they have to offer. Want to skip the carbs from the bread? No problem. Remove the avocado pit and put your optional additions into the center of the avocado and enjoy!

DIRECTIONS:

1. Remove pit and scoop avocado meat into a large bowl. Mash with a fork or mashed potato masher.

2. Spread evenly over your favorite morning slice of bread. There are a variety of non-preserved sprouted breads made with wholesome ingredients found in the freezer section of most grocery stores.

3. Top with a variety of toppings and find your favorite mix!

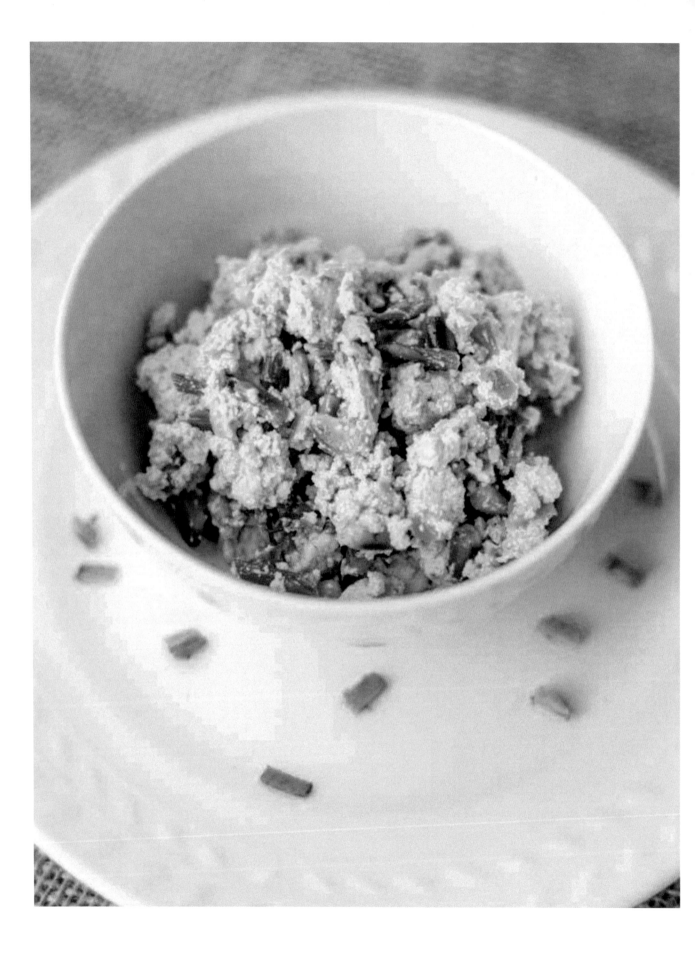

tofu scramble with asparagus and basil

INGREDIENTS:

2 tbsp. olive oil

1/2 cup finely diced shallots

1 cup asparagus tips, cut into bite-size pieces

1 block of organic non-GMO extra-firm tofu

6-8 sundried tomatoes ready to eat or soaked in water

4 tbsp. nutritional yeast

2 tbsp. Nama Shoyu or wheat-free tamari

1 tsp. turmeric powder

A pinch of sea salt & freshly ground black pepper

Sliced basil leaves

I'm not a huge fan of tofu in certain dishes, but keeping dairy and meat products out of my fridge, I am! In order to get the texture of eggs without the use of faux meat products, this tofu recipe certainly mimics that feeling. I'm a savory lover, so this is right up my alley for a delicious breakfast.

DIRECTIONS:

1. Remove tofu from packaging. Drain tofu and set on a plate lined with paper towels. Press to remove excess water.

2. Add oil to sauté pan on medium heat. Add shallots and reduce heat to low. Sauté until fragrant and translucent.

3. Add asparagus, sun-dried tomatoes, and crumbled tofu. Cook on medium-high heat for 3 minutes.

4. Add nutritional yeast, tamari, sea salt, turmeric, and black pepper, toss and turn heat off.

Before serving, add a handful of fresh basil.

meatless meals

PLATE SHIFTING

What is Plate Shifting? Plate Shifting is a concept that attempts to introduce new foods to the plate not found in the category of meat, dairy, grains, or fruits but in the category of vegetables, more specifically, leafy greens. The shift comes in direct proportion to the meat. In order to make more room for the vegetables, something needs to move, and that means the meat. The suggestion is for the meat to be eaten in smaller portions, more aptly to the size of the palm of your hand. The purpose of plate shifting is to achieve a healthier way of eating by introducing a vegetable side dish while minimizing the meat portion. Using plate shifting as a first step towards minimizing animal protein is more appealing than radically adjusting the diet by expecting the immediate elimination of meat.

WHY GO MEATLESS?

Going meatless may reduce your risk of chronic preventable conditions like cancer, cardiovascular disease, diabetes, and obesity. Going meatless can also help reduce our carbon footprint and save precious resources like fossil fuels and fresh water.

So, if going meatless for you is not an option, try Meatless Monday instead and make it a practice! A weekly reminder to restart healthy habits encourages success!

If you feel by going meatless, you will be missing out on the day's protein needed for energy and muscle rebuilding, have no fear. There are numerous plant-based foods that contain the right quantity of eight essential amino acids to satisfy a complete protein!

Try incorporating these high protein plant foods every Monday:

Almonds	Mung Bean Sprouts
Lentils	Rye
Sesame	Soybeans (tofu,
Sunflower Seeds	tempeh)
Chia	Walnuts
Buckwheat (doesn't	Amaranth
contain wheat)	

Want a complete protein? Add these foods into your diet:

Spirulina	Sunflower
Hemp Seeds	Pea
Quinoa	Wheatgrass

The push for plants stems from the notion that meat is highly acidic and promotes inflammation, especially red meat. Meat is also high in cholesterol (as is chicken, even the white breast). Since we eat our meat cooked, the natural digestive enzymes found in abundance in raw or fermented meat is killed off. The digestive process involved in breaking down animal proteins takes an arduous toll on our digestive system.

High-protein may also bring on gout, increase cholesterol and triglyceride levels, stress the heart, may damage the liver, cause constipation due to the excessive use of fiber-poor animal foods, can wash minerals and vitamins out of the body, and increase the risk of certain types of cancer.

The American diet is overloaded with meat consumption. So by giving Meatless Monday a try, you are not only benefitting yourself, the environment but the animals too.

If I eliminate meat from my diet, where will I get my iron?

If one increases the consumption of plant-based foods, it is easy to consume more iron. These plant-based foods offer the most amount of iron:

Lentils	Beets
Mung Bean	Parsley
Sesame	Sunflower
Almonds	

Additionally, more consumption of dietary fiber from whole foods and beans provides for better elimination. When trying to obtain iron from plant-based foods, the absorption is best when consumed with vitamin C.[177, 178]

Since our digestive tract is designed to consume vegetables, fruits, seeds, and nuts, it is our recommendation for optimal digestive health.

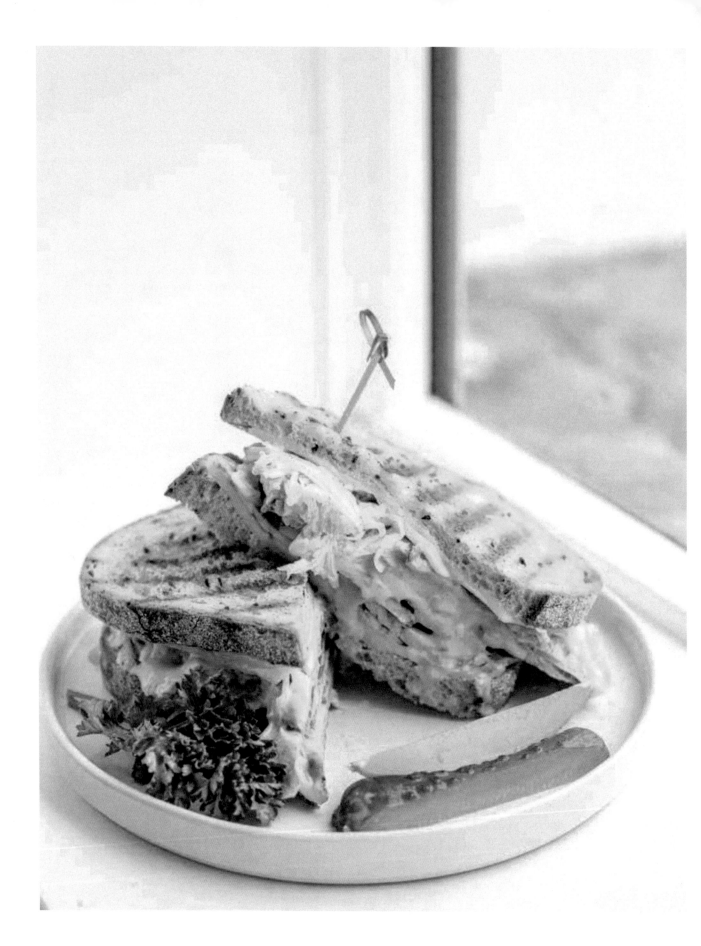

tempeh reuben

INGREDIENTS:

8 oz. unflavored tempeh (soy, adzuki, or other bean), sliced into strips

$1/4$ cup Bragg's liquid aminos

1 onion, quartered

2 cloves garlic, peeled

1 bay leaf

Raw fermented, plain sauerkraut

Traditional rye seeded bread

$1/4$ cup Vegenaise

3 tbsp. relish

2 tbsp. ketchup

Vegan swiss or Monterey Jack Cheese

Vegan butter

We wanted to start out changing up dinner meals with comfort foods. What better way to transition away from meats than to stick with foods that give us that very same "satisfying" feeling after each bite. This tempeh Reuben certainly does the trick! For best results, it's important to get traditional rye bread with seeds and lather up the outer sides with vegan butter like Earth Balance. Be sure to heat in a panini maker. If you don't have one, no problem! Just heat in a pan as if you were making a grilled cheese!

DIRECTIONS:

1. Slice tempeh. Add to medium-sized sauté pan with Bragg's liquid aminos, onion quarters, garlic, and bay leaf. Simmer for 10 minutes until softened and aromatic. Cover and let cool.

2. Prepare Thousand Island dressing by mixing together mayonnaise, relish, and ketchup in a small bowl.

3. Spread vegan butter on one side of each piece of bread. Set in sauté pan or panini maker to brown. Layer with thousand island dressing, sauerkraut, tempeh, and cheese. Layer other side of bread with thousand island dressing and combine. Pan fry or heat until cheese is melted, turning once.

4. Slice in half and serve with your favorite naturally fermented pickle.

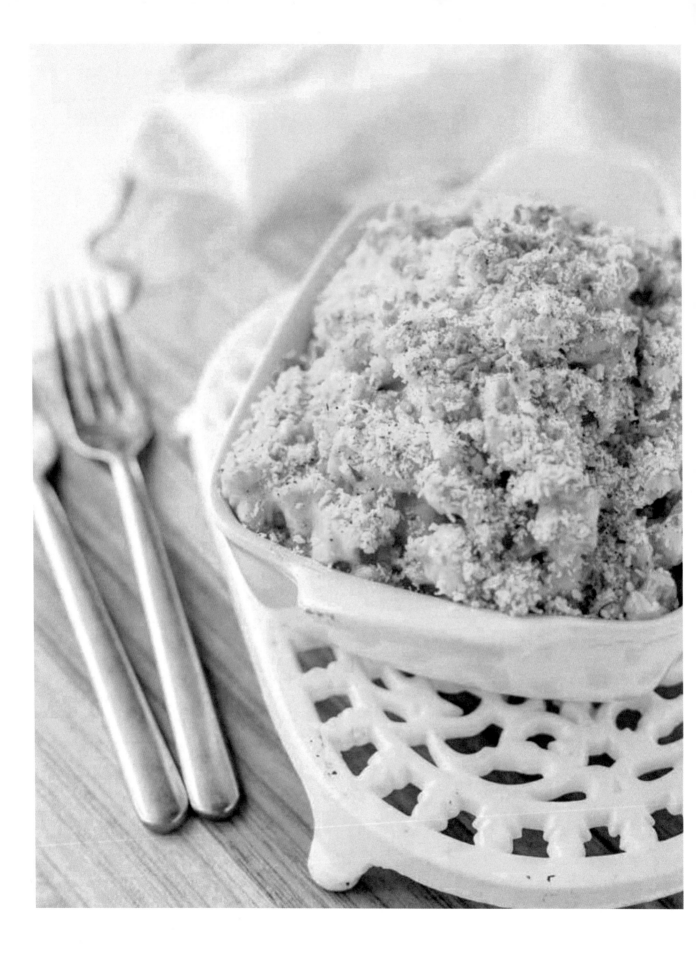

vegan mac-n-cheez

INGREDIENTS:

1 box pasta shells, cook as directed

2 organic Russett potatoes - skin peeled and cubed (soak cubes for 1 hour)

$\frac{1}{2}$ cup carrots (approx. 2 large carrots)

2/3 cup red onions coarsely chopped

1 $\frac{1}{2}$ cup cashews (soaked for 1 hour)

$\frac{1}{2}$ cup vegan butter

1 tsp. Dijon mustard (preferably Maille)

2 tbsp. lemon

3 cups water

4 cloves garlic (peeled)

$\frac{1}{2}$ tsp. ground turmeric (for color only)

$\frac{1}{4}$ tsp. paprika (for color only)

Salt and pepper to taste

Italian seasoned Panko breadcrumbs

Mac-n-cheez without fillers or artificial ingredients? You bet! It's creamy and delicious!

DIRECTIONS:

1. Set pot of water on high to boil. Follow directions on pasta box and cook for only half that time. Drain in colander and rinse with cold water.

2. Peel potato skins, chop into cubes, and let potato soak covered in water for 1 hour, rinsing occasionally.

3. Soak cashews in a separate bowl, covered with water for 1 hour. Rinse thoroughly once soaked.

4. Peel carrot skins and chop into half-moons

5. Coarsely chop red onion.

6. Juice lemon. Set aside.

7. Next, add to blender: vegan butter, dijon mustard, lemon, soaked cashews, and set aside.

8. Steam in large sauté pan: rinsed potatoes, carrots, onions, water, garlic until tender and water is reduced, leaving a creamy consistency.

9. Add turmeric, paprika, salt, pepper, and turn off heat.

10. Let stand 5 min to cool. Add sauté mixture to existing ingredients in blender and blend on high until creamy and smooth.

11. Add cheezy sauce and pasta to bowl and mix together.

12. Transfer cheezy mac to a baking dish and top with Italian seasoned panko breadcrumbs.

13. Bake in oven at 350°F for 30 minutes.

Serve hot and Enjoy!

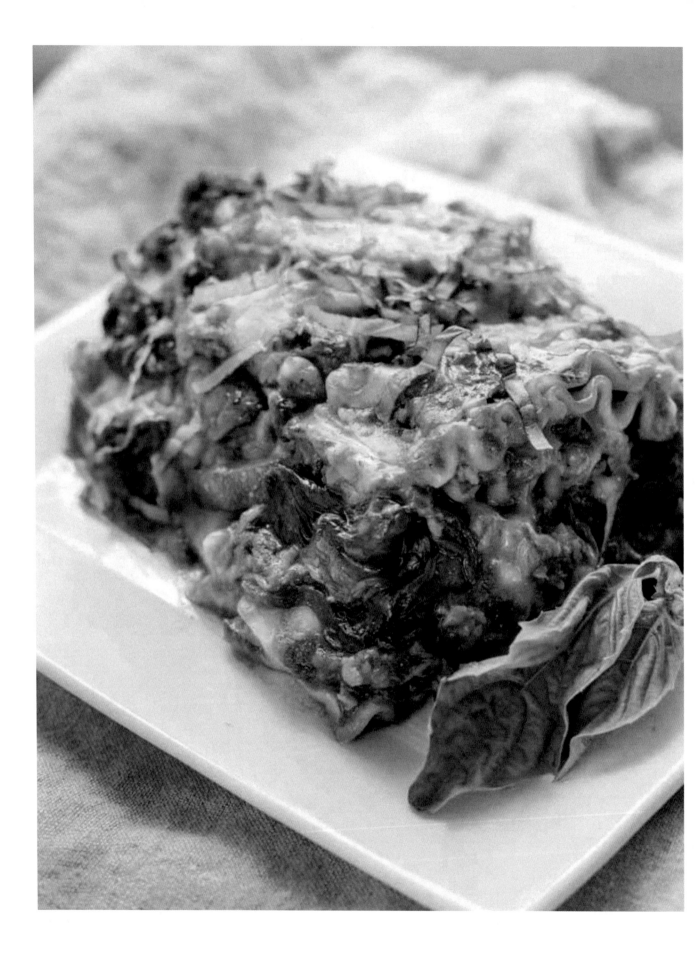

vegan lasagna with spinach, mushroom, and zucchini

WHAT YOU'LL NEED:

16 oz. box lasagna shells

2, 8" x 4" x 2" glass baking dishes

INGREDIENTS:

4 oz. white button mushrooms, sliced

1 small zucchini, quartered

2 tbsp. olive oil

8 oz. package baby spinach

Meatless ground beef (we used Gardein, but there are countless others)

Vegan mozzarella shreds (we used Violife)

Vegan parmesan (we used Follow Your Heart parmesan shredded cheese)

32 oz. ready-made marinara sauce

4 oz. basil leaves

DIRECTIONS:

1. Remove meatless ground beef from freezer the night before and store in refrigerator.

2. Prepare the pasta: Boil all lasagna pasta sheets al dente. Prepare ice bath for lasagna sheets. Turn heat off. Remove lasagna sheets with tongs and set in ice bath.

3. Prepare the vegetables: In a large skillet over medium heat, warm the olive oil. Once shimmering, add the mushrooms, zucchini, spinach and package of meatless ground beef. Cook until wilted and most of the moisture is gone. Remove vegetables from heat and set in a small holed colander or large sieve to drain excess liquid. Season with salt and pepper.

4. Preheat oven to 425°F.

5. Layer the bottom of both dishes and spread tomato sauce evenly over the bottom. Layer lasagna noodles (cut ends to fit) and overlap if necessary. Top with more tomato sauce. Add strained vegetable mixture Layer with the mozzarella shreds, parmesan shreds, and add another layer of lasagna sheets. Repeat steps above – tomato sauce, veggie mixture, mozzarella, and parmesan. Add more sauce and top with parmesan.

6. Rub olive oil on aluminum foil before wrapping taut around the edges of the glass baking jar.

7. Bake covered for 25 minutes, then remove cover, rotate glass by 180°, and continue to cook for about 5-10 more minutes until steaming and corners are bubbling.

8. Remove from oven and set out to cool for about 10 minutes before serving.

9. Top with fine basil threads.

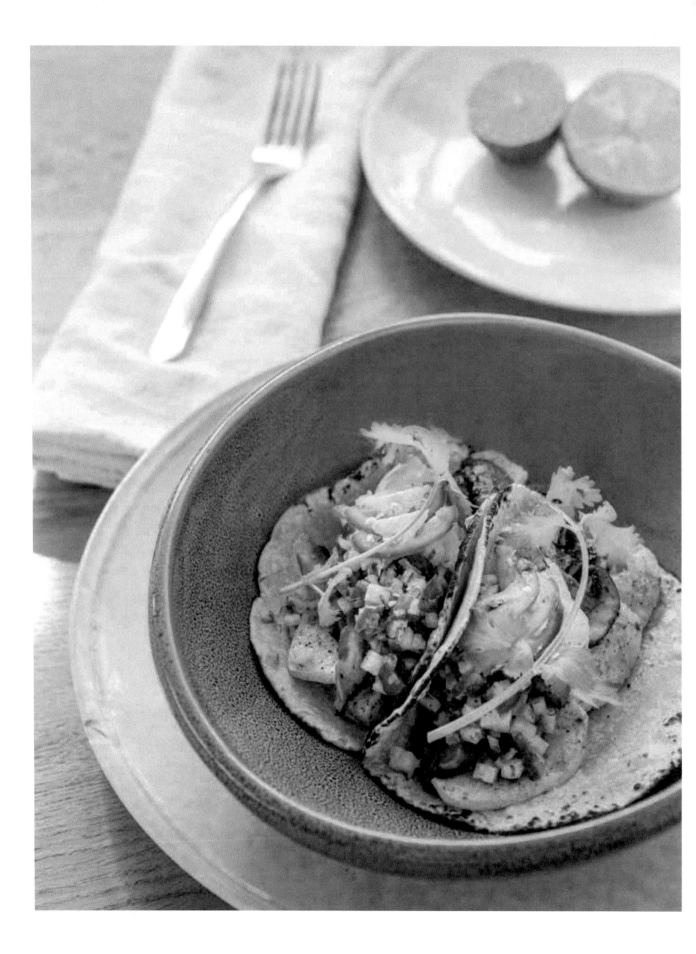

chayote and kabocha tacos with jicama slaw & pepita cream

INGREDIENTS:

Jicama Pico de Gallo, pg. 267

Pepita cream, pg. 267

Mushroom marinade:

1 cup tamari, gluten-free soy sauce

$1/2$ tsp. cumin

1 tbsp. chopped cilantro

$1/2$ tbsp. onion powder

$1/2$ tbsp. garlic powder

$1/2$ cup vegan Worcestershire sauce

2 tbsp. olive oil

1 chayote squash, peeled and cut into thin strips

$1/2$ kabocha squash, seeded and sliced into thin strips

$1/2$ lb. oyster mushrooms

1 jalapeno, sliced into rounds

Cilantro

Organic corn & flour tortillas

Chayote (pronounced chi-yote) is a type of summer squash native to Mexico. It has the crunchy texture of a pear with a mild cucumber-like flavor. It is high in antioxidants, vitamins B and C, potassium, and even amino acids! Here we roast it to complement the bacopa marinated mushrooms. These tacos give the feel of eating meat, leaving you to wonder if it's 100% plant-based!

DIRECTIONS:

1. Soak pepitas about 8 hours prior to prepping tacos.
2. Make the mushroom marinade. In a medium-sized sauté pan on medium heat, add marinade and sliced oyster mushrooms. Once softened, remove from heat and let stand.
3. Meanwhile, heat oven to 350°F. Line a sheet pan with oiled kabocha and chayote squash. Sprinkle with salt and pepper. Cook until just tender, approximately 20 minutes.
4. Prepare jicama pico de gallo and set aside in small bowl to dress tacos.
5. Prepare pepita cream and set aside in small bowl to dress tacos.
6. Slice jalapeno and pull cilantro leaves from stems.
7. Warm tortillas in a towel in the oven set to OFF.
8. Layer tortillas with squashes, pico de gallo, pepita cream, and top with jalapeño rounds and cilantro.

Serve warm.

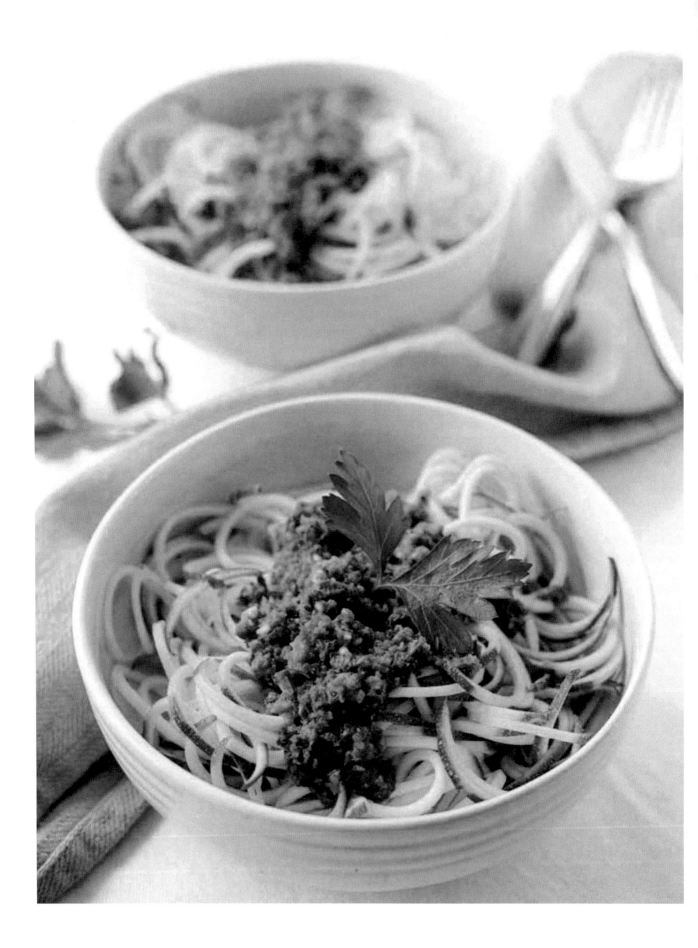

zucchini spirals with cool red pepper marinara

INGREDIENTS:

4 cups chopped red peppers

1/2 red onion roughly chopped

1 bunch fresh basil, chopped

1 clove garlic

1 tbsp. fresh oregano

2 tsp. fresh thyme

1/4 cup extra virgin olive oil

1 tsp. fresh-squeezed lemon juice

4 medium-sized zucchini

dash Nama Shoyu

A no-cook, essentially raw dish, will satisfy like no other! Red peppers are used in this dish to keep with Food Combining principles you'll find at the very end of this book. Tomatoes, in the holistic health world, are considered a fruit and not a vegetable. Red peppers pack the most nutrition because they've sat on the vine the longest, hence the term vine-ripened! And if it's been vine-ripened, it's better for you! The life span of a pepper goes from green to yellow to orange then red. Red peppers, by comparison, contain 11 times more beta-carotene than their former self, and one and a half times more vitamin C.[179] Zucchini is rich in antioxidants, so we thought we'd skip the pasta on that note!

DIRECTIONS:

1. Press zucchini through a spiralizer to make your "spaghetti."

2. In a food processor, combine all ingredients above except for zucchini.

3. Mix marinara in with zucchini pasta.

Serve at room temperature and enjoy!

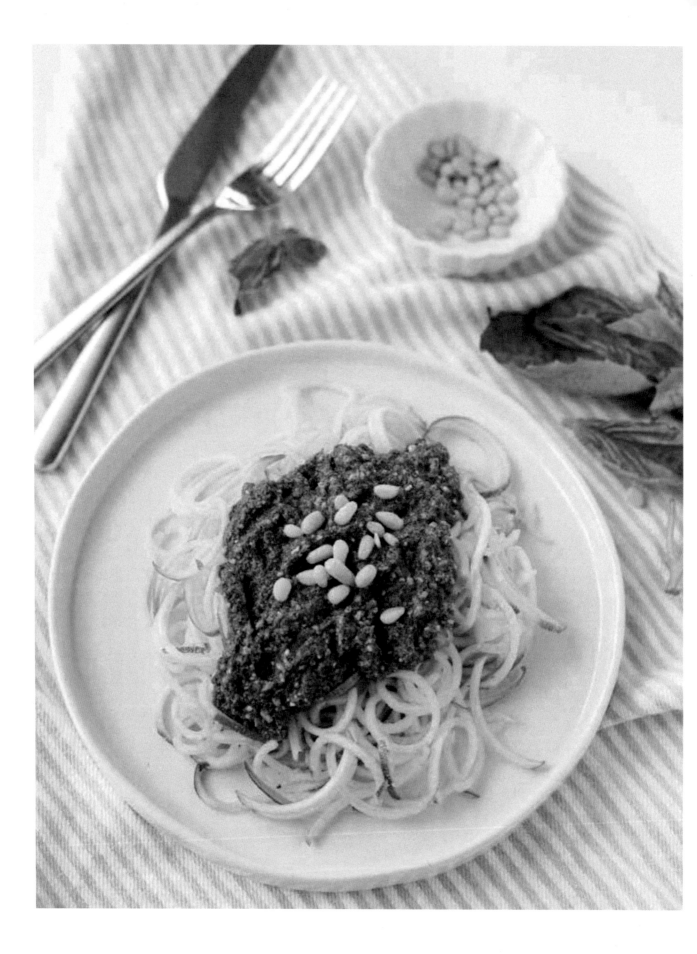

zucchini noodles with basil pesto

INGREDIENTS:

For the pesto:

Blend in a small food processor or blender

4 cups fresh basil leaves

juice from one fresh lemon (approx. $1/4$ - $1/2$ cup)

3 garlic cloves finely chopped

$1/2$ c. pine nuts

4 tablespoons olive oil

Himalayan salt and pepper

For the zucchini pasta:

4 medium zucchini

Sweet basil, the common use in Italian dishes, offers more than just a delectable flavor. The purported health benefits of basil include: reducing memory loss associated with stress and aging, reduce depression related to chronic stress, reduce blood pressure in people with hypertension and protect against aspirin's damage to the gut lining and preventing certain cancers, including breast, colon, and pancreas.[180]

Eat warmed or at room temperature. If heating, sauté zucchini in a little bit of olive oil and drain moisture before serving. Enjoy another heart-healthy, heart-warming meal!

DIRECTIONS:

1. Remove basil leaves from stems and set aside.
2. Place basil, olive oil, and garlic in food processor or blender and pulse until a paste. Add in $1/2$ of lemon juice and pine nuts and process until smooth.
3. Add in remaining lemon juice.
4. Season with salt and pepper.
5. Press zucchini through a spiralizer to make zucchini "spaghetti" or shave zucchini over a cheese grater.

Serve at room temperature.

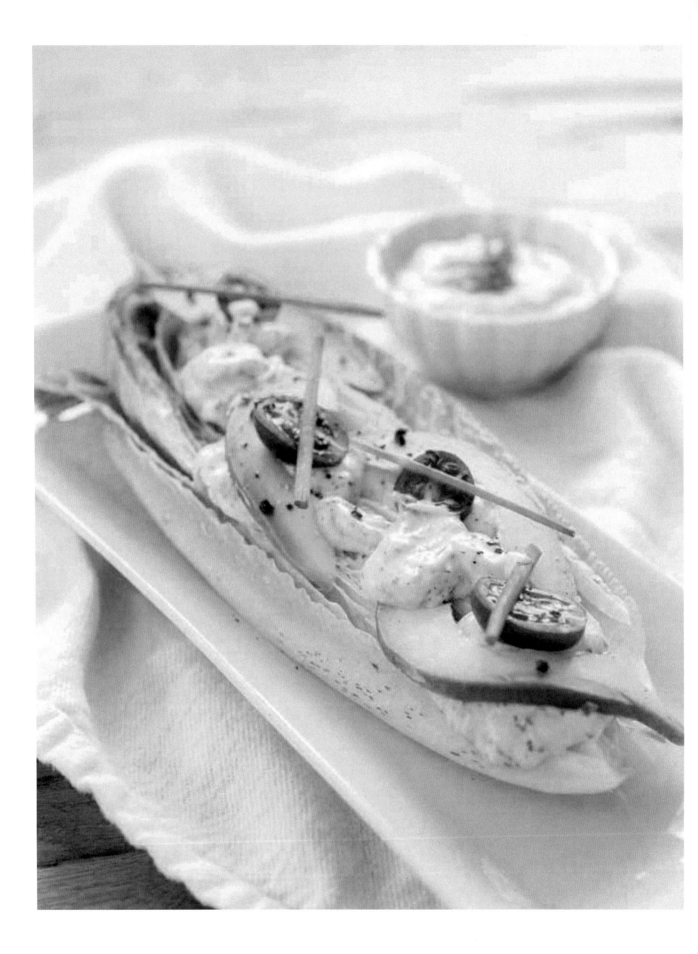

dressings

Salad dressings are easy to make and can last for several weeks in the refrigerator, depending on what has been added to your dressings. Fruits and veggies will give it a shorter shelf life, but you should be able to keep dressings for up to 7-14 days.

When it comes down to flavor and health, bottling your own is best.

Current trends are moving away from inflammatory and genetically modified vegetable oils like soybean and vegetable oils. Oils commonly used in bottled dressings are highly refined, turning your healthy salad into a horror.

There are plenty of healthy alternatives. Try these on for size:

Olive	Flax
Hemp	Avocado
Coconut	Grapeseed

The key to making a dressing is offsetting the oils with acid. Acid can come from citrus fruits, vinegars, and mustards.

Vinegar used in salad dressings slows digestion, so if embarking on a holistic healing diet, a better option would be to use lemon or any of the low sugar fruits found in the citrus family.

Asian dressings are a fantastic use for bitter greens, cabbages, and sea veggie dishes. The sweet and salty flavors of these dressings are a perfect complement to the bitter and pungent flavor of these greens. Many of the Asian dressings call for sesame tahini or miso paste and can be offset with lemon, lime, or rice wine vinegar.

Make as much or as little as needed, store in glass containers, and you have a perfect "go-to" dressing made from the freshest ingredients!

buttermilk ranch dressing

INGREDIENTS:

$\frac{1}{2}$ cup dairy-free buttermilk (2 tsp. fresh lemon juice added to $\frac{1}{2}$ cup organic plain soy milk)

1 cup Vegenaise

1 tsp. dried dill

$\frac{1}{4}$ cup freshly chopped parsley

4 tbsp. freshly chopped chives

1 tsp. crushed garlic

$\frac{1}{2}$ tsp. sea salt

$\frac{1}{4}$ tsp. freshly ground black pepper

1/8 tsp. cayenne

$\frac{1}{2}$ tsp. white vinegar

You may not be a believer, but you will be after you try this dressing. It rivals real buttermilk dressing and may *possibly* taste *even* better! For the best meatless meal, put a dollop of dressing on a southwest veggie burger. We love Sunshine Burgers! Top with red pepper, hearty romaine, and spinach, and you've got yourself a nutrient-dense, satisfying meat-free, dairy-free meal right before your very eyes!

DIRECTIONS:

1. Mix lemon juice and soy milk and set aside to curdle for 10 minutes. For a more sour flavor, leave at room temperature overnight.

2. Crush or finely dice garlic, chop parsley, and chives. Add to a medium-sized bowl. Mix in Vegenaise and dried dill.

3. Add cayenne, white vinegar, vegan buttermilk to mix. Top with salt and pepper.

Dressing can be stored in refrigerator for up to 10-14 days.

Enjoy on your favorite southwest salad!

meyer lemon vinaigrette

INGREDIENTS:

3 tablespoons fresh Meyer lemon juice

3 tablespoons olive oil

salt and black pepper to taste

DIRECTIONS:

1. Whisk all ingredients together.

Dressing can be stored up to one week if it lasts that long!

miso peanut ginger dressing

INGREDIENTS:

2 tbsp. Ume Plum vinegar

6 tbsp. water

2 tablespoons mellow white miso

1 tablespoon agave (or other sweetener)

1 tablespoon mirin (Japanese Sweet white wine)

1-1$\frac{1}{2}$ tbsps. finely chopped peeled fresh ginger

1 tbsp. smooth peanut butter (substitute Sun Butter or organic sesame tahini if peanut allergy)

DIRECTIONS:

1. Blend in a blender or whisk together to avoid separation.

Can be stored for up to one week.

japanese style ginger dressing

INGREDIENTS:

1 cup peeled, roughly chopped carrots

1/4 cup chopped sweet white onion

2 tbsp. ginger minced

1 tbsp. sweetener of choice

1/4 cup Nama Shoyu or organic soy sauce

1/2 cup rice vinegar

1/2 tsp. salt

1/2 cup organic raw sesame oil

1/4 cup organic grapeseed oil

DIRECTIONS:

1. Blend ingredients all together in a high-speed blender.

Can be stored for up to one week.

shallot vinaigrette

INGREDIENTS:

1/4 c. olive oil

1 shallot, minced

2 tablespoons good quality red wine vinegar

1 tablespoon chopped fresh parsley

salt and pepper, to taste

DIRECTIONS:

1. Cook the shallots under tender and translucent.

2. Let cool.

3. In a high-speed blender, combine the shallot mixture with the remaining ingredients and blend on high.

Can be stored up to one week in the refrigerator.

roasted cherry tomato vinaigrette

INGREDIENTS:

1-pint organic or heirloom cherry tomatoes (not grape)

3 tbsp. olive oil, plus 1 tbsp.

1 shallot, finely chopped

1 tbsp. red wine vinegar

2 tbsp. chives (garnish)

Salt and pepper to taste

Directions:

1. Rinse, pat dry, then score cherry tomatoes.
2. Pre-heat oven to 350°F.
3. In a baking pan, add the tomatoes, shallot, and olive oil in the oven for 20 minutes.
4. Remove from oven and let cool. Once cool, remove tomato skins.
5. Add tomatoes, their juices, and red wine vinegar to a high-speed blender adding 1 tbsp. oil while blending to emulsify dressing.

Store in refrigerator for up to one week.

remoulade

INGREDIENTS:

1 cup vegan mayonnaise (Vegenaise)

1 tbsp. ketchup

1 tbsp. Dijon mustard (preferably Maille)

1 tsp. hot sauce

1 tsp. vegan Worcestershire sauce

Juice from 1 lemon

2 tsp. small capers

2 tsp. chopped shallot

2 tsp. chopped curly parsley

2 tsp. chopped red bell pepper

DIRECTIONS:

1. Place all rémoulade ingredients in a food processor and mix well. Set aside or store, covered, in the refrigerator for up to 1 week.
2. We use this remoulade as a dressing for crab cakes and accompanying salad. It's more than just a sauce!

fishless fridays - sea veggies

Sea veggies?

The second part of our meatless meals section is what we call our Fishless Fridays, which instead adds a significant amount of sea vegetables, known as seaweeds! All plants of the sea, like nori, wakame, kombu, dulse, arame, and Irish moss are multicellular algae. Some are green, others are brown, or red, and some are even translucent!

Seaweeds take up the majority of their nutrients from the medium they live in; seawater. They absorb nutrients directly into their tissues. There are over 79 minerals and trace elements in seaweed, including a significant amount of iodine necessary for optimal thyroid production. They are high in iodine and contain minerals, protein, and lignans, plant compounds with cancer-protective properties.

Seaweeds are ancient superfoods that are loaded with nutrition! In fact, the phytonutrients present in them are so concentrated that you only need to eat a small amount to get their health benefits. Most health food stores will either carry a variety of dried seaweeds in bulk or ready-to-use seaweed salad mixes that are kept hydrated and in salt in a plastic bag.

The toxicity risks of sea vegetables can be controlled by purchasing certified organic. They are easy to find as they can be purchased online and shipped. Once at home, store them in the pantry and reconstitute with filtered water when ready to use. Three personal favorites are Maine Coast Sea Veggies and SeaVegi™ brands. My favorite seaweed mix comes dried and is sold by SeaSnax.

So, what seaweeds do I familiarize myself with?

Let's start with **nori**, the one you have probably tried if you've ever gone out for sushi. Nori is rich in iron, potassium, magnesium, vitamin A, C, B2, and of course, iodine. It's also a good source of protein.

Wakame is another one you might have encountered since it's most commonly used in miso soup that is also served in Japanese restaurants. Wakame is high in B vitamins and essential fatty acids, which means it's very good for your skin.

Kombu, a brownish-green sea vegetable, is used to treat thyroid conditions and is very rich in minerals and folate.

Dulse has a beautiful deep rosy-purple color and is also commonly added to soups or, in a powder form, used as a thickening agent. It's exceptionally high in iron, magnesium, beta carotene, and protein!

Arame is a mild tasting sea vegetable that can be added to salads and almost anything else you wish to try it with. The dark brownish strands are rich in calcium, iron, zinc, manganese, folate, and vitamins A and K.

Irish moss is most commonly used to thicken foods, especially desserts. It's yellowish-brown and is rich in vitamin A, minerals, and protein but especially rich in sulfur, which means it's good for decalcification.

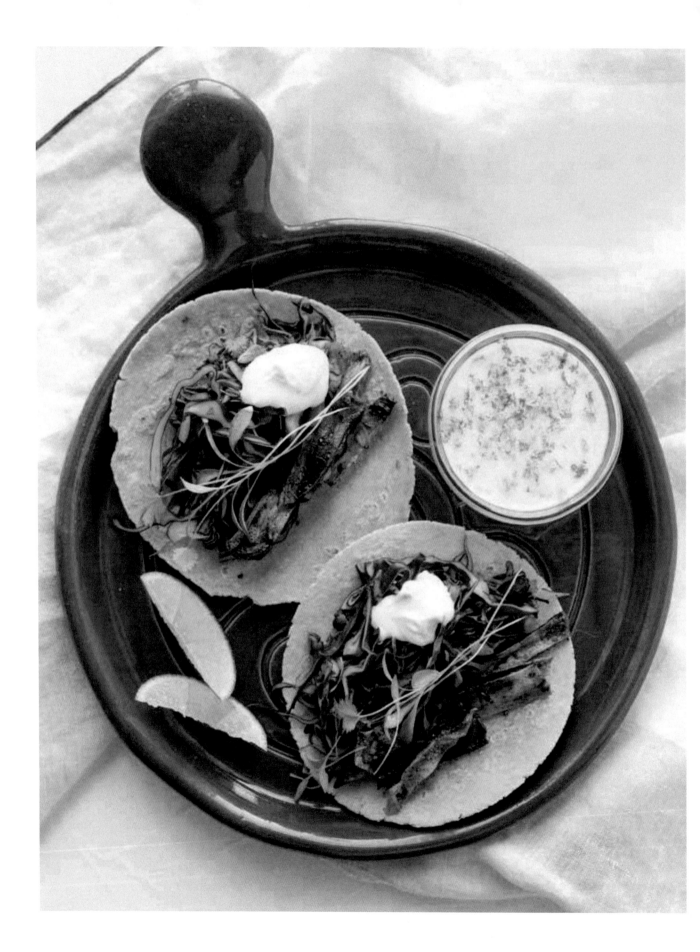

jackfruit tacos with cabbage slaw and coconut lime crema

INGREDIENTS:

Fresh jackfruit, sliced at an angle.

For the blackening seasoning:

1 ½ tsp. onion powder

1 tsp. smoked paprika, garlic powder, dried thyme, black pepper

½ tsp. cayenne pepper

For the cabbage slaw:

½ small purple cabbage thinly sliced

1 14.5 oz. can drained, rinsed black beans

Juice from one lime

½ cup cilantro, leaves only

Salt and pepper

Coconut lime crema, pg. 266

Organic corn and flour mini tortillas

Organic canola oil

Cast iron pan

The flesh of young unripe fruit, or green jackfruit, has a texture similar to pulled pork and is extremely versatile in cooking. Instead of tackling this monstrous and sticky fruit, the most convenient way to prep jackfruit is to purchase brined in a can.

DIRECTIONS:

1. Prepare coconut lime crema from pg. 266 and set in refrigerator to thicken.

2. For the cabbage slaw: Cut cabbage in half. Cut and remove white stem by cutting in a triangle. Slice cabbage at an angle, cutting thin, long strips.

3. Mix together in a bowl sliced cabbage, black beans, lime juice, and cilantro. Set aside.

4. For the jackfruit: Drain and rinse jackfruit. Slice jackfruit triangles into three sections. Set in a medium-sized bowl.

5. Pre-heat oven to 250°F for soft tortilla shells.

6. Prepare the blackening seasoning. Mix blackening seasoning in with jackfruit making sure to completely cover and saturate with herbs and spices.

7. Add 3 tbsp. of canola oil to cast iron pan on medium heat over flame or on grill, leaving in cast iron skillet until blackened. Cook until dark and softened. Be sure to use a sturdy potholder when removing cast iron skillet as the handle will be as hot as the pan. Let cool.

8. Warm flour/corn tortillas in oven wrapped in a potato cloth or paper towels for 2-3 minutes.

9. Remove tortillas and assemble tacos with blackened jackfruit, cabbage slaw, coconut lime crema and top with a sprig of cilantro.

Serve immediately.

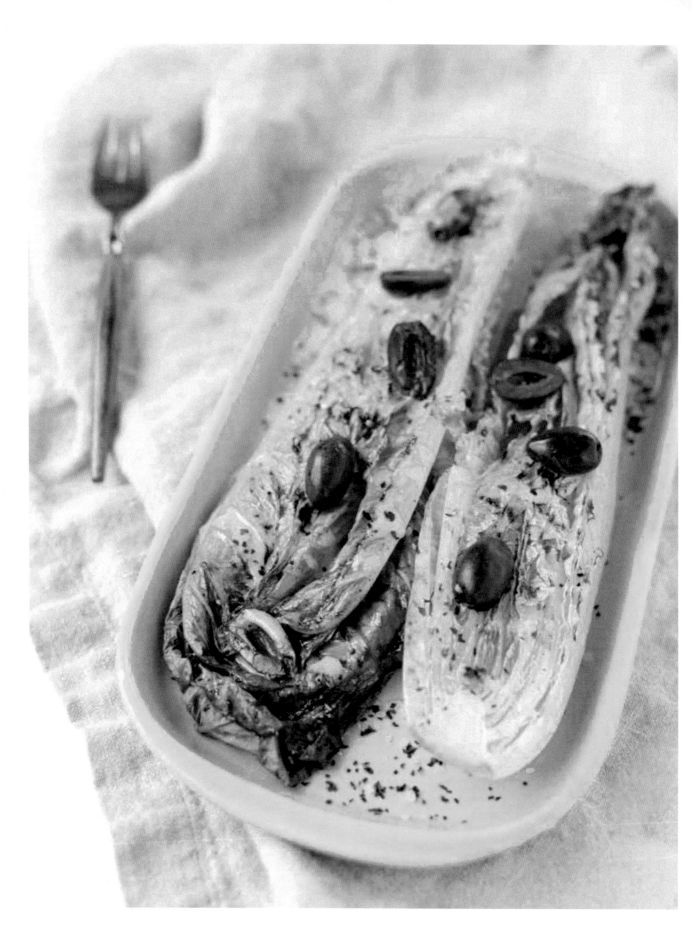

grilled romaine with caesar dressing

FOR THE DRESSING:

$3/4$ cup extra-virgin olive oil plus 2 tbsp.

$1/2$ cup filtered water

1 tbsp. fresh lemon juice

1 tbsp. apple cider vinegar

1 tsp. Vegan Worcestershire sauce

$1 1/4$ tsp. whole grain mustard

$1/2$ tablespoon ground chia seeds

4 cloves fresh garlic

4 tablespoons vegan parmesan cheese

Himalayan salt and white pepper

For the salad:

2 heads of romaine lettuce cut in half lengthwise

$1/2$ cup wild or organic capers

$1/4$ cup raw hemp seeds

$1/2$ cup vegan parmesan cheese

$1/4$ cup dulse flakes

DIRECTIONS:

1. To make the salad dressing, add all ingredients to a blender and process on high speed for 20-30 seconds until very smooth and creamy. Add a slight amount of additional lemon juice or water to thin to your desired consistency. Set aside.

2. Rub the inner edges of the romaine with olive oil.

3. Wash the heads of romaine lettuce and dry with a kitchen towel (do not break apart the individual leaves – leave the heads fully composed).

4. Turn grill to lowest setting. Put romaine oil side down for 5 minutes, then remove and let cool.

Liberally drizzle the dressing over the top of each romaine head.

In a pinch, this dressing can be used over raw romaine. It doesn't need to be cooked. It provides a heartier meat-like flavor when cooked, but it's the dressing that mostly provides the health benefits in this instance.

This happens to be our favorite go-to salad and is incredibly filling and satisfying. We hope you like it too! The faux vegan cheese we find works best is Follow Your Heart parmesan shreds, which tastes most like the real thing. It's mostly organic and 100% non-GMO, which is alright with us!

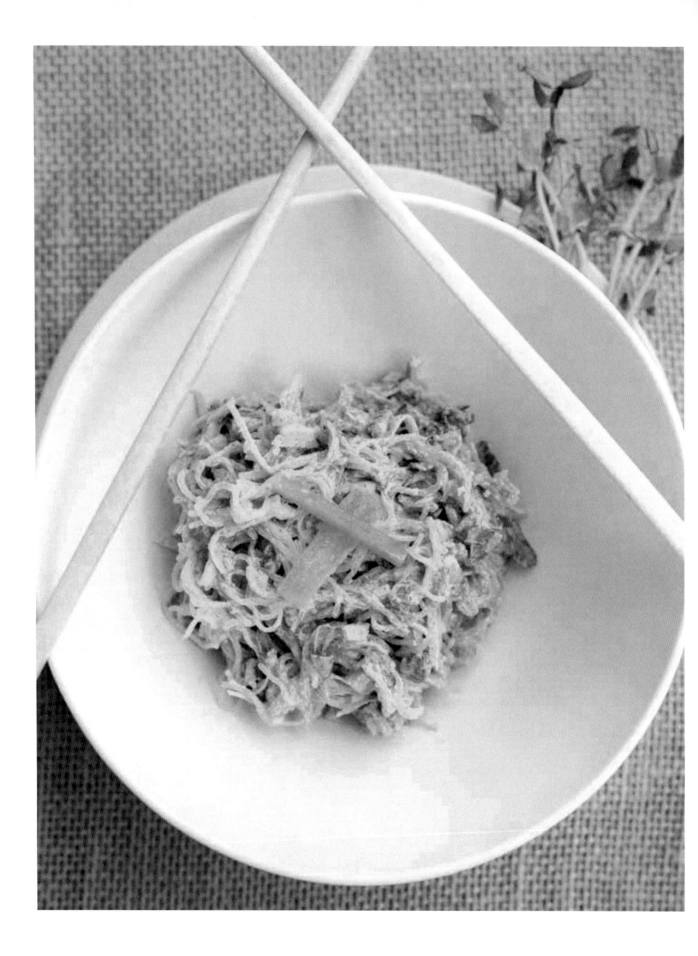

pad thai noodle salad

INGREDIENTS:

1 cup almond butter

1 pkg. kelp noodles

$1/2$ cup shredded carrots

5 scallion bottoms sliced or $1/8$ onion sliced

$1/2$ cucumber sliced into thin strips

jicama sliced into thin strips

$1/2$ cup roughly chopped cilantro

For the Sauce:

3-4 oz. freshly squeezed lemon juice

$1/2$ in. fresh ginger chopped

1 tbsp. kelp or dulse powder

2 celery ribs

3 cloves garlic

$1/4$ tsp. cayenne

1 juicing carrot

2 tbsp. Nama Shoyu

$1/4$ cup cilantro, coarsely chopped

Kelp is considered a valuable source of iodine, a trace mineral, and essential nutrients that play an important role in thyroid function and metabolism.

The clear kelp noodles used in this recipe must be rinsed thoroughly to rid the salty liquid it has been packaged in, which also helps to separate them. The noodles themselves are incredibly long, so it is best to cut them with kitchen shears.

DIRECTIONS:

1. Mix together in a bowl: kelp noodles and sauce.
2. Toss in shredded carrot, scallions, cucumber, jicama.
3. Lightly sprinkle cilantro.
4. Serve as a main dish.

For the sauce:

Add almond butter, freshly squeezed lemon juice, ginger, dulse flakes, celery, garlic, cayenne, carrot, and Nama Shoyu to blender and blend until smooth.

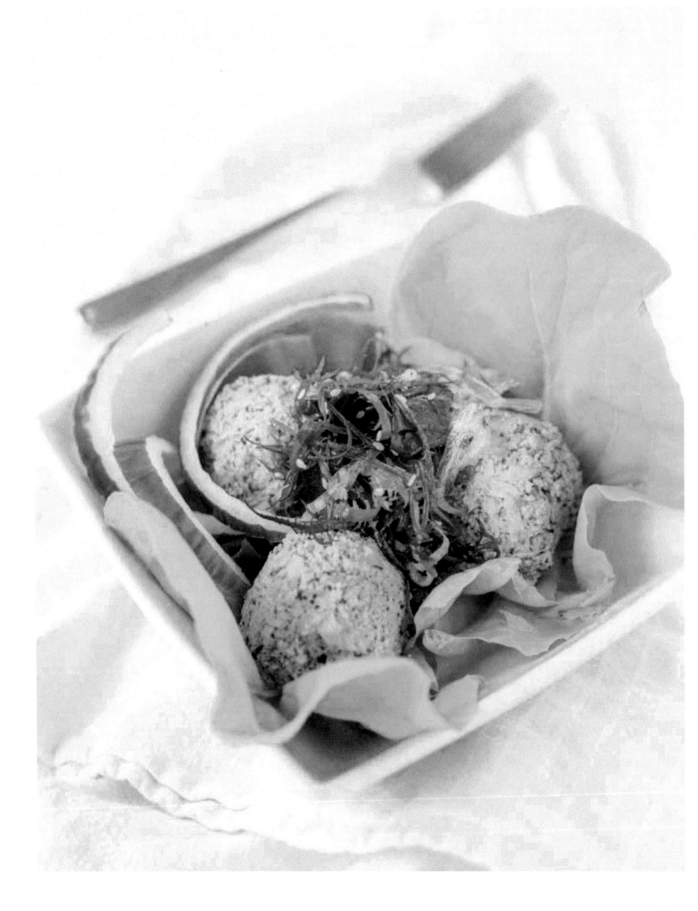

faux salmon & seaweed salad

INGREDIENTS:

1 cup walnuts (soaked overnight)

2 celery ribs

2 tbsp. red bell pepper

1 tbsp. fresh dill

1 tbsp. fresh lemon juice

Generously sprinkle with Himalayan salt and freshly ground pepper

2 heads Bibb lettuce or butter lettuce leaves

For the seaweed salad:

1 (6 oz.) package seaweed mix, preferably dried.

2 green onions

2 tbsp. sesame oil

2 tbsp. rice vinegar

2 tsp. white sesame seeds

1/2 tsp. red pepper flakes

Nama shoyu to taste

The fresh sea flavors in this dish give you all of the nutrients without all of the harmful contaminants found in marine life. The seaweed mix we use for this dish is SeaVegi's Seaweed Salad Mix containing: wakame, agar, suginori, tsunomata, and mafunori. The veggie mix has been verified to be non-GMO by the Non-GMO Project. The faux salmon, well, you will be surprised by its taste and texture, and the combo is a fantastic Fishless Friday meal.

DIRECTIONS:

1. Blend the soaked walnuts in a food processor until a creamy consistency.

2. Add the celery, onion, herbs, lemon juice, salt, and pepper and set aside.

3. Using an ice cream scoop, add to lettuce

4. Serve with seaweed salad (optional)

For the Seaweed Salad:

1. Rinse seaweed, then soak for 15 minutes. Soaking will rehydrate your dried seaweed. Drain the seaweed and set in a medium-sized bowl

2. In a separate dish, mix the oil and vinegar, soy sauce, and sweetener. Pour the dressing over the seaweed and mix well.

3. Add sesame seeds and chili flakes.

4. Top with sliced green onion.

5. Add to faux salmon pate over Bibb lettuce.

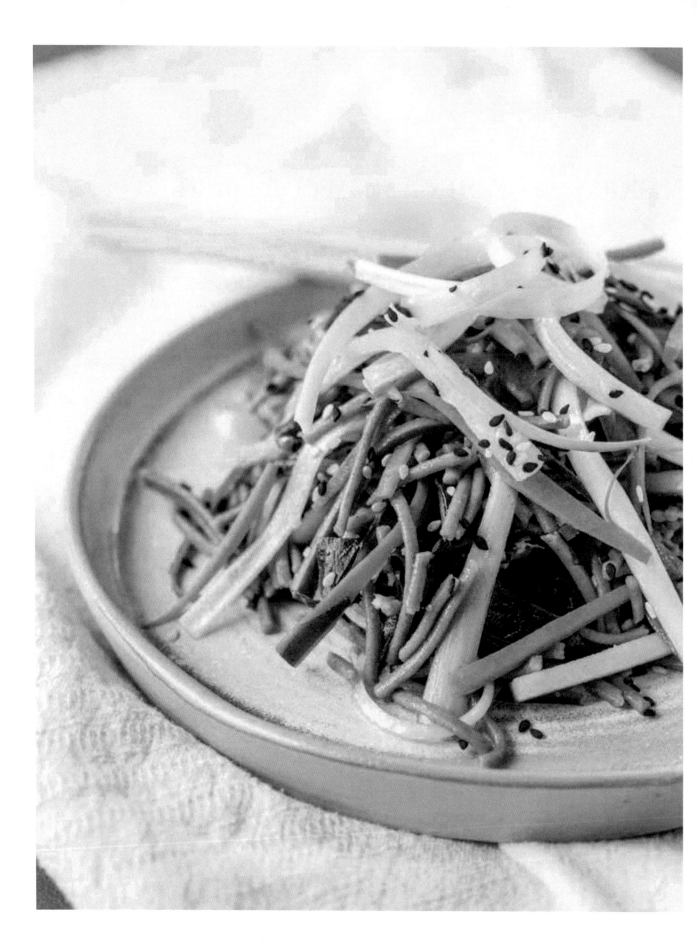

thai soba noodle salad with vegetables and wakame

INGREDIENTS:

1/4 cup wakame, soaked in cold water for 10-15 minutes, until softened

1 small box of soba (buckwheat) noodles

1 cucumber, seeded and julienned

1/2 cup carrot matchsticks or shredded carrots

2 tbsp. white sesame seeds

1 small bunch scallions, white part only

2 in. of fresh ginger, grated

4 garlic cloves, crushed

3 tbsp. toasted sesame oil

1 lime, juiced

1 tsp. Nama Shoyu or Bragg's liquid aminos

Soba is the Japanese word for buckwheat. Soba noodles generally are a combination of wheat and buckwheat flour. For a gluten-free option, make sure to purchase 100% buckwheat soba. Wakame typically comes dried in packages found in the Asian section of supermarkets. Emerald Cove, a popular non-GMO brand, is the brand we use. Another substantial yet delectable meal!

DIRECTIONS:

1. Cook the soba noodles. Follow directions on box. Drain and drizzle with sesame oil to keep noodles from sticking.

2. Prepare the wakame according to the directions on package.

3. Julienne the cucumbers and scallions.

4. Grate the ginger and crush the garlic and set aside in a small bowl with Bragg's liquid aminos.

5. Mix garlic, ginger, and Bragg's into noodles. Toss in vegetables and wakame.

Sprinkle with sesame seeds and serve.

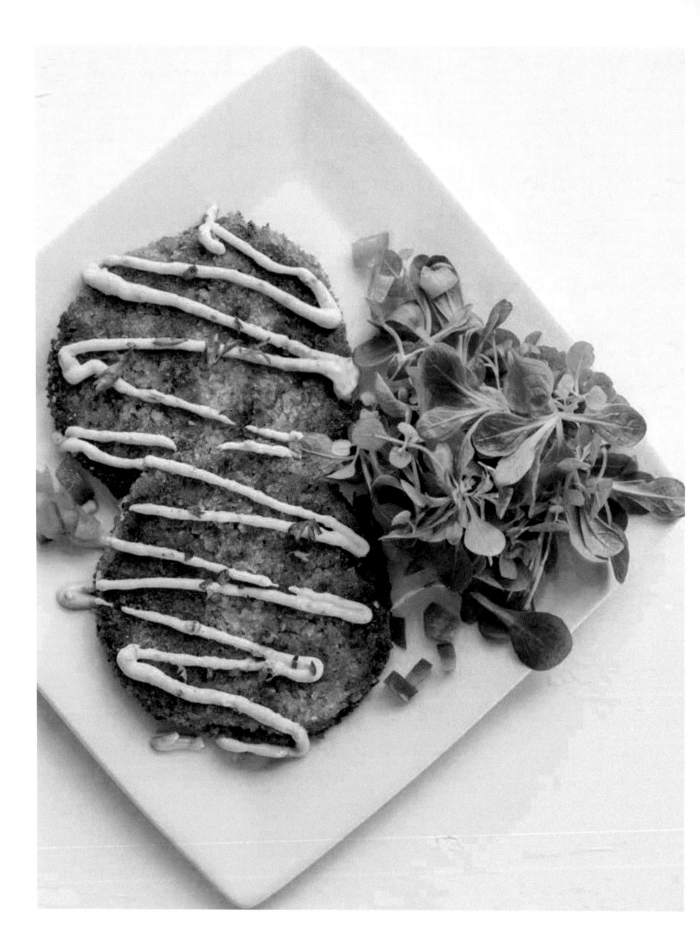

vegan crab cakes with remoulade

INGREDIENTS:

For the crab cake:

1 toasted nori sheet

Two, 14-ounce cans hearts of palm, rinsed set in towel to dry

1/2 cup olive oil

1/2 cup organic canola oil

1/4 cup finely diced red onion

1/4 cup finely diced red bell pepper

3 tbsp. Vegenaise (soy version)

2 tsp. Old Bay seasoning

1 tbsp. nutritional yeast flakes

2 tsp. arrowroot powder

Salt and pepper to taste

2 cups panko breadcrumbs

This recipe can also be made using frozen artichoke hearts and shredded potatoes. This recipe, hands down, is a sure-fire hit with both young and old alike.

DIRECTIONS:

1. Grind the nori using a spice grinder or a coffee grinder. Break the nori into pieces, place it in the grinder, and pulse until powdered or purchase in flakes.

2. Drain and rinse the hearts of palm and press in a towel to dry them. In a food processor, gently pulse until it looks like the consistency of crabmeat.

3. Place a small sauté pan on medium heat. Add 1 teaspoon of oil and heat for 30 seconds. Sauté the onion and bell pepper until soft, 3 to 5 minutes.

4. In the bowl of a food processor, add to the hearts of palm, 1 cup of Panko crumbs, sauteéd onion, bell pepper, Vegenaise, 1 teaspoon Old Bay seasoning, nori flakes, nutritional yeast flakes, arrowroot powder, and salt and pepper. Pulse and then blend until incorporated. Cover and refrigerate for 30 minutes.

5. Scoop with an ice cream scoop to portion and flatten into small cakes. Coat the small cakes with breadcrumbs. Form and let sit in the refrigerator for 1 hour or until firm.

6. To cook Crab Cakes: Place a sauté pan on medium-high heat. Add a mixture of organic canola and olive oil and heat for 2 minutes. Working in batches, sauté the cakes (make certain that the oil comes about halfway up the sides of the cakes) until browned on both sides and heated through, 2 to 3 minutes on each side.

7. Remove the cakes to a baking sheet lined with parchment paper and place in a warm oven (275° F) until all of the cakes are completely cooked.

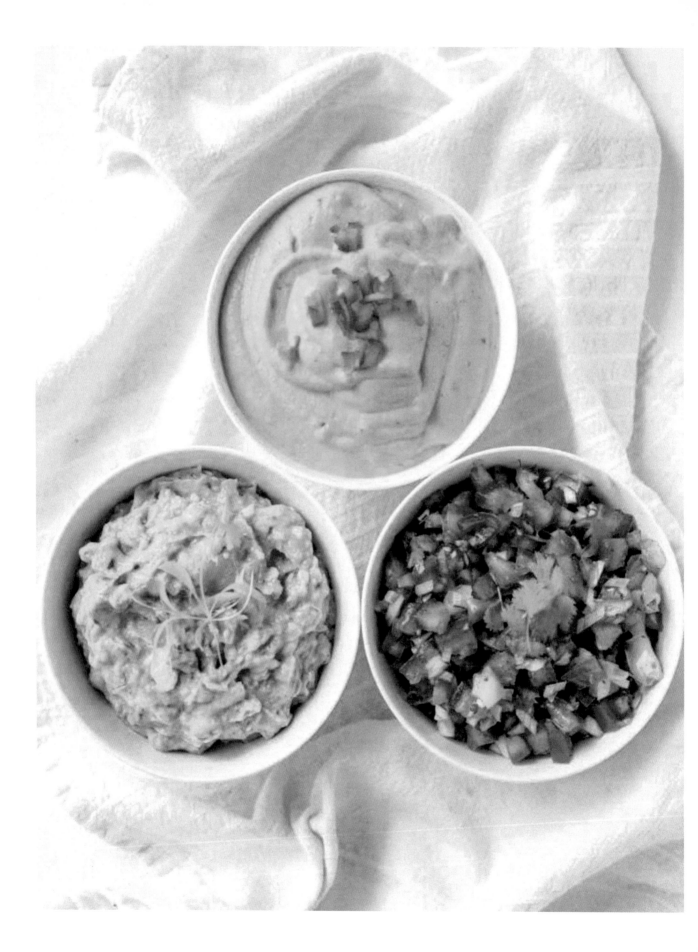

dips and sauces
delicious guacamole

INGREDIENTS:

5 medium-sized ripe avocados or 4 large avocados

1 bunch cilantro, tough stems discarded

1 jalapeño

3 limes

1 tomato (optional)

pinch of cayenne pepper

DIRECTIONS:

1. Remove pit and scoop avocado meat into a large bowl. Mash with a fork or mashed potato masher.
2. Finely chop ½ bunch of cilantro leaves.
3. Seed jalapeño and finely chop.
4. Juice 2 limes
5. Coarsely chop tomato, drain liquid

Mix together all ingredients and drizzle juice of 1 lime on top to preserve color. Sprinkle with cayenne. Serve immediately.

fresh tomato salsa

INGREDIENTS:

2 ½ - 3 lbs. organic slicer or multicolored heirloom cherry tomatoes

1 bunch cilantro, tough stems discarded

¼ cup diced red onion

1 jalapeño, seeded and finely chopped

1 lime

DIRECTIONS:

1. Chop tomatoes into bite-size pieces. Drain the liquid from the tomatoes in a sieve (or strainer).
2. Use ½ bunch of cilantro and finely chop.
3. Add finely chopped onion, jalapeño, and juice of 1 lime.
4. Season with salt and pepper

Stir and let sit in the refrigerator for several hours or overnight.

raw vegan cheddar cheese

INGREDIENTS:

1 cup raw cashews, soaked for 4 hours and rinsed

1/2 large red bell pepper

1/4 cup water

2 tbsp. lemon juice

2 tbsp. nutritional yeast

1 tbsp. tahini

1/4 teaspoon sea salt (add more to taste)

1 clove garlic

2 tsp. onion powder

DIRECTIONS:

1. In a high-speed blender, blend all ingredients until creamy and completely smooth.

2. Add more water if it is too thick.

coconut lime crema

INGREDIENTS:

1 (13.5 oz.) can full-fat coconut milk or 1, 6-oz. can coconut cream

1/2 tsp. lime juice

1/4 tsp. arrowroot powder

1/4 tsp. tapioca starch

DIRECTIONS:

1. Open can of coconut and skim cream and drain excess liquid. Reserve liquid for smoothies or other recipes.

2. Put coconut cream in blender and blend with lime juice, tapioca starch, and arrowroot powder.

3. Refrigerate for at least one hour to thicken.

4. Crema is ready to serve.

Refrigerate any unused portion.

pepita cream

INGREDIENTS:

¹/₂ cup raw pepitas (pumpkin seeds) soaked overnight

¹/₄ cup lime juice

¹/₄ cup filtered water

³/₄ teaspoon salt to taste

DIRECTIONS:

1. Rinse pepitas thoroughly. Transfer to a high-speed blender.
2. Add lime juice, water and blend until smooth and creamy.
3. Pepita cream is ready to eat.
4. Store in refrigerator.

jicama pico de gallo

INGREDIENTS:

¹/₂ cup jicama

2 limes, juiced

1 cup diced tomatoes

¹/₄ tsp. garlic powder

2 tsp. chopped cilantro

2 tbsp. diced red onion

Salt and pepper to taste

DIRECTIONS:

1. Peel jicama, slice, and dice into small pieces.
2. Core tomato and chop into a small dice.
3. Juice 2 limes. Set aside.
4. In a mixing bowl, add jicama, tomato, lime juice, garlic powder, onion, cilantro and salt and pepper, and mix.
5. Allow pico de gallo to rest to allow flavors to meld.

chipotle vegan queso

INGREDIENTS:

2 tbsp. olive oil

1/2 medium yellow onion, chopped

4 cloves garlic, minced

1/2 tsp. paprika

1/2 tsp. ground chili powder

1/2 tsp. cumin

1 cup peeled, cubed Russet potato soaked in water

1 1/2 cups water

1/2 cup cashews soaked 4 hours

1 1/2 cups filtered water

1 sundried tomato, rehydrated

1 tbsp. pickled jalapeño

1/2 dried chipotle rehydrated, seeded

This dip is a must "have on hand." It can accompany any southwestern meal or used as a dipping sauce with tortilla chips. Its unique flavors give this queso dip a double thumbs up!

DIRECTIONS:

1. Prep Russet potato first to allow starches to leach into water. Drain water, rinse, repeat about 3 times while prepping other queso ingredients.

2. Drain and rinse cashews.

3. Sauté onion and garlic in olive oil in skillet just until fragrant.

4. Add paprika, cumin, and chili powder. Let flavors meld, approximately 1 minute.

5. Add the soaked and rinsed cashews, potatoes, and 1 1/2 cups water to pan. Let the mixture come to a simmer avoiding a rapid boil, occasionally stirring until the potatoes are soft approximately 5-6 minutes.

6. Remove from heat.

7. Add to a high-speed blender: rinsed sundried tomato, rinsed chipotle pepper, and salt. Pour in queso base from skillet and blend on high until creamy.

8. Add water if too thick. Adjust consistency accordingly.

9. Transfer to a serving bowl and add pickled jalapeños.

cashew cream cheese

INGREDIENTS:

2 cups cashews, soaked approximately 8 hours

$3/4$ teaspoon vegan probiotic (make sure probiotic capsule is vegan)

$3/4$ cup tepid water

For the flavoring:

2 tablespoons nutritional yeast

$1/2$ tablespoon onion powder

$1/4$ teaspoon fresh ground nutmeg

$1/2$ teaspoon Himalayan salt freshly ground pepper

Cheesecloth for covering

Used as the accompanying dish to our dehydrated flax crackers, this cheese is an easy-to-make recipe for those just getting started with raw food or dairy-free cheeses. Make sure to purchase raw cashews (not roasted/salted) and make certain the probiotic, including the capsule, is completely vegan as many probiotics use a lactase starter culture. An alternative to using a probiotic would be chickpea miso. The toppings can be subbed out with fresh herbs and spices like chives, oregano, and thyme or just plain salt and pepper and nutritional yeast.

DIRECTIONS:

1. In a high-speed blender, blend soaked cashews, water, and probiotics until smooth. Transfer to a medium glass bowl, and allow to sit, covered with cheesecloth on counter for 24 hours to culture.

2. In a small bowl, combine nutritional yeast, onion powder, nutmeg, and 1 teaspoons salt. Set aside until cheese spread has cultured.

3. Once cheese has cultured, mix in spices and refrigerate up to 7 days.

Use as a dip or spread.

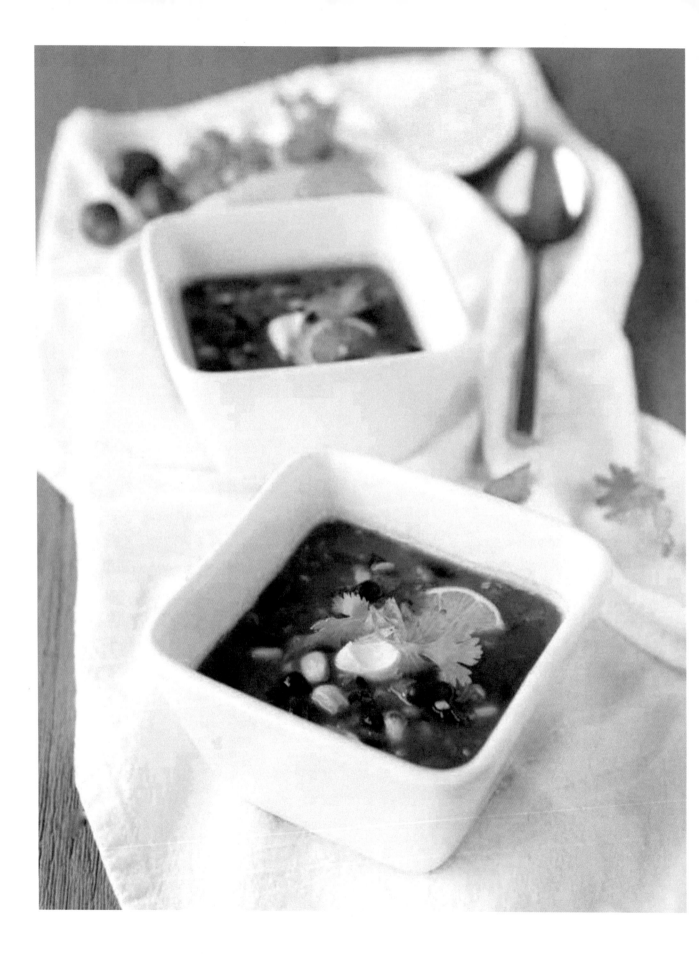

soups & stews
souping

For starters, and not meaning appetizers, "souping" was the trend for 2016.

Why would souping replace juicing in the quest of those seeking optimal health?

The appeal of souping, in part, is that it promises an easier detox than a juice cleanse. Those that decidedly prefer souping claim that juices being absent of fiber to whisk away toxins and the absence of the need to chew makes juicing just about as difficult as water fasting.

Souping is gaining traction and has a much higher appeal due to its high fiber content, which has a multitude of benefits that juicing lacks. So while soups are thicker, more nourishing, and more nutrient-dense, it seems "souping" is the better alternative to juicing when it comes to cleanses. However, souping too, has its drawbacks. When cooked, reheated, or put in the microwave, the nutrient value of heat-sensitive vitamins like D, E, and K is significantly diminished.

A SOUP CLEANSE?

The juice cleansing trend started from a good place and evolved into something that's not so healthy. Many juice cleanses that are offered contain a significant amount of sugar (sometimes more than soda) and not enough nutrients that the body needs for an extended period of time, for instance, fat necessary for attention, focus, and energy.

All in all, both juices and soups are fantastic support tools to aid with digestive repair.

By feeding your body with adequate nutritious whole foods, drinking water, and moving throughout the day—your body has everything it needs. By consuming daily soups that are rich in vegetables and superfoods, your body can receive a ton of vitamins and nutrients without forcing the digestive system to work as hard.

Soups can include other ingredients like legumes and nuts, providing nutrients like healthy fats and protein. And because you're consuming this all in the form of soup—the total volume of liquid alone will make you feel fuller on fewer calories.

Maintaining a healthy weight and keeping your body strong enough to do things like detox naturally are processes that require learning and practicing lifelong healthful behaviors. No soup-cleanse can compete with a lifestyle change, but what soups can do is support the lifestyle change if consumed with juicing daily.

Souping for more than one full day at a time is not advised. Our lungs, kidneys, liver, and skin are wondrous organs that naturally detox when we engage in healthy behaviors.

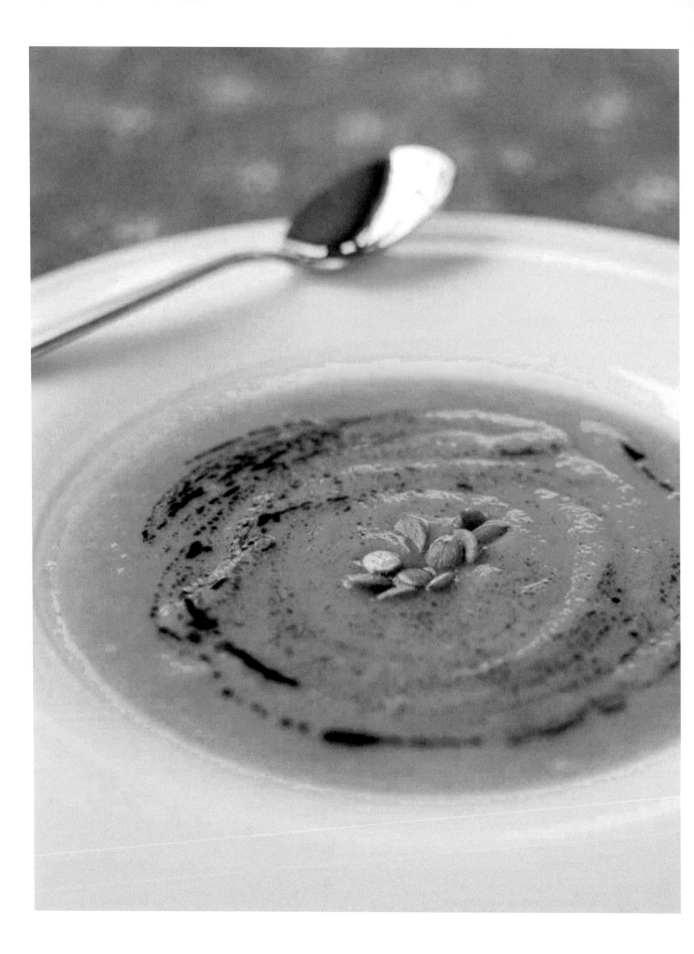

spiced pumpkin soup with toasted pumpkin seeds

INGREDIENTS:

1 tsp. whole coriander, toasted and ground

1 tsp. sweetener of choice

1/8 tsp. cayenne pepper

$1/2$ lb. butternut squash, peeled and cut into 2-inch cubes (or 2 bags frozen butternut squash)

1 can unsweetened pumpkin puree

2 tablespoons olive oil

1 cup hot water

2 tsp. toasted pumpkin seed oil

$1/4$ tsp. toasted pumpkin seeds (optional)

$1^{1}/_{2}$ cup diced sweet onion

$1/4$ cup sherry wine

1 teaspoon Himalayan salt

DIRECTIONS:

1. Preheat the oven to 475 degrees

2. In a bowl, add the butternut squash and olive oil.

3. In a small bowl, mix the coriander, sweetener, cayenne, and 2 tsp. salt. Pour onto squash and mix well with hands.

4. Transfer squash to a glass or ceramic roasting pan and roast for 35 minutes, occasionally turning until tender and browned.

5. In a sauté pan, sauté onions in 1 tbsp. olive oil until translucent. Add sherry wine and turn heat on high until liquid is cooked down and thickened. Add pumpkin puree and mix well.

6. Remove butternut squash from oven and transfer squash to a food processor or blender. Add the water, pumpkin puree, and blend until smooth. Transfer the soup to a saucepan, season with salt, and keep warm. If storing, add to a glass container and let cool. Cover when cool.

7. Sprinkle with salt. Drizzle toasted pumpkin seed oil and top with toasted pumpkin seeds.

split pea soup

INGREDIENTS:

4 cups low-sodium vegetable broth, divided

1/2 medium yellow onion, chopped

2 small cloves garlic, finely chopped

scant · teaspoon smoked paprika

1/8 cup sundried tomatoes (not packed in oil), chopped

1/2 pound dried green split peas, rinsed (a little over 1 cup)

Freshly ground black pepper

The smoked paprika and sundried tomatoes give this vegan rendition the same hardiness and richness that has traditionally given split pea soup its flavor from using ham or pork.

Considered a starchy vegetable like potatoes, corn, and squash, they are part of the legume family. They boast an impressive nutrient profile and contain just about every nutrient and mineral you need, including fiber!

DIRECTIONS:

1. In a large pot, bring 1/4 cup broth to a simmer over medium-high heat. Add onion and garlic and cook about 6 minutes or until onion is translucent and tender.

2. Stir in smoked paprika and cook 1 minute. Add tomatoes, peas, remaining 3³/₄ cups broth, and 1 cup water and bring to a boil. Reduce heat to low, cover, and simmer about 40 minutes or until peas are tender.

3. Purée soup with a hand-held immersion blender or in a blender or food processor until smooth and creamy. Return to heat and simmer 5 minutes more, stirring occasionally.

4. Season with black pepper and serve.

oriental sweet potato and carrot soup

INGREDIENTS:

4 medium carrots cut into 2 in. pieces

1 pound white-fleshed oriental sweet potatoes, peeled and cut into 1 in. pieces

4 tbsp. organic, unrefined coconut oil

1 medium sweet onion, thinly sliced

48 oz. vegetable stock or low-sodium broth

1 tbsp. fresh lemon juice (from a squeezed lemon)

2 tbsp. finely chopped flat-leaf parsley

The flavors in this soup are sure to surprise. An oriental or Japanese sweet potato is slightly sweeter than a traditional yam and contains white flesh and garnet-colored skin. When cooked, it retains its shape and firmness but results in a creamy flavor making it a natural choice for this soup.

DIRECTIONS:

1. Melt 2 tbsp. of coconut oil in a medium saucepan. Add the onion, cover and cook over moderately high heat, occasionally stirring, until softened but not browned. Add the carrots and sweet potatoes, cover, lower temperature to sweat the vegetables as they are just beginning to soften about 5 minutes.

2. Add the vegetable stock and bring to a soft boil.

3. Cover partially and cook over moderate heat until the vegetables are tender about 15 minutes.

4. In a blender, puree batches until smooth. Return to the saucepan.

5. When ready to serve, stir in the lemon juice and parsley.

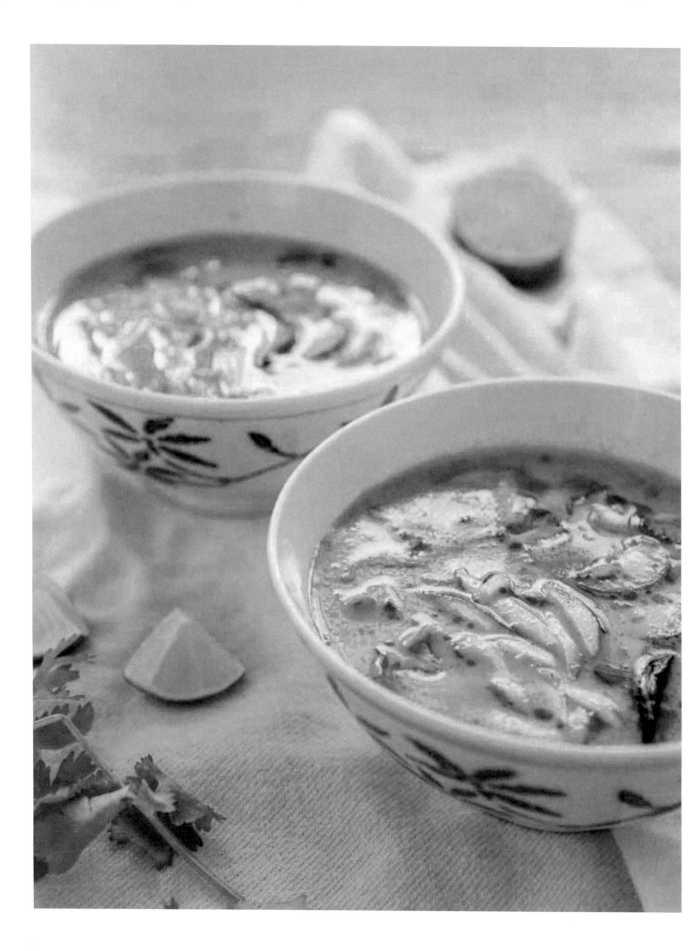

tom kha gai with tofu

INGREDIENTS:

6 cups Ocean's Halo sea vegetable broth

2 stalks fresh lemongrass

8 kafir lime leaves

1, 14-oz. can coconut milk

2 cloves garlic sliced

1-inch ginger, peeled and sliced

1 shallot diced

8 oz. shiitake mushrooms, stems removed, caps thinly sliced lengthwise

2, dried Thai bird chilies, seeds removed

2 tbsp. red curry paste

14 oz. extra-firm tofu, cubed

1 lime

1 tsp. sugar

Chili oil (optional)

cilantro for garnish

1 tbsp. oil

DIRECTIONS:

1. Dice shallots, slice garlic and ginger.

2. Slice lemongrass lengthwise, outer layers discarded.

3. Prepare Thai bird chilies. (Chilies can be left whole, sliced, diced, or chopped. The seeds add spice and can be removed for less intense heat.)

4. Drain water from tofu and press with paper or kitchen towel. Cube tofu into bite-size pieces.

5. In a saucepan, sauté shallots, garlic, ginger, lemongrass, red curry paste, and lime leaves in 1 tbsp. oil just until fragrant.

6. Add the broth and simmer for about 7-10 minutes to let the broth infuse.

7. Add the tofu and mushrooms, and simmer for 5 more minutes.

8. Slice lime into wedges.

9. Add in the coconut milk, chilies, and sugar.

Adjust flavoring by adding a pinch of salt and lime juice from lime wedges. Divide soup among bowls. Serve with chili oil, cilantro, and lime wedges.

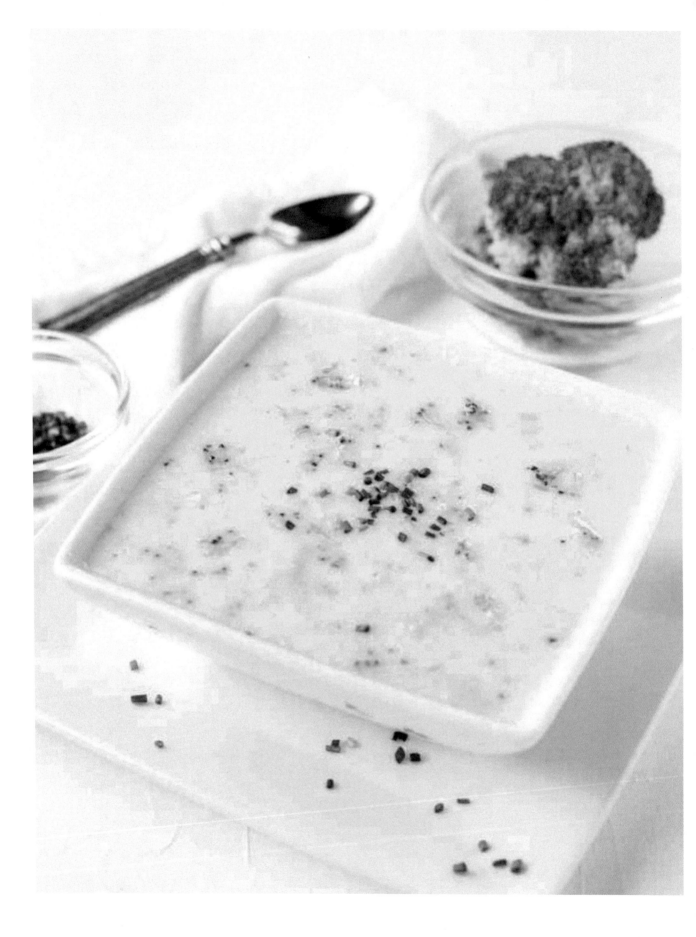

creamy broccoli leek soup

INGREDIENTS:

2 large heads of broccoli chopped (using all the florets and one stem)

2 large leeks, white and light green part only, rinsed

4 cloves garlic (chopped)

48 oz. no-chicken broth (or vegetable broth)

1 bunch chives finely chopped

3 tbsp. olive oil

1 cup cashews; soaked 4 hours

Creamy is an understatement! The stems from the broccoli give the thickness the soup needs, and the cashews provide the creaminess making it a close comparison to traditional cream of broccoli soup!

DIRECTIONS:

1. Cut dark green leaves of leeks. Keep white and light green parts only. Slice down center and rinse inner leaves. Slice into thin rounds on the bias.

2. Chop broccoli into bite-size pieces and one stem. Set one stem aside.

3. Chop garlic and set aside.

4. Heat 3 tbsp. olive oil in pan and sauté leeks approximately 3-4 minutes until translucent. Do not burn.

5. Add in garlic and sauté 1-2 more minutes.

6. Add sliced broccoli stem and toss with the leeks and oil to coat.

7. Pour in 48 oz. of broth. Turn to high to bring to a slight boil then lower to simmer. Do not cover.

8. Simmer for 5 minutes, then turn heat off.

9. Drain and rinse cashews. Add cashews and broccoli floret to the soup.

10. Let soup cool slightly.

11. Add soup to blender and fill 2/3 way full. Turn on high and pour into serving bowl. Add another batch if necessary and blend.

Ladle into serving size bowls. Season with salt and pepper.

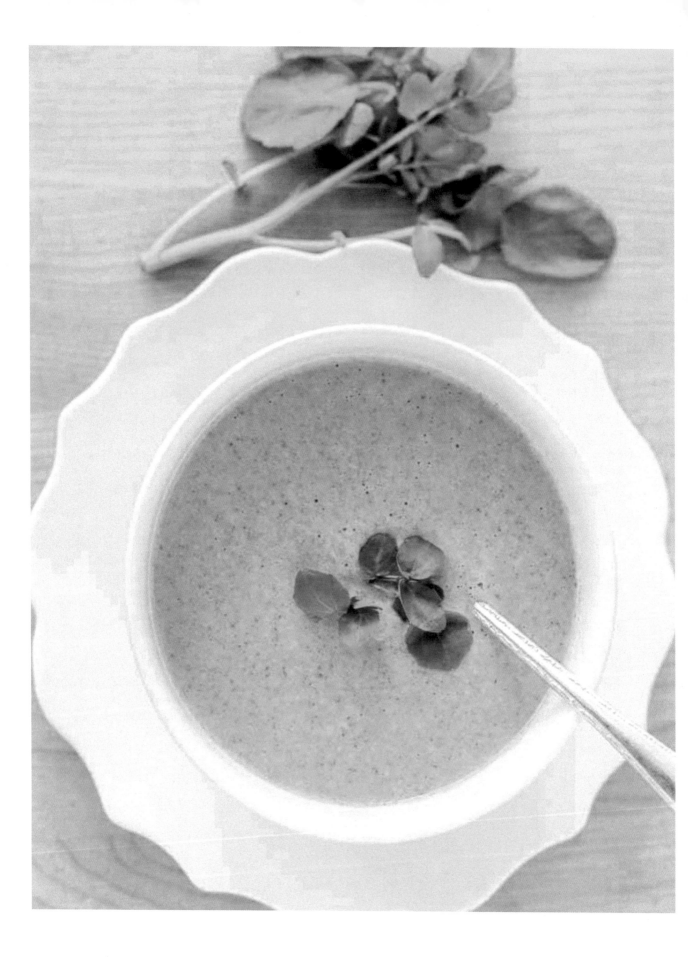

zucchini & watercress soup with black garlic

INGREDIENTS:

2 tablespoons extra virgin olive oil

4 black garlic pods

1 medium sweet onion, diced

3 medium zucchini, roughly chopped

$\frac{1}{4}$ cup almond butter

1 qt. vegetable broth

2 cups watercress, stems removed, coarsely chopped

salt and black pepper, to taste

Plant lovers beware. This soup is sure to get you hooked. The almond butter is disguised, allowing the peppery watercress to shine and the black garlic giving way to the umami flavors.

DIRECTIONS:

1. In a large saucepan, heat the oil over medium heat.

2. Add the onion and black garlic and cook for 5 minutes until tender.

3. Add the zucchini and sauté another 3 minutes.

4. Add the almond butter and vegetable stock and bring to a boil.

5. Reduce the heat to low and simmer for 5 minutes until the zucchini is tender. Do not cover.

6. Add the watercress and cook for 3 more minutes, then turn off the heat.

7. Using a slotted spoon, transfer the vegetables to a blender with about a cup of stock and blend until smooth.

8. Pour back into the saucepan and combine.

9. Season with salt and pepper.

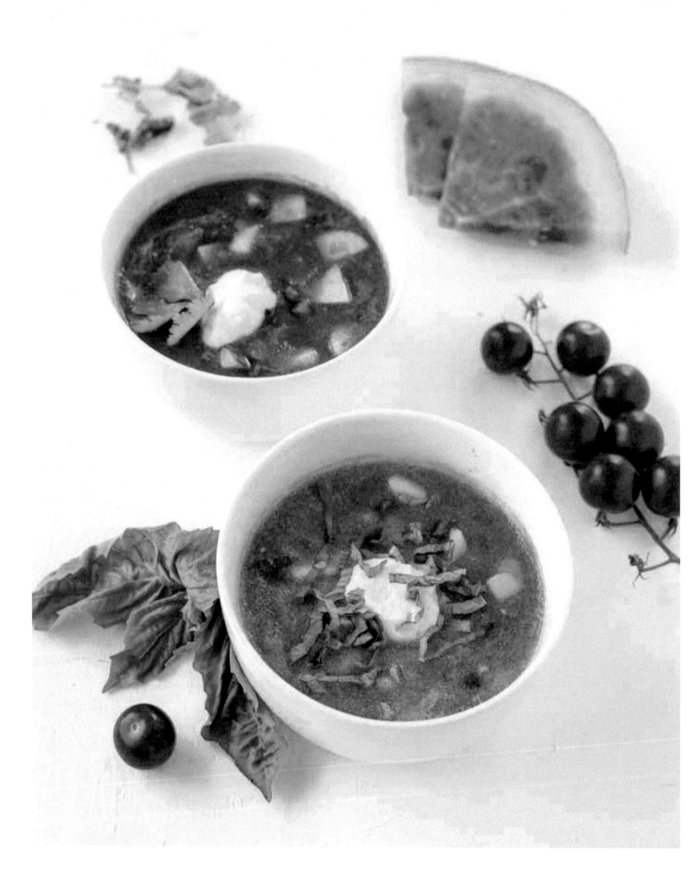

traditional & watermelon gazpacho

INGREDIENTS:

For the tomato gazpacho:

5 lbs. (8-10) tree-ripened tomatoes (beefsteak or heirloom)

1 English (seedless cucumber), peeled and coarsely chopped

1 red bell pepper, finely chopped

1 jalapeño, seeded and finely chopped

1/4 cup sherry or balsamic vinegar

1/3 cup extra-virgin olive oil

Handful fresh basil

Salt and freshly ground pepper

For the watermelon gazpacho:

6 cups seedless watermelon

Cilantro

Avocado

DIRECTIONS:

1. Core and mark an X at the bottom of each tomato. Bring a pot of salted water to a boil.

2. Prepare an ice bath for the tomatoes. When water comes to a boil, drop tomatoes in to blanch for 1 minute. Use a slotted spoon to remove tomato from water and set in the ice bath. Let cool.

3. Meanwhile, prepare all of the vegetables and set aside.

4. Remove tomatoes and drain the ice bath. Set a sieve over bowl. Peel skins from tomatoes and remove seeds over sieve to collect liquid. Deposit tomatoes into a blender.

5. Puree the tomatoes, and add olive oil and sherry vinegar.

6. In a large bowl, combine pureed tomatoes and vegetables.

7. Top with basil threads, add a dollop of vegan crème fraîche Season with salt and pepper and serve.

To Make the watermelon gazpacho:

Scoop the insides of a seedless watermelon and put in a blender, and blend on low until smooth. Pour into a large bowl.

Cut avocado in half. Remove pit and skins. Cut into cubes.

Pull cilantro leaves from stems.

Seed jalapeño, chop red bell pepper into bite-size pieces. Cut cucumber into small dice.

Add avocado, jalapeño, red bell pepper, cucumber, avocado, and cilantro to watermelon. Top with a dollop of vegan crème Fraiche and garnish with cilantro leaves.

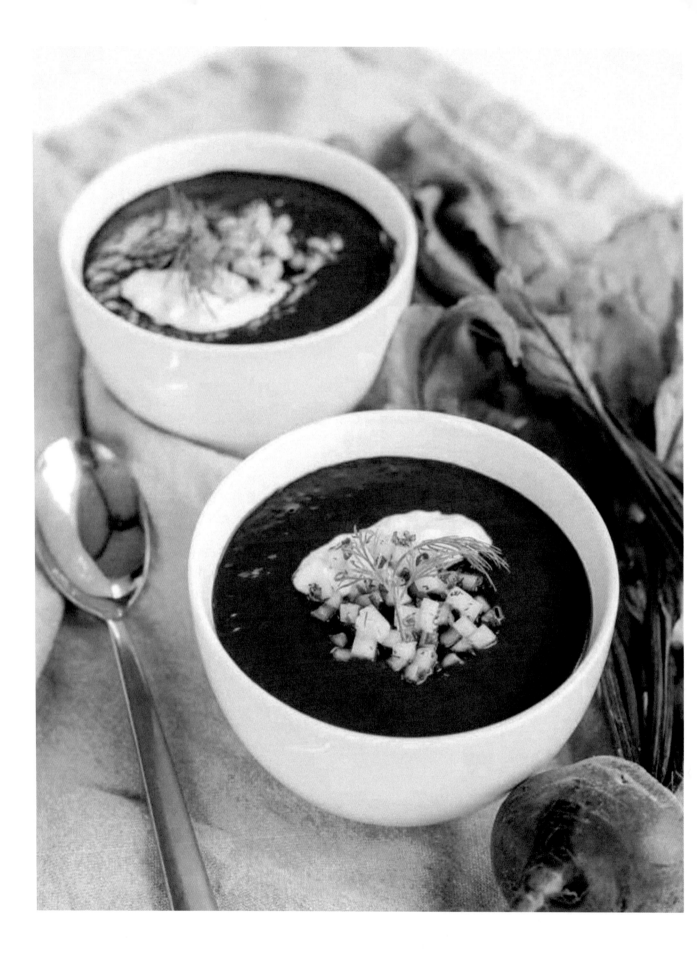

lithuanian borscht soup with forager cream

INGREDIENTS:

4 medium-sized beets

1 container Forager brand vegan sour cream

2 tbsp. fresh dill plus 1 tsp. for garnish

2 tbsp. finely chopped chives, plus 1 tsp. for garnish

1 small cucumber coarsely chopped, skin on if organic

Himalayan or sea salt to taste

One of my favorite soups of all time, I had to give it up for almost ten years until I stumbled upon a great sour cream/buttermilk alternative. I use the Forager brand, a coconut-based creamery, with minimal ingredients and an awesome organic USDA label, which gives me the go-ahead to use! It has an incredibly familiar sour cream taste and blends incredibly well, making this soup one of my all-time favorites soups again!

DIRECTIONS:

1. Cut stems off of beets and wash thoroughly with water. Place in a glass baking dish with 2 cups water. Cover with aluminum foil and place in oven at 350º F for 1 hour. When finished, take out of oven and set out to cool. Save reserve water.

2. In a large bowl, add finely chopped cucumber, chives, dill, and mix together.

3. When beets cool, skin beets. The skins will slide off nicely, or they can be peeled. Remove top and bottom edge of beets.

4. Cut 3 beets in half and cut the 4th beet into cubes.

5. Add 3 whole beets and Forager brand sour cream to a blender and blend until smooth.

6. Pour into a large serving bowl. Add in vegetables and herbs mix, as well as diced beets from 1 beet.

7. Garnish soup with dill, chives, and a dollop of Forager vegan sour cream.

ginger & turmeric in warm coconut milk

INGREDIENTS:

2 inches fresh ginger, grated

2 small shallots, diced

2 large garlic cloves, sliced

2 inches fresh turmeric, grated (or 1 tablespoon dried)

1 tablespoon fresh lemongrass, sliced lengthwise

2 dried red chilies, sliced

1 teaspoon dried coriander

2 (13$\frac{1}{2}$-ounce) cans coconut milk

Zest of 1 lime or two Kaffir lime leaves

1 tablespoon lime juice

2 star anise, whole

1 tablespoon brown sugar

1 tablespoon soy sauce

1 bunch of mizuna greens, bok choy or spinach (about 2 cups), chopped

1 large russet potato, peeled and cubed (about 1 cup)

2 medium carrots, thinly sliced at an angle (about 2 cups)

2 cups no-chicken broth

2 cups water

DIRECTIONS:

1. Place the ginger, shallot, garlic, turmeric, lemongrass, chilies, and coriander in a food processor with 3 tablespoons of coconut milk. Puree until finely blended.

2. In a large pot over medium heat, add this mixture and cook for 3–5 minutes. Add the lime zest/Kaffir lime leaves, lime juice, star anise, brown sugar, soy sauce, and salt. Continue to cook for another 1–2 minutes, until the sauce becomes fragrant.

3. Add the remaining coconut milk, mizuna greens, potato, carrots, no-chicken broth, and water. Continue to simmer over medium heat until the carrots and potatoes are tender.

4. Taste the soup and adjust seasonings. There should be a nice balance of salty, sweet, sour, and spicy heat.

Serve while hot.

vegan southwest soup with cilantro lime crema

INGREDIENTS:

1 cups black beans

4 ears of organic corn or 1 bag, frozen

1 Vidalia onion, diced

8 celery ribs, coarsely chopped

1 large red bell pepper

5 cloves of garlic, finely chopped

2 oz. cilantro, tender leaves only

1 whole tomato

2 tbsp. cumin

2 tbsp. chili powder

1 tsp. red pepper flakes

2 quarts of filtered water

1 bunch scallions, white and light parts only

One of the best southwestern soups every made, we have been able to enjoy playing around with shredded cheese alternatives and conversely using some of our amazing coconut crema for a creamier version or a side of chipotle queso to dip our tortilla chips in. It will not disappoint!

DIRECTIONS:

1. Remove husks and cut corn off of the cob by placing end of cob on sturdy surface like a plate or cutting board, holding pointed edge firmly with one hand. Slice down the cob with a sharpened knife, allowing kernels to fall onto the surface.

2. Peel and seed tomato (remove seeds and juices).

3. In a large pot, sauté onions, garlic, celery, and peppers on medium heat with olive oil.

4. Once the vegetables are soft, add the water, corn, black beans, cilantro, tomato, and all other seasonings.

5. Bring to a boil and then reduce heat to a low simmer. Let the soup simmer for 30 minutes.

6. Slice scallions across the bias.

7. Add salt and pepper to taste.

8. Serve with a dollop of vegan sour cream, crispy tortilla strips, and scallions on top.

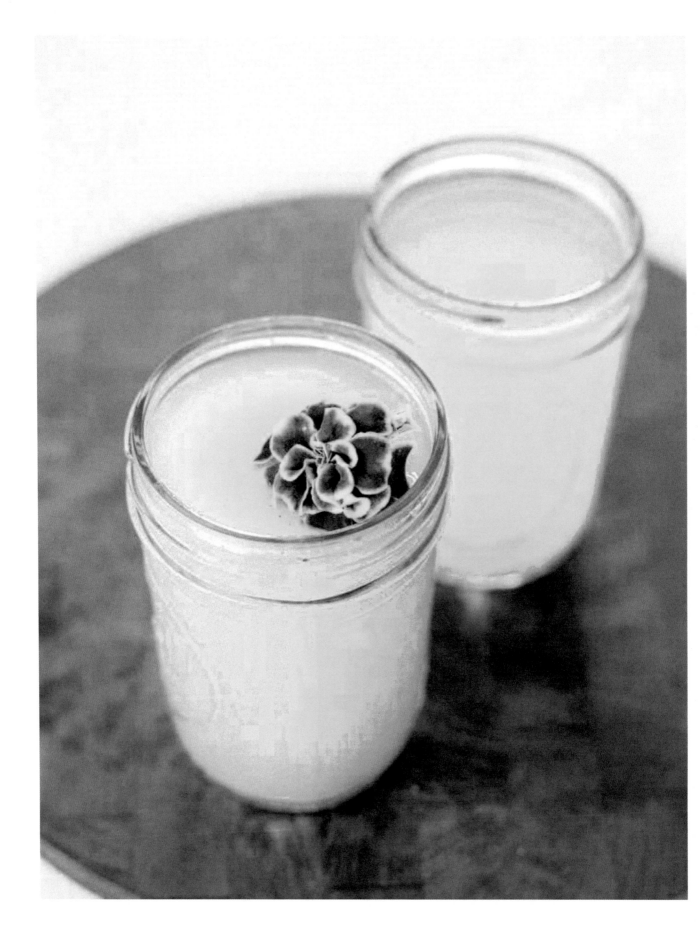

elixirs and tonics

Elixirs are healing remedies; they address situations of imbalance and symptoms of illness. Also, elixirs are made with delicious flavoring agents, flowers, and healthy sweeteners, as well as use a different ratio of medicinal potency.

Tonics, on the other hand, promote overall good health and balance; they fortify your system and keep you feeling fit and well. Tonics teach the body to continue on with the particular chemistry the formula contains. They fortify the system with healing blocks that actually remain within. Ideally, the body continues producing the chemical reaction without the assistance of the herbs.

An elixir is used to treat a headache or cold or cramps while a tonic might be used to improve immunity, boost energy, or relieve chronic stress.

Both elixirs and tonics are delivered to our bloodstreams in liquid form, making them efficient vehicles for healing and restoration when consumed on an empty stomach. Traditionally, they both are efficient at delivering potent nutrition directly into the bloodstream.

They are powerful reminders that we have the power to heal from within.

loving liver elixir

- Fresh garlic: 3 to 5 cloves
- 2 apples, cored
- Dash of Ceylon Cinnamon

Send all ingredients except cinnamon through a juicer.

bragg's alkaline elixir

- 2 tbsp. raw apple cider vinegar
- 1 tbsp. fresh lemon juice
- 1 tsp. raw honey
- 1 cup filtered water
- Dash cayenne pepper

Shake to mix.

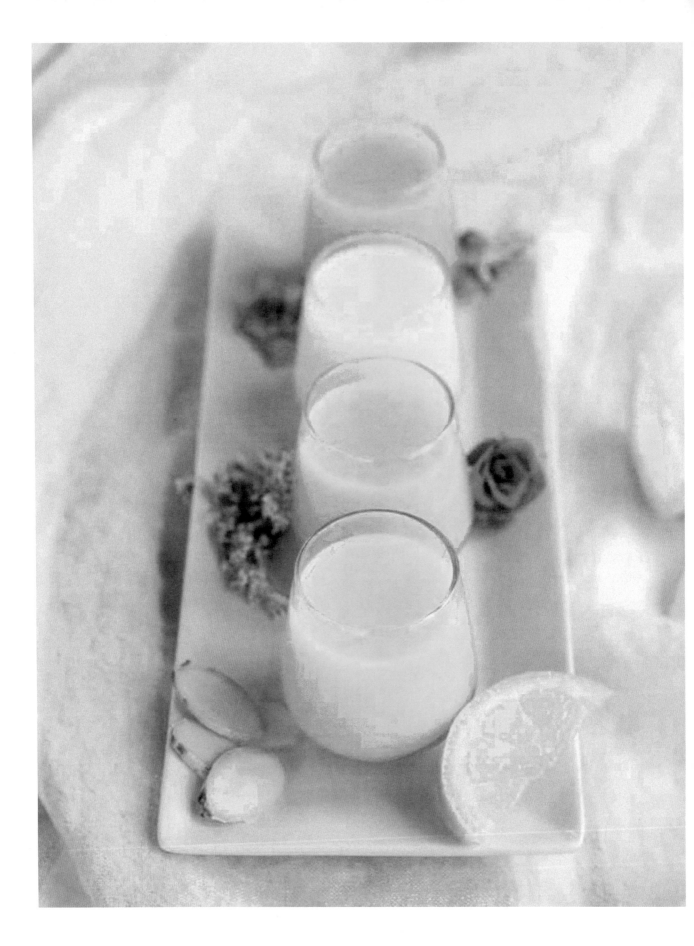

elixirs

Both elixirs and tonics are delivered to our bloodstreams in liquid form, making them efficient vehicles for healing and restoration when consumed on an empty stomach.

DIRECTIONS:

Send all roots, shoots, and citrus through a juicer. While the pith and rind of citrus fruits may be bitter, they contain the highest amount of disease-fighting properties, so it's best to send through the juicer with skins and pith intact. Since we are consuming the skins, make sure your roots, shoots, and citrus are all organic.

All food grade oils, extracts, vinegars, pepper, powders are added at the end.

From Front to Back:

Calm

$1/2$ Lemon, $1/2$ red apple, 1 knuckle ginger, 1 in. fresh turmeric, 1 drop Lemongrass Oil & Lavender Oil

Immune Defense

$1/2$ Lemon, 1 knuckle ginger, dash of cayenne, 4 drops Pau D'Arco Extract, 1 drop Oregano Oil

Super Hero!

2 in. fresh turmeric, 1 knuckle ginger, $1/2$ grapefruit, 1tsp. Manuka honey, $1/4$ tsp. black pepper and dash of cayenne.

Digest Ease

$1/2$ Lemon, $1/2$ Grapefruit, 2 tsp. Apple Cider Vinegar with the mother, 1 drop Peppermint Oil, dash of Cayenne

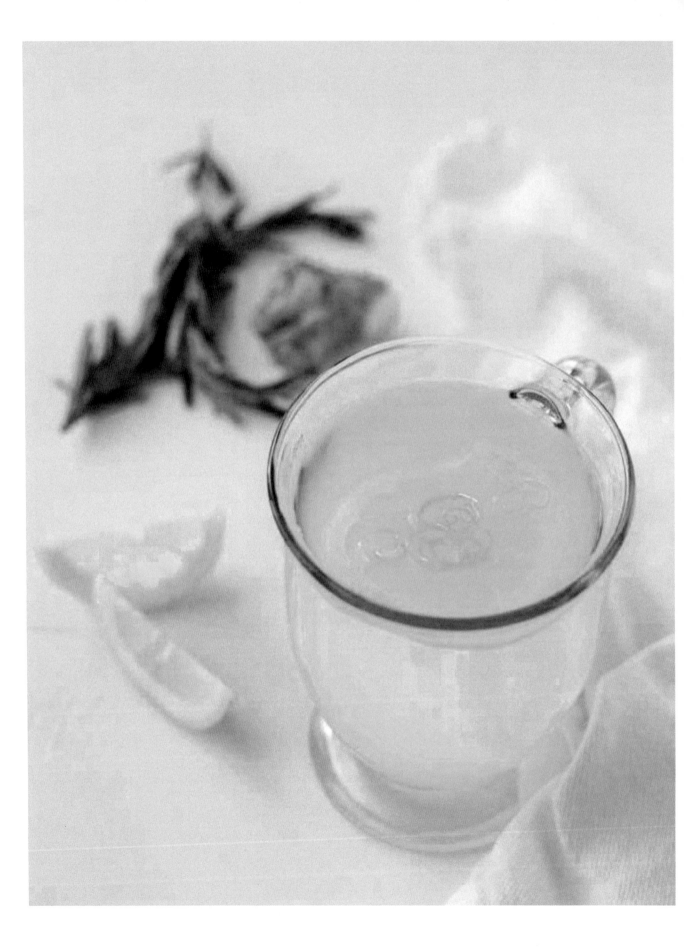

golden sunshine tonic

INGREDIENTS

- Peel and juice of 1 lemon
- 1, 2-inch piece fresh ginger, peeled and grated or chopped
- 1 inch freshly juiced turmeric
- 1 tsp honey or other sweetener
- 2 drops food-grade lemon-balm extract (also called Melissa)
- 1 sprig rosemary, optional

The anti-inflammatory herbs turmeric and ginger offer a tangy, slightly sweet flavor that pleases the palette while getting to work on the healing process. Lemon balm, the "it" herb for alchemists, has been found to have antimicrobial, antioxidant, and antianxiety properties.

DIRECTIONS

1. In a small saucepan over high heat, cook the lemon peel, ginger, turmeric, and 1 cup of water until the water just begins to boil, 1 to 2 minutes. Remove from heat.

Stir in lemon juice, honey, and lemon-balm extract, and then strain into a mug, reserving peels. Garnish with a couple of 2-inch pieces of cooked lemon peel and sprig of rosemary

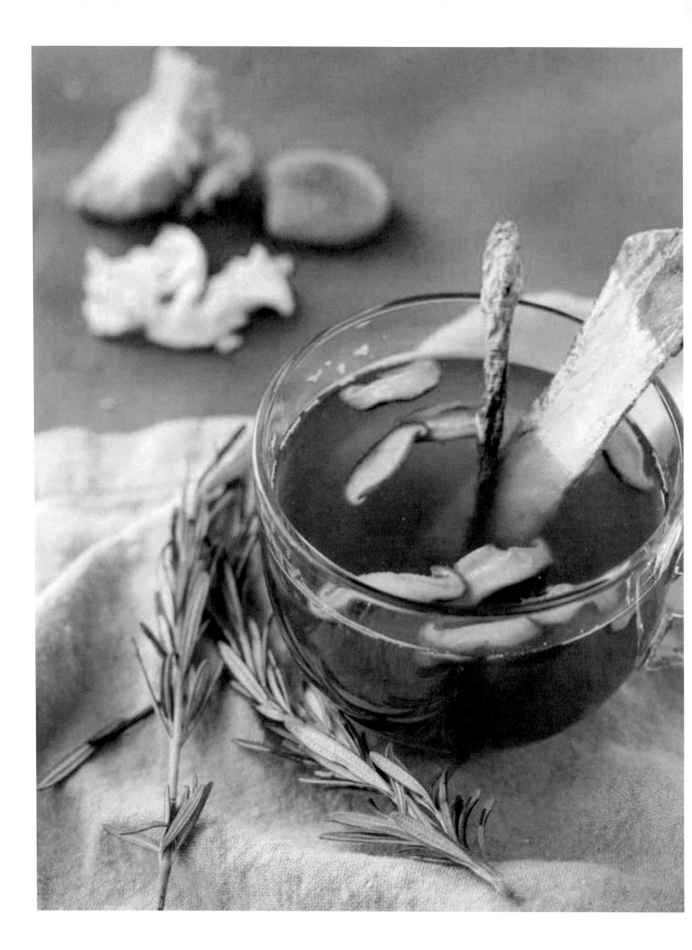

the immune-slayer tonic

INGREDIENTS

- 4 thinly-sliced mushroom caps, such as shiitake
- codonopsis and astragalus roots
- 2 chopped, frozen, and thawed artichokes (or canned in water)
- 2 reishi mushroom teabags
- Juice of $\frac{1}{2}$ lemon
- 2 tsp. balsamic vinegar
- 1 sprig rosemary, optional

Get a wellness boost with the immunity-enhancing mushrooms in this rich, savory drink. Incorporating codonopsis and astragalus root supports the digestive system and nutrient assimilation. It is also an excellent blood tonic. The artichoke has been shown to work as a potent antioxidant that also breaks down lipids (fat) in the liver

DIRECTIONS:

1. In a small saucepan over high heat, cook mushrooms, mushroom roots, artichokes, and 16 ounces of water until the mixture just starts to boil, 1 to 2 minutes.
2. Turn off the heat and add the tea bags; steep 15 minutes.
3. Stir in lemon juice, balsamic vinegar, and a pinch of salt, then transfer into a mug.
4. Garnish with rosemary or cilantro.

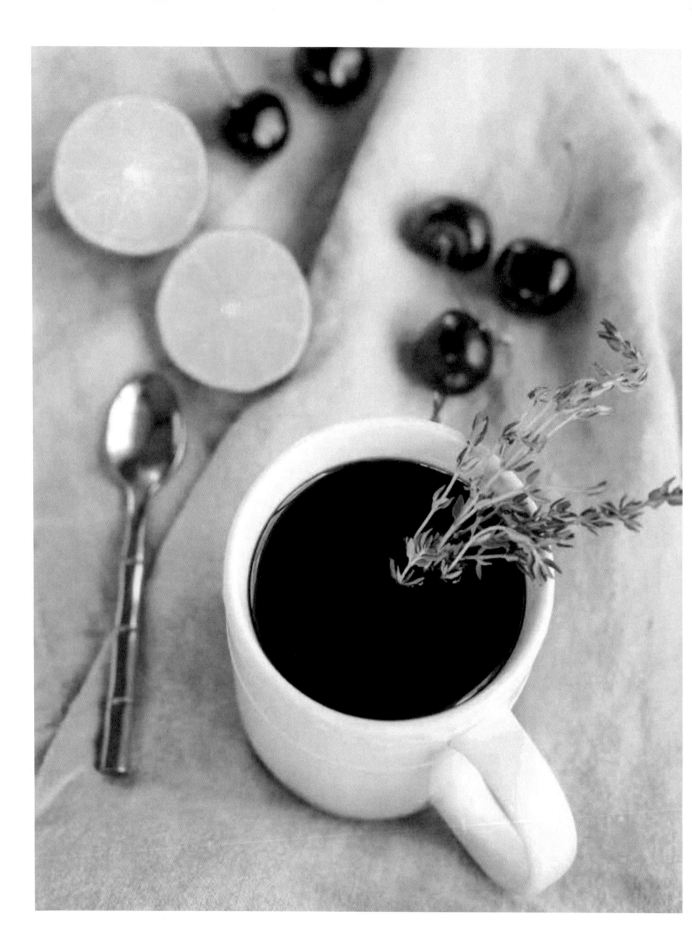

cheery cherry tonic

INGREDIENTS

- 1 tsp fresh thyme leaves
- 2 organic green tea teabags
- $\frac{1}{2}$ cup unsweetened tart cherry juice
- Juice of $\frac{1}{2}$ lime, plus 1 or 2 slices lime for garnish
- 1 tsp stevia powder or 2 tsp honey

Put some zip in your sip with revitalizing green tea. You'll benefit from its antioxidant-rich catechins, plus receive a mild dose of caffeine and theobromine, the latter of which improves blood flow and lightens your mood without the jitters. A big plus: Tart cherry juice can reduce inflammation and soothe sore muscles.

DIRECTIONS:

1. In a small saucepan over high heat, cook thyme leaves and 1 cup of water until water just begins to boil, 1 to 2 minutes.
2. Turn off the heat and add tea bags; steep for 4 minutes.
3. Add cherry or cranberry juice, lime juice, and stevia or honey, then transfer into a mug.
4. Garnish with lime and thyme sprig.

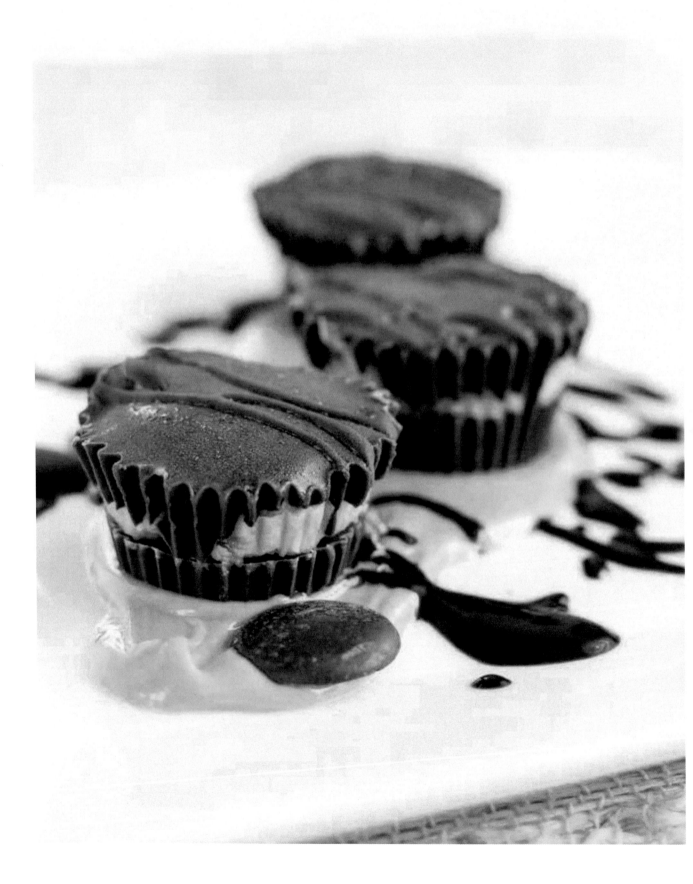

desserts

This section is for the sweet tooth and the chocolate lover! These desserts are divine, and the best part is they're easy to make. Desserts do not go hand-in-hand with an optimal holistic diet, but they definitely go hand-in-hand with emotional eating, cravings, and just being in love with sweet foods.

You will find these desserts satisfying and nourishing and, best of all, naturally free from gluten! We definitely don't count calories or count anything else (except grams of sugar) as it's entirely unnecessary when consuming plant-based whole foods, but regardless of source, desserts should be kept to a minimum in the weekly diet.

If consuming sweets on a regular basis, you may want to switch over to stevia and limit the use of sweeteners even though some sweeteners have been dubbed "healthy." Sugar is sugar, regardless of source. If consumed in isolation from the plant, the fiberless sugar just gives your body the extra job of leveling out blood sugar levels. There's no other way to spin it.

If stevia is not a big hit in your book, then try soaked medjool dates, figs, or even add a bit of honey (whoa! not vegan, but you get my drift) to your desserts.

TIP

Many grain-free, dairy-free, and vegan desserts use nuts as creamers or avocados as flavorful thickening agents, and for good reason! They're creamy and delicious! When using avocado, it's important to note that an avocado needs to be perfectly ripe. If it is under-ripe, it will not blend nor taste sweet. If it's overly ripe or contains brown spots, the dessert will be overpowered by the avocado's apple-like richness. It's best to stick avocados in the refrigerator when there's a slight give to the flesh (but not mushy to the touch) to slow the ripening process.

Don't forget when adding nuts to desserts that the nuts have been soaked overnight in filtered water, then given a vigorous rinse to eliminate the phytic acid.

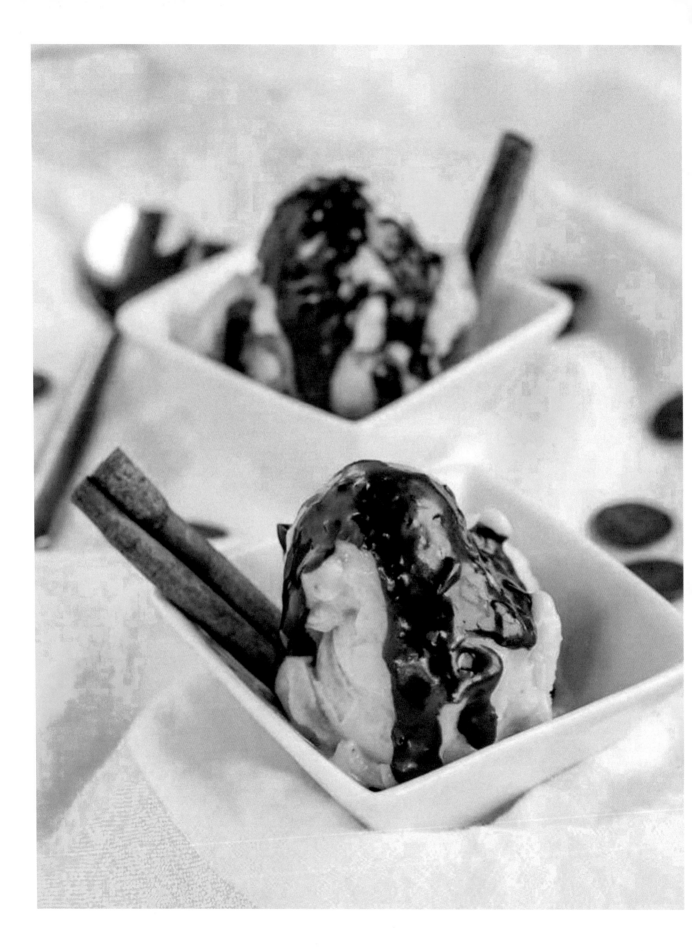

banana ice cream with chocolate sauce

FOR THE ICE CREAM:

Peel and freeze 5 bananas.

FOR THE CHOCOLATE SAUCE:

$1/2$ cup dates, pitted and roughly chopped

$1 1/2$ teaspoon Ceylon cinnamon

1 tablespoon raw cacao powder

$1/2$ teaspoon Madagascar bourbon vanilla or 1 vanilla bean with insides scraped

$1/2$ cup water, and more to thin as needed

1 tbsp. sweetener of choice

If using a masticating Juicer:

If using an Omega juicer, add the attachment without the screen.

If using a blender or food processor:

When freezing bananas, slice into small pieces first.

Thaw frozen bananas out for about 5 minutes and then place into blender or food processor.

DIRECTIONS:

1. Soak dates for approximately 1 hour in $1/2$ cup water
2. In a blender, combine all ingredients except bananas. Blend well and season to taste. Add more water to adjust consistency.
3. Send bananas through juicer or blend in food processor.
4. Store extra banana ice-cream in freezer and thaw before serving.

Top banana "ice cream" with chocolate sauce. Serve immediately.

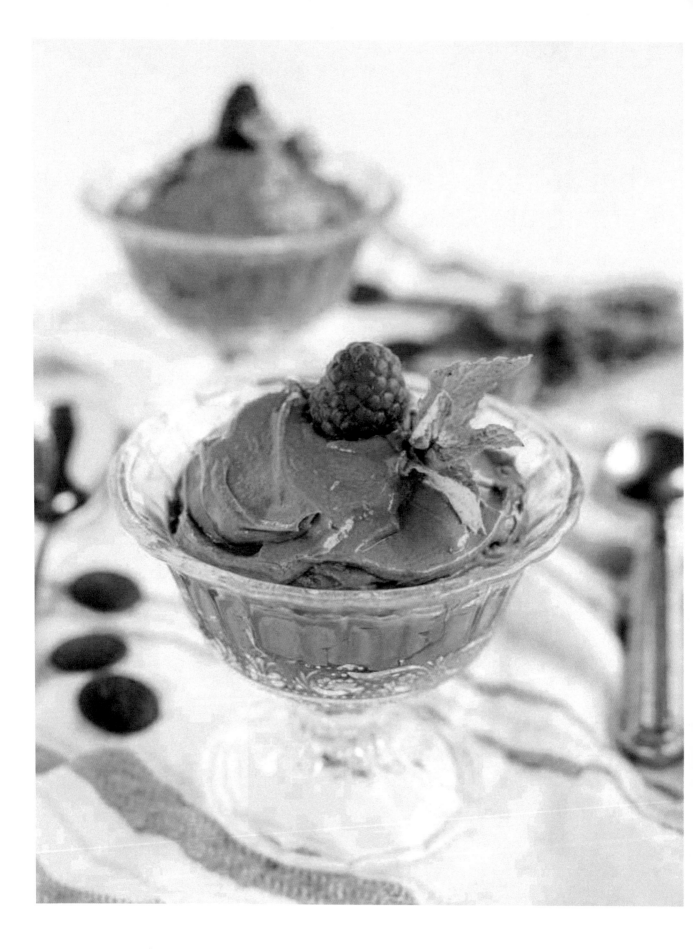

raw chocolate mousse

INGREDIENTS:

flesh from 1 ripe avocado (not too ripe; not too hard; discard brown spots)*

$1/2$ cup raw cashews, soaked 4 hours

$1/4$ c. raw cacao powder

$3/4$ c. raw cacao butter

2 tbsp. organic coconut oil, liquid consistency

6 tbsp. Dark Amber Agave

pinch of Himalayan or sea salt

filtered water for consistency

raw cacao chips (optional)

fresh berries and mint for garnish (optional)

You will never look at chocolate mousse the same way again....! I promise.

DIRECTIONS:

1. In a blender, process all ingredients, adding water as necessary until you have a smooth consistency.

2. Refrigerate for a few hours before serving.

3. Garnish as desired.

*Store avocado in refrigerator at just the right softness to retard any further ripening.

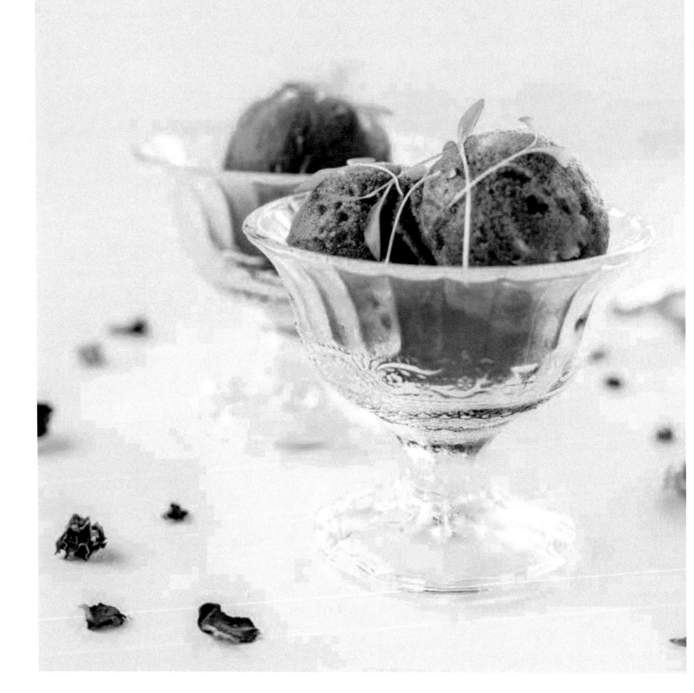

raspberry mousse

INGREDIENTS:

1 large avocado

2 cups of frozen raspberries

Juice of 1 lime

1 teaspoon vanilla extract

$\frac{1}{4}$ cup powdered sweetener or 3 tbs. liquid sweetener such as agave

Micro cilantro

Not your average everyday mousse. It's kid-tested and holistic health approved. Once frozen, natural ice creams without the use of fillers tend to take more time to thaw as opposed to traditional store-bought frozen desserts. Give yourself some extra time with this dessert resting at room temperature so that it has enough time to thaw...that is if you have any leftover to freeze!

DIRECTIONS:

1. Put all ingredients together in a food processor or into a high-speed blender

2. Process only until the mixture is well combined.

3. Serve as you would ice cream.

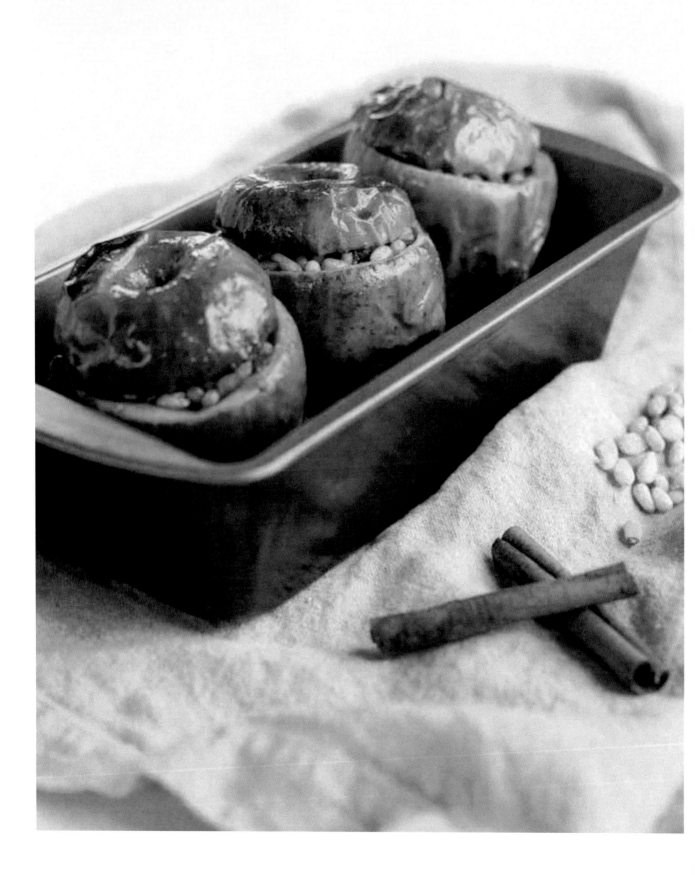

sweet and tangy baked apples

INGREDIENTS:

4 tart apples such as Pippin or Granny Smith

$1/2$ tsp. coconut oil

2 tsp. ground pine nuts

1 tsp. cinnamon

1 tsp. maple syrup

$1/4$ tsp. ground ginger

$1/4$ cup apple juice

These freshly baked apples are the best! They remind me of fall while living in Vermont, making freshly baked desserts after apple picking. Another amazing plant-based dessert to bring to the Thanksgiving table!

DIRECTIONS:

1. Preheat the oven to 400°F

2. Grind the pine nuts in a mini food processor.

3. Cut the top of the apples about $1/3$ of the way down. Cut out a 1-inch piece of the center core.

4. Mix the coconut oil, ground pine nuts, cinnamon, maple syrup, and ginger together and put in the well in the center of the apples. Place in a baking dish with the apple juice, cover with foil, and bake about 20 minutes.

5. Uncover, baste with apple juice, and bake until soft – about 10 more minutes or until desired consistency.

Let apples cool before serving.

chocolate almond butter cups

Middle Layer

¹/₂ cup smooth no-stir almond butter

1 tsp. Madagascar vanilla extract

1 tbsp. coconut oil

4 tbsp. agave

Top/Bottom Layer

¹/₂ cup extra-virgin coconut oil

1 cup raw cacao powder

1 ¹/₂ tsp. Madagascar vanilla extract

4 tbsp. agave

To make the middle layer:

Combine all of the ingredients above: almond butter, vanilla, and sweetener in a small bowl and mix until smooth.

Make the top and bottom layer:

1. Combine all of the ingredients in a small bowl and mix until evenly incorporated.

2. Set 15 mini baking cups in mini muffin pans. Pour about one tablespoon of the bottom layer mixture into each baking cup. Place on a flat surface in the freezer for approximately 15 minutes until the chocolate has hardened.

3. Remove the pan from the freezer and add one tablespoon of almond butter mixture to each individual cup. Put the tray back into the freezer and chill for another 10 minutes.

4. Remove tray from freezer and finish almond butter cup with the remaining chocolate and freeze until the chocolate layer has hardened.

Store the almond butter cups in the freezer for up to 30 days.

Makes 15 cups

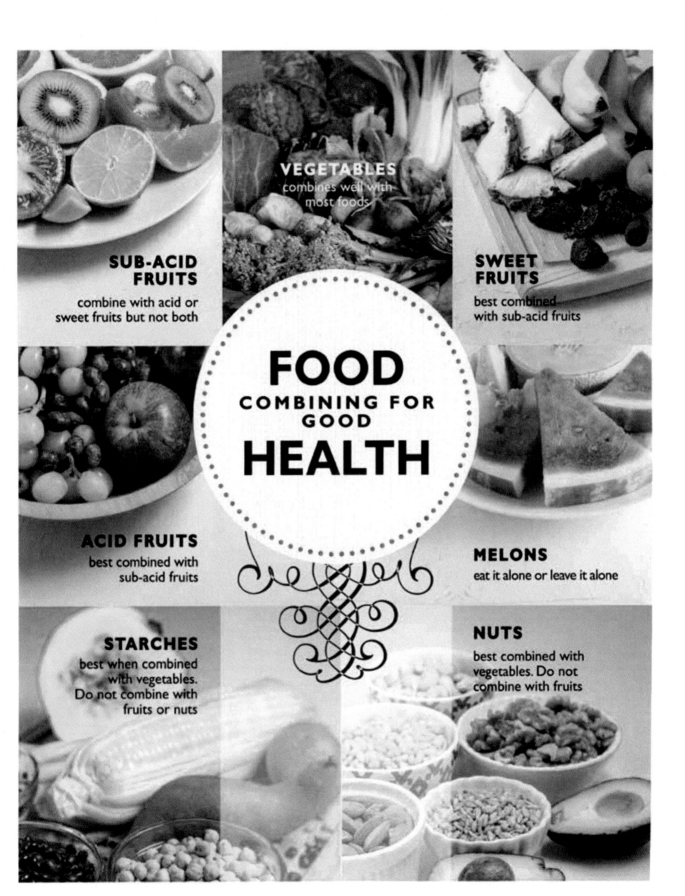

VEGETABLES
combines well with
most foods

**SUB-ACID
FRUITS**

combine with acid or
sweet fruits but not both

**SWEET
FRUITS**

best combined
with sub-acid fruits

FOOD
COMBINING FOR
GOOD
HEALTH

ACID FRUITS

best combined with
sub-acid fruits

MELONS

eat it alone or leave it alone

STARCHES

best when combined
with vegetables.
Do not combine with
fruits or nuts

NUTS

best combined with
vegetables. Do not
combine with fruits

optimal digestion through food combining

FOOD COMBINING – THE DIRECT LINK TO OPTIMAL DIGESTION

It's interesting to note that in days past, food combining didn't exist, not because the science wasn't invented yet because it didn't need to be. Our hunter-gatherer ancestors naturally combined their foods in such a way where optimal digestion occurred without a concerted effort. Prior to the age of agriculture, at no point did our ancestors consume cow's milk) nor did they eat cereal grains. Today, we have so many meal choices, as well as so many packaged "non" foods that we need to pay more attention to not only "what" we put into our bodies, but how much and in what combination. The latter is what we now call the art of food combining.

According to Hippocrates Health Institute, there are two Food-Combining Principals:

1. ***All Foods contain natural chemicals*** – and chemicals react with each other. The same philosophy applies to our bodies. Many meals and store-bought foods contain so many ingredients, that when put together in one sitting, can be very difficult for our bodies to digest, which can lead to fermentation in the gut.

2. ***We digest food at various rates in various acid/alkaline environments.*** Have you ever eaten a piece of fruit right after a large dinner? Usually, the result is indigestion or bloating because fruit, which digests the fastest, runs into the previous meal, which is much slower to digest. The result is what we like to call a digestive back up!

The poorer your digestion, the more affected you could possibly be from improper food combining. As we discussed in the first chapter, the stomach's job is to break down your food with gastric acid. Remember, low acid means a slower and less efficient digestive movement. Food combining focuses solely on digestive wait times. Different nutrients digest at different rates. For example, carbohydrates, like fruit, digest the fastest, then protein and then fat. We discuss this in more detail in just a bit.

Why should you food-combine? Because optimal digestion equates to optimal health. The end result? Better absorption, which in turn leads to more energy, feeling lighter, ease when eliminating, and the distinct possibility for weight loss!

According to Donna Gates, a well-known expert on digestion, states that "When you eat foods that don't combine correctly, the digestive system gets mixed signals about which digestive juices and enzymes to release. Food remains in the digestive tract longer than it should, and...forms a landscape that only viruses, cancer cells, and parasites can tolerate..." Okay, Donna, so let's now understand how to avoid that mess!

Let's talk about what the Food Combining Groups are and how to combine them properly.

- **Proteins:** Nuts and seeds. The average time for protein foods to digest is 3-4 hours, but for some, it can be as many as 6-12, and that most certainly includes meats.

- **Starches:** Starches also include sprouted grains (like quinoa, millet, and buckwheat) and starchy vegetables (like squashes, root vegetables, and potatoes). The average digestion time for starches is 2-3 hours.

- **Vegetables:** Sprouted greens, microgreens, and green leafy vegetables such as kale and spinach.

- **Fruits:** Fruits can also be broken down into two categories: acid and sub-acid fruits.

- **Acid fruits** take 1· hours to digest and include fruits like grapefruit, pineapple, lemons, and oranges.

- **Sub-Acid** fruits also take 1· hours to digest and include fruits such as apples, most berries, peaches, mangos, kiwi, pears, cherries, and grapes.

THE FIVE BASIC RULES – HOW TO PUT THEM TOGETHER:

Now, Food Combining can get pretty complicated, but since we do not want to drive you crazy, or add unnecessary stress, here are the basic rules to follow:

1. Fruit: Eat it alone or leave it alone. Make sure fruit is ripe and try to eat locally and seasonally. Many fruits that have to travel far are picked unripe.

2. Do not eat starchy foods with fats (like nuts and avocados). We call it the slow and sluggish event!

3. Fruits and nuts should not mix. That's a surefire way to increase the bloat and burp!

4. Vegetables can combine with everything except fruit. Truly, a happy meal!

5. The fewer the ingredients, the better. The more ingredients a food or meal is comprised of, the increased likelihood it will contain an unwanted combination.

THE 80/20 PRINCIPLE

Most of us just eat way too much food. It's okay to indulge once in a while, but if we overeat too often, it puts a significant strain on our digestive systems. Try to remember the 80/20 principle, which states: Eat only until your stomach is 80% full.

Eating slowly helps as well because it takes time for the full signal to reach our brain.

Also, try to eat in a stress-free environment and, most importantly, eat while sitting, not standing. If you can, try to avoid those seats in the car or at your office desk!

The 80/20 principle can also be thought of in relation to plant-based foods. Try to aim for 80% plant-based and 20% animal products. However, the ideal amount is zero.

And once you reach the 80/20 plant-based ratio, try 80% raw and 20% cooked, *all* plant-based! Not ready to commit? Try it for 21 or 30 days! Don't forget, the helpful little digestive agents are known as food enzymes. You know, the ones that are so important in the digestive process are eliminated when heated above 110 degrees.

WATER AND ENZYME DILUTION

Drinking water during meals can dilute digestive enzymes, so try not to drink water at least 30 minutes before meals or wait about an hour after eating.

REMOVING ENZYME INHIBITORS BY SOAKING NUTS, SEEDS, AND BEANS

Nuts and seeds and beans should be soaked before consumption because they naturally have an enzyme inhibitor that inhibits them from sprouting. As discussed in Chapter 4, some of those inhibitors are antinutrients and may work against your digestive tract. By soaking most nuts overnight, they become easier to digest.

Think that it takes too much time? Don't sweat. There are numerous "packaged" (but incredibly healthy, I might add) products on the market that have taken all of the proper steps for you. Here are identifying terms you'll want to look for when buying packed nuts and seeds: sprouted, dehydrated, living, soaked, but maybe not all or in that order. When nuts and seeds are manufactured to no longer contain enzyme inhibitors, it makes snacking on nuts that much healthier. Buying "raw" does not mean it has undergone the sprouting process.

SAUERKRAUT AND FERMENTED FOODS

Try to include some fermented foods in your diet each day. A couple of tablespoons of sauerkraut or fermented veggies like kimchi contain a plethora of good bacteria that are beneficial for gut flora. Sauerkrauts and fermented foods are not raw fermented if the container contains vinegar. Vinegar is an acid that will "cook" your fermented veggies, killing off the beneficial bacteria. In this case, look for "raw" or "fermented."

DIGESTION BEGINS IN THE MOUTH

The goal is to liquify your solids and chew your soups. Definitely challenging, but try to aim for chewing 30-60 times before you swallow. If your teeth can do more of the prepping, which stimulates the release of enzymes in the saliva, it helps to alleviate the stress and pressure on your pancreas to release digestive enzymes.

REFRAIN FROM EATING REFINED GLUTEN (AKA PROCESSED AND PACKAGED FOODS)

Gluten is the protein in wheat, but over the years, it has been hybridized numerous times within such a short time span that the protein content has been increased exponentially. Excess protein can lead to gut inflammation, which then leads to digestive issues. Some surmise "leaky gut" stems from the wheat protein zonulin.

TAKE DIGESTIVE ENZYME SUPPLEMENTS

As Dr. Howell's theory suggests, we are born with a certain number of digestive enzymes that diminish with age and poor lifestyle habits. Digestive enzymes help digest meals more efficiently so that the nutrients from your food are broken down and can be better absorbed through the villi in the small intestine. Again, there are multiple digestive enzyme products on the market that you can take just prior to eating a meal to help facilitate the breakdown of foods you consume. Don't forget we list a few of the more common digestive enzymes in Chapter 1, like protease, lipase, and amylase.

EXERCISE AND DIGESTION

Our bodies were meant to move. Light exercise that increases breathing and gets the heart rate up can help move the bowels and reduce heartburn. Also, light forms of exercise can help alleviate stress, which again helps with efficient digestion and swift elimination.

ALLOW TIME IN BETWEEN MEALS TO THOROUGHLY DIGEST

And lastly, try to give your body time to digest between each meal; at least 3 hours if possible, and stay away from eating late in the evening. Give yourself at least 3 hours between your last meal and going to bed.

Remember: The path to optimal digestion takes time and persistence, but the results are well worth it! You've come so far!

CULMINATING THOUGHTS AND IDEAS FOR DAILY PRACTICE

If you can't always prepare your foods or just need to keep things simple, remember these basic steps:

1. Drink warm lemon water upon awakening. As the liver detoxes the body during sleep, the lemon water further assists with toxin removal.

2. Buy as much organic produce as possible as organic farming practices nourish the soil, which in turn produces a higher quality product than conventionally grown. It's not just about pesticides!

3. Use coconut oil. The chemical composition is much more stable during high heat cooking

than other oils. Of course, it's best raw and contains heart-healthy omega-9s.

4. Consume red/orange vegetables as they contain a significant amount of beta-carotene, the primary source of Vitamin–A. That means great for your skin, nails, hair, and any mucosal lining in the body.

5. Remember to eat your green leafy vegetables. Despite being loaded with nutrients like folic acid, Vitamin K, iron, and calcium, leafy greens even contain water!

6. Many of the red/blue fruits contain flavonoids and antioxidants, which are essential for optimizing health.

7. Try quinoa. Quinoa is not a grain but rather a seed and contains eight essential amino acids that make it a great source of plant-based protein.

8. Make green juices or smoothies at home. Green drinks are the best fast food. They are a great way to get an abundance of greens in the body that one normally couldn't consume in one sitting. Be wise when blending because calories can add up if food besides fruits and vegetables are added. Drink juices on an empty stomach for rapid absorption.

9. Eat daily plant-based omega-3 fats like chia, flax, and hemp seeds. Not sure what to do with them? Top cereals or salads with these healthy fats or freely add them to smoothies.

10. Locate local sprouts and microgreens. While two entirely separate species and growing methods, sprouts and microgreens offer a significant amount of nutrients. Babies, as I refer to them, contain more disease-fighting compounds than their mature counterparts.

11. And best of all, proper food combining can leave us feeling healthy and satisfied.

index

Açai	204, 207
Acidifying foods	23
ALA	60
Algae	67, 188, 204
Algal oil	92
Alkaline	16-20, 289-310
Allium	49-50
Amylase	15
Ann Wigmore	41
Antioxidants	47, 51-52
Bee pollen	66, 72
Beta-carotene	39-40, 44, 52
Biosolids	34
BMAA	67, 95
Brian Clement	14, 53, 63, 96
Bt toxin	27-28
Cacao	66, 204
Calcium	88-89
Cancer	62, 73
Chlorella	66, 68, 118, 204
Chlorophyll	40-43, 66, 73, 143
Coconut	69-70, 203, 205
Coconut oil	58, 70, 313
Concentrace	106-107
Cruciferous	44, 129-130
DHA	60, 63, 92
Digestion	11-12, 15, 17, 310-313
Digestive enzymes	13, 313
Dioxins	94
Distilled water	107
Dulse	88, 250
Ellegic acid	49
Endocrine disruptors	93
Enzymes	12-15, 313
Field crop rotation	33
Flavonoids	48-49
Food enzymes	13
Free radicals	43-44, 51
Garlic	49
GMO seed	27, 29, 35
HDL	20, 70
Heart disease	59
Hemp	72, 203-204, 245
Hemp seed	66, 72, 83, 230
Hippocrates Health Institute	2, 14, 41, 53, 63, 66, 310
Hormones	81, 87, 90, 93, 96
Hybridization	78
IGF-1	87
Immune	18, 289
Indoles	50
Iron	38
Isoflavones	50
Jeffrey Smith	29

Juicing 143-148
Kale 20-22, 88, 115-116, 129-130, 137
Kelp 68, 88, 257
LDL 20, 49, 58-59, 159
Lemon 19, 160, 311, 313
Lipase 13
Lutein 52
Lycopene 52
Maca root 66, 72, 204
Magnesium 41
Manure 81
Mercury 94
Milk 27, 87-90, 102
Monounsaturated fats 187
Monsanto 26-30, 87
National Bioengineered
Food Disclosure Standard 25
Omega 9 20, 60, 187
Organic Farming 33-34
Oxygen 37-38, 41
Pasture-raised 89
PBDEs 95
PCBs 27, 93-94, 103
pH 16-19, 88, 104, 107, 109
Phytochemicals 47-51, 159-160
Polyphenols 48
Polyunsaturated fats 60, 188

Protein 42, 82, 204, 230
Quinoa 83, 115-116, 204, 230
rBGH 87
Reverse osmosis 106
S. 764 federal standard for food labeling 30
Saturated fats 58-59, 187
Sea vegetables 67-68, 250-251
Selenium 52, 191
Soy 31, 53-55
Spirulina 66-68, 204
Superfood 65-66
T. Colin Campbell 84
Tap water 103-104, 109
The China Study 84
Tilapia 97
Toxaphene 95
Transfats 57
Transgenic modification 27
USDA 27, 30, 89-90
USDA Organic label 27
Vitamin A 39-40, 52, 59-60
Vitamin B5 35, 39
Vitamin C 20-21, 44, 52
Well water 107-108
Wheatgrass 42-45, 66-67, 230
Xenoestrogens 93
Zilmax 82

references

1. Dr. Edward Howell, Enzyme Nutrition

2. Read more: http://www.livestrong.com/article/111402-alkaline-vs.-acidity-body/#ixzz29hsdnqCw

3. http://www.livestrong.com/article/111402-alkaline-vs.-acidity-body/#ixzz29hsQm83l

4. Ibid

5. Read more: http://www.livestrong.com/article/111402-alkaline-vs.-acidity-body/#ixzz29hsutstH

6. https://liveenergized.com/alkaline-foods-2/the-7-most-alkaline-foods/

7. https://www.greatfallstribune.com/story/money/2016/04/05/embargoed---food-firms-start-labeling-gmo-products-vermont-law-looms/82511830/

8. http://www.justlabelit.org/right-to-know-center/labeling-around-the-world/

9. https://www.usda.gov/media/blog/2013/05/17/organic-101-can-gmos-be-used-organic-products

10. "The 2010 Eurobarometer on the life sciences." Nat. Biotechnol. 29 (2): 113-14. Doi:10.1038/nbt.1771. PMID 21301431.

11. https://www.nongmoproject.org/gmo-facts/

12. https://responsibletechnology.org/gmo-education/articles-about-health-risks-by-jeffrey/

13. https://www.usda.gov/media/blog/2013/05/17/organic-101-can-gmos-be-used-organic-products

14. http://www.monsanto.com/newsviews/pages/gm-seed-accidentally-in-farmers-fields.aspx

15. http://arstechnica.com/tech-policy/2013/06/organic-farmers-cant-fight-monsanto-patents-in-court/

16. http://responsibletechnology.org/michelle-perro-interview/

17. http://responsibletechnology.org/irtnew/wp-content/uploads/2017/11/Summary-Improved-Health-by-Eliminating-GMOs-by-Jeffrey-Smith.pdf

18. https://www.sciencemag.org/news/2016/07/us-senate-passes-gm-food-labeling-bill

19. Ibid

20. https://www.nongmoproject.org

21. Ibid

22. https://www.nongmoproject.org

23. Ibid

24. http://www.dripirrigation.org/organic_agriculture.html

25. http://www.ecfr.gov/cgi-bin/text-idx?SID=176b3a9b699c02c4f14d234b7dfa54f8&node=7:3.1.1.9.32.3.354.4&rgn=div8

26. http://www.iatp.org/files/Sewage_Sludge__Food_Safety.htm

27 http://www.ecfr.gov/cgi-bin/text-idx-?SID=176b3a9b699c02c4f14d234b7dfa54f8&node=7:3.1.1.9.32.3.354.4&rgn=div8

28 https://rodaleinstitute.org/blog/10-ways-organic-improves-soil-health/

29 http://www.mightygrow.com/resources/trace-minerals-organics/

30 http://www.fda.gov/Food/ResourcesForYou/Consumers/ucm261680.htm

31 https://growingnaturals.com/2016/05/is-non-heme-iron-better-for-you/

32 How to Find Vitamin B-12 in Foods | eHow.com http://www.ehow.com/how_2258990_vitamin-b_12-foods.html#ixzz29QXkIcCS

33 Which Foods Contain Vitamin B5? | eHow.com http://www.ehow.com/facts_5201963_foods-contain-vitamin-b5_.html#ixzz2DLMojpoY

34 Foods Containing B6 | eHow.com http://www.ehow.com/about_5286042_foods-containing-b.html#ixzz29QVxBXaH

35 http://www.livestrong.com/article/320841-foods-high-in-abscisic-acid/#ixzz2BlGttrDc

36 Foods to Fight Cancer, by Richard Believeau, Ph.D and Denis Gingras, Ph.D

37 Foods to Fight Cancer, by Richard Believeau, Ph.D and Denis Gingras, Ph.D

38 Foods to Fight Cancer, by Richard Believeau, Ph.D and Denis Gingras, Ph.D

39 Ibid

40 http://nccam.nih.gov/health/antioxidants/introduction.htm

41 https://www.statista.com/statistics/217108/level-of-genetically-modified-crops-in-the-us/

42 An Evidence Based Approach to Phytochemicals and Other Dietary Factors by Jane Higdon, Ph.D. and Victoria Drake, Ph.D

43 http://articles.mercola.com/sites/articles/archive/2010/02/25/saturated-fat-is-not-the-cause-of-heart-disease.aspx

44 https://articles.mercola.com/sites/articles/archive/2020/07/11/saturated-fat-myth.aspx?cidsource=dnl&cid_medium=email&cid_content=art1HL&cid=20200711Z1&mid=healthrtlucm20200711z1&rid=914164014

45 https://articles.mercola.com/sites/articles/archive/2016/09/11/omega-3-from-plants-vs-marine-animals.aspx

46 http://www.whfoods.com/genpage.php?tname=nutrient&dbid=84

47 https://www.fredhutch.org/en/news/releases/2013/07/omega-three-fatty-acids-risk-prostate-cancer.html

48 https://www.ncbi.nlm.nih.gov/pmc/articles/PMC4303825/

49 https://www.livestrong.com/article/463401-wheatgrass-vs-chlorella-vs-spirulina-vs-barley-grass/

50 https://www.drweil.com/diet-nutrition/food-safety/is-spirulina-safe/

51 https://www.ncbi.nlm.nih.gov/pubmed/1906616

52 https://raysahelian.com/chlorella.html

53 Ibid

54 http://www.whfoods.com/genpage.php?p-friendly=1&tname=foodspice&dbid=135

55 https://www.ncbi.nlm.nih.gov/pmc/articles/PMC2763764/

56 https://www.naturalscience.org/topics/health/glyconutrients/

57 http://www.ehow.com/about_5047377_benefits-aloe-vera.html

58 https://www.medicalnewstoday.com/articles/318591#contains-healthful-compounds-

59 https://www.leaf.tv/articles/difference-between-aloe-vera-gel-juice/

60 https://www.leaf.tv/articles/difference-between-aloe-vera-gel-juice/

61 https://coconutoils.com/lauric-acid/

62 http://www.ehow.com/about_5063723_nutritional-benefits-coconut.html

63 http://www.ehow.com/about_5063723_nutritional-benefits-coconut.html

64 https://www.livestrong.com/article/510928-coconut-oil-medium-chain-triglycerides/

65 https://www.health.harvard.edu/staying-healthy/coconut-oil

66 http://www.ehow.com/about_5063723_nutritional-benefits-coconut.html

67 https://www.ncbi.nlm.nih.gov/pmc/articles/PMC5796020/

68 http://www.webmd.com/balance/goji-berries-health-benefits-and-side-effects

69 https://www.healthline.com/health/goji-berry-facts#use

70 http://www.extremehealthusa.com/Goji-Articles/GojiStory.aspx

71 https://www.ncbi.nlm.nih.gov/pmc/articles/PMC5920423/

72 https://www.webmd.com/sex-relationships/features/the-truth-about-maca#1

73 https://www.ncbi.nlm.nih.gov/pmc/articles/PMC3614604/

74 https://zerbos.com/top-5-maca-root-benefits-and-nutrition/

75 https://www.ncbi.nlm.nih.gov/pmc/articles/PMC4377380/

76 https://www.healthline.com/nutrition/6-health-benefits-of-hemp-seeds

77 https://www.ncbi.nlm.nih.gov/books/NBK92757/

78 https://www.emedicinehealth.com/reishi_mushroom/vitamins-supplements.htm

79 http://www.livestrong.com/article/374745-cordyceps-benefits/

80 http://www.livestrong.com/article/518116-cordyceps-for-adrenal-fatigue/

81 https://www.ncbi.nlm.nih.gov/books/NBK92758/

82 https://www.livestrong.com/article/403273-side-effects-of-the-chaga-mushroom/

83 http://www.livestrong.com/article/403273-side-effects-of-the-chaga-mushroom/

84 https://thecowdocs.wordpress.com/2017/06/20/grazing-cattle-is-more-than-having-grass/

85 https://www.lhf.org/learning-fields/crops/hay/

86 https://www.history.com/news/dust-bowl-migrants-california

87 https://livinghistoryfarm.org/farmingin-the30s/crops_17.html

88 https://www.historylearningsite.co.uk/modern-world-history-1918-to-1980/america-1918-1939/farmers-and-the-new-deal/

89 https://www.nature.com/articles/s41599-018-0152-2

90 https://livinghistoryfarm.org/farmingin-the40s/machines_08.html

91 Congressional Record, March 9, 1966, page 5491

92 Ibid.

93 https://livinghistoryfarm.org/farmingin-the50s/crops_01.html

94 https://livinghistoryfarm.org/farmingin-the50s/crops_01.html

95 https://www.challenge.org/knowledgeitems/the-dangers-of-monoculture-farming/

96 https://livinghistoryfarm.org/farmingin-the50s/crops_01.html

97 https://www.ncbi.nlm.nih.gov/books/NBK305168/

98 The China Study, T. Colin Campbell

99 https://www.nytimes.com/2008/01/27/weekinreview/27bittman.html

100 http://www.livinghistoryfarm.org

101 Michael Pollen, Food Inc.

102 Michael Pollen, Food Inc.

103 https://www.nrdc.org/sites/default/files/cesspools.pdf

104 https://www.ncbi.nlm.nih.gov/pmc/articles/PMC3489133/

105 https://www.nrdc.org/sites/default/files/cesspools.pdf

106 Michael Pollen, Food Inc.

107 http://www.ibtimes.com/livestock-steroids-regenerate-water-trenbolone-may-pose-environmental-risk-1411950

108 The China Study, T. Colin Campbell

109 http://www.livestrong.com/article/339269-foods-that-create-mucus/

110 https://detox.net.au/mucoid-plaque-and-mucus/

111 http://www.ncbi.nlm.nih.gov/pubmed/6940487

112 http://www.vrg.org/nutrition/iron.php

113 http://fooddemocracy.wordpress.com/2007/08/28/artificial-hormones/

114 http://articles.mercola.com/sites/articles/archive/2010/11/25/finally-huge-victory-against-monsanto-milk.aspx

115 http://www.ncbi.nlm.nih.gov/pubmed/17448154

116 Colon Plaque - Mucoid Plaque - by Dr. Richard Anderson, ND., N.M.D.

117 United States Department of Agriculture (USDA) National Nutrient Database for Standard Reference, Release 18

118 http://www.livestrong.com/article/32887-calcium-rich-plant-foods/

119 https://detox.net.au/mucoid-plaque-and-mucus/

120 https://www.fsis.usda.gov/wps/portal/fsis/topics/food-safety-education/get-answers/food-safety-fact-sheets/food-labeling/meat-and-poultry-labeling-terms/meat-and-poultry-labeling-terms

121 https://www.nhlbi.nih.gov/news/2019/say-what-scientists-claim-red-meat-an36d-white-meat-can-have-equal-effects-blood

122 http://www.banderasnews.com/0510/hb-eatfish.htm

123 https://ods.od.nih.gov/factsheets/Omega3FattyAcids-HealthProfessional/

124 https://ods.od.nih.gov/factsheets/Omega3FattyAcids-HealthProfessional/

125 https://www.researchgate.net/publication/298352359_Case_Study_A_PROMISING_ALTERNATIVE_TO_FISH_OIL_SOURCE_OF_OMEGA_3_PRODUCTION_ROLE_OF_ALGAE

126 https://www.webmd.com/vitamins-supplements/ingredientmono-1565-ALGAL-OIL.aspx?activeIngredientId=1565&activeIngredientName=ALGAL+OIL&source=0

127 http://www.vnv.org.au/Articles/Fish.htm

128 Killer Fish, Dr. Brian R. Clement, PhD, NMD, LN, p.1

129 https://www.webmd.com/diabetes/endocrine-system-facts

130 https://www.hormone.org/diseases-and-conditions/autoimmune-disease

131 https://www.niehs.nih.gov/health/topics/agents/endocrine/index.cfm

132 http://www.nytimes.com/2009/06/28/opinion/28kristof.html?_r=0

133 https://pubs.usgs.gov/fs/fs095-01/fs095-01.html

134 https://www.ncbi.nlm.nih.gov/pmc/articles/PMC3514464/

135 http://www.banderasnews.com/0510/hb-eatfish.htm

136 https://www.westonaprice.org/health-topics/environmental-toxins/mad-as-a-hatter/

137 Killer Fish, Dr. Brian R. Clement, PhD, NMD, LN

138 https://www.riverkeeper.org/campaigns/stop-polluters/pcbs/

139 https://www.sfpe.org/general/custom.asp?page=FPE_2015_Q4_4

140 http://www.ncbi.nlm.nih.gov/pubmed/16767233

141 Killer Fish, Dr. Brian R. Clement, PhD, NMD, LN

142 Ibid.

143 Ibid

144 https://www.nationalchickencouncil.org/about-the-industry/statistics/broiler-chicken-industry-key-facts/

145 http://www.foodsafetynews.com/2013/01/why-we-havent-seen-inside-a-broiler-chicken-factory-farm-in-a-decade/#.VAheXOuWsds

146 http://money.cnn.com/2012/11/27/news/economy/farming/

147 https://www.chickencheck.in/blog/con-fusing-chicken-labels/

148 https://www.post-gazette.com/news/health/2008/02/07/Chicken-feed-additive-may-pose-danger/stories/200802070475

149 https://duq.edu/news/releases/human-health-risk-linked-to-arsenic-additive-in-chicken-feed

150 http://www.ewg.org/tap-water/report-findings.php

151 www.cancer.org

152 http://www.ewg.org/tap-water/report-findings.php

153 http://www.ewg.org/tap-water/report-findings.php

154 http://www.ewg.org/tap-water/report-findings.php#sthash.1BdXuvUx.dpuf

155 www.about.com/environment

156 http://environment.about.com/od/healthenvironment/a/tap_water_safe.htm

157 http://environment.about.com/od/healthenvironment/a/tap_water_safe.htm

158 Ibid

159 www.nrdc.org/water/drinking/qbw.asp

160 www.filteredwatersolutions.com

161 http://www.mercola.com/article/water/distilled_water.htm

162 http://www.wisegeek.org/what-is-distilled-water.htm

163 http://www.mercola.com/article/water/distilled_water.htm

164 http://water.epa.gov/drink/info/well/index.cfm

165 http://EzineArticles.com/7112384

166 http://www.epa.gov/ttn/atw/hlthef/chlorofo.html

167 https://www.globalhealingcenter.com/natural-health/what-are-phytochemicals/

168 https://www.healthline.com/nutrition/okra-health-benefits#section4

169 https://www.medicalnewstoday.com/articles/265853#benefits

170 https://www.medicalnewstoday.com/articles/284765#benefits

171 https://www.medicalnewstoday.com/articles/276714#benefits

172 https://www.medicalnewstoday.com/articles/325000#heart-health

173 https://www.medicalnewstoday.com/articles/309369#benefits

174 https://www.medicalnewstoday.com/articles/269468#benefits

175 https://www.drweil.com/diet-nutrition/food-safety/is-carrageenan-safe/

176 https://greatist.com/health/burn-fat-and-control-appetite-cayenne-pepper#1

177 http://www.ncbi.nlm.nih.gov/pubmed/6940487

178 http://www.vrg.org/nutrition/iron.php

179 https://www.webmd.com/diet/peppers-health-benefits#1

180 https://www.healthline.com/nutrition/basil#benefits

Made in the USA
Columbia, SC
03 May 2021